Atlas of Clinical Cases in Rhinoplasty

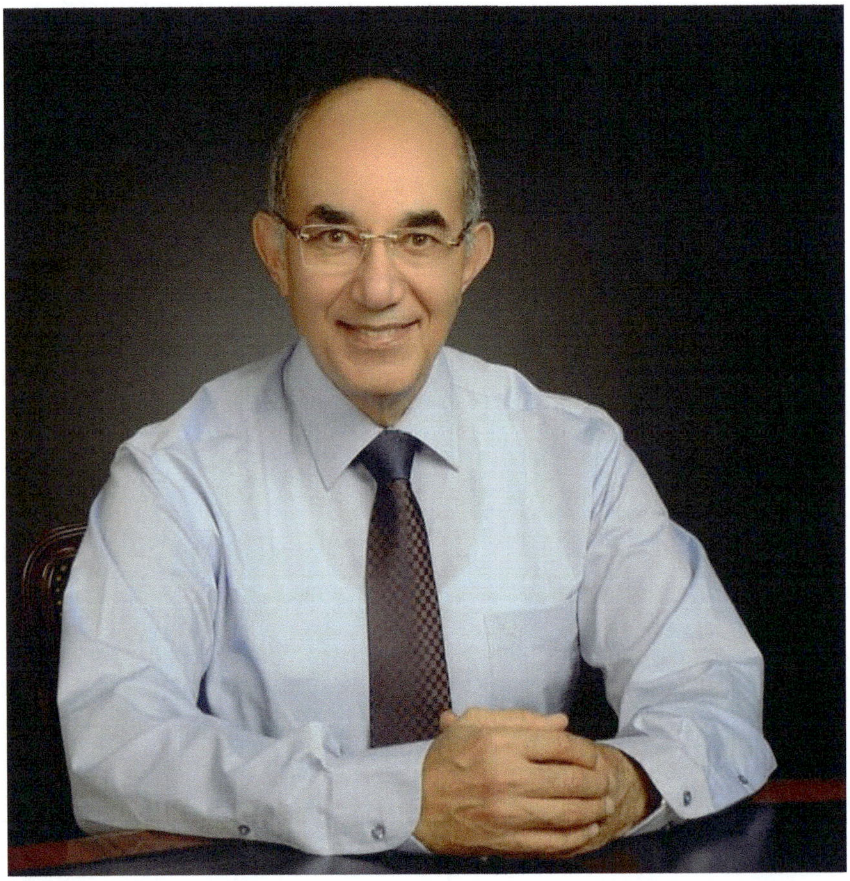

Motaz H. A. Shafy

Atlas of Clinical Cases in Rhinoplasty

Volume I

Springer

Motaz H. A. Shafy
Shafy's Clinics
Al Nakheel Center
Jeddah, Saudi Arabia

ISBN 978-3-031-07506-3 ISBN 978-3-031-07504-9 (eBook)
https://doi.org/10.1007/978-3-031-07504-9

This Springer imprint is published by the registered company Springer Nature Switzerland AG
The registered company address is: Gewerbestrasse 11, 6330 Cham, Switzerland

Acknowledgements

I would like to acknowledge and give special thanks to the following people without whom the following textbook and atlas would not have been possible. As a medical professional, I see surgery, specifically Rhinoplasty, as a work of art as well as a scientific endeavor. Every artist has their muse, or inspiration, for me this person was Mr. Tony R. Bull, F.R.C.S Consultant E.N.T Surgeon who was my mentor at the Royal National Throat, Nose and Ear Hospital in London. Mr. Bull's creative approach, passion, and devotion towards the field of Rhinoplasty was what inspired me to develop my own innovative surgical techniques. Mr. Bull was also one of the people who has seen my early work and encouraged me to take my research further turning it from a research article to a full-fledged book.

I would also like to thank my great friend and colleague, Mr. Bahir Skinner A.B.I.P.P, Medical Photographer, for his professional advice regarding medical photography and other technical details.

Furthermore, I would like to show my gratitude towards Elia Anis Ishaak, M.Sc. Ph.D., Professor of Pathology, and Solafa Amin AbdulAziz, MD, Professor of Pathology who work at Cairo University for their help in the histology of the Inferior Vestibular Bands and the Vestibular Septum.

Additionally, I am thankful towards Dr. Mohamed Saad Lotfy, CEO of Viral Media, his team, and Engineer Roshdy Al Bahlool, B.Sc. from Menoufia University of Egypt, for their technical expertise in conducting the medical artistic illustrations evidenced in this book.

Moreover, I would like to thank Dr. Soliman Fakeeh and Dr. Mazen Fakeeh for providing their hospital's facilities, including their O.R. and pathology department, where I conducted my Ear, Nose, and Throat surgeries.

I would like to thank Eisel M. Monton, R.N.B.S.N for her diligent efforts in her secretarial assistance.

I would like to thank Ms. Elizabeth Pope, Editor at Springer, for her professional guidance regarding the writing and reviewing of this book taking it to new heights.

Last but not least, I would like to give a special thanks to my family, without whose support this book would not have been possible.

Contents

About the Author

Motaz H. A. Shafy F.R.C.S. holds the following degrees: MBBCh, Cairo University; FRCS RCPSG (Glasgow); and FRCS (Edinburgh). Throughout his career, he has undertaken training and held consultancy posts in the United Kingdom, the Kingdom of Saudi Arabia and Egypt. Dr. Shafy's previous roles included: House Surgeon and Physician, Cairo University Hospitals; Senior House Officer in ENT Surgery, Stobhill General Hospital, Teaching Hospital Glasgow University; Registrar, Senior Registrar, The Royal National Throat Nose and Ear Hospital, London; Consultant ENT Surgeon positions at Chase Farm Hospital, London; Consultant ENT Surgeon King Abdul Aziz University Hospital and Daghastani Hospital Kingdom of Saudi Arabia; Consultant ENT Surgeon in Shafy Clinics, Kingdom of Saudi Arabia and Shafy Center, Giza, Egypt. Dr Shafy's main areas of clinical interest are the preservation of Aesthetic Rhinoplasty and Examination.

Part I
Introduction

Introduction to the Atlas

1

The concept of an Atlas is ideal for the surgery of Rhinoplasty. In this Atlas more than 4600 photographs of a wide range of clinical conditions that present for Rhinoplasty are displayed. These varieties of noses include; the large, the bulky, the crooked, the deviated, the oblique, the fractured, finesse, secondary, ethnic, pediatric and special clinical conditions. In each case the nose and face are looked at from multiple different angles through the standard and the newly introduced specialized photographic views.

In the specialized views, each of the four anatomical subdivisions of the nose is clearly illustrated. Twenty-nine (29) photographs are taken to the nose and face pre-operatively and the same post operatively.

A guide is written for assessment of the pre-operative photographs followed by the analysis of the post-operative photographs.

Successes, difficulties as well as pitfalls are discussed and illustrated photographically.

The art of displaying the pre-operative and post-operative **photographs** must be simple and easy for the eyes in order to clearly and immediately see the results. The aim that all photographs can be **seen at a glance**. **The text** must be well organized, simple, scientific and stereotyped so that it can be **read at a glance.** The principle theme of the Atlas is:

SAG—Seen at A Glance

RAG—Read at A Glance

1. **The Seven Gold Standard Steps for Successful Rhinoplasty are**
   I. Correct Clinical and Psychological Assessment
   II. Correct Photographic Documentation
   III. Correct Photographic Display
   IV. Correct Pre-Operative Surgical and Photographic Assessment
   V. Correct Surgical Planning
   VI. Correct Surgical Techniques
   VII. Correct Post-Operative Analysis

2. **The Necessity of Photography**
   Photographs in Rhinoplasty are necessary for the following two important reasons:
   1. **Medicolegal Documentation**.
   2. **Photographic Anatomy**: A method designed to enhance diagnosis and improve surgical planning.

The photographs highlight certain **anatomical areas** in the nose and face that are missed and could not be seen by the surgeon's eyes at the time of the clinical examination in the first interview with the patient.

Not all informations could be seen live. The surgeon needs time to study and absorb more facts. This can only be achieved by having the fixed documentations of the photographs.

In a way this is similar to the **forensic investigators** who take photographs of the scene of an incident or a crime to critically and carefully study them later. They discover many details that were overlooked at the time of their first inspection of the place. Both sides, of the face and nose, could be seen at the same time e.g. two lateral, two oblique views, basal and over head views.

3. **Normal Individuals and NOT Patients**

People seeking Rhinoplasty are not sick individuals. They cannot be called or referred to as a patients. They only becomes a patients if and when surgery is indicated. Dealing with these cases by the surgeons is partly informal and partly formal.

A lady with a large nose is very much like a pregnant lady. Both are not sick. They cannot be called patients. They become patients if and when surgery is indicated i.e. when they sign the consent for surgery.

M. H. A. Shafy, *Atlas of Clinical Cases in Rhinoplasty*,
https://doi.org/10.1007/978-3-031-07504-9_1

4. The Unpleasant Terms and Patients' Psychology

Some terms are commonly used among Rhinoplasty surgeons to describe certain nasal deformities e.g. "polly beak", "Parrot beak" and "pig snout".

These terms are written in many of the renowned Rhinoplasty books. To the surgeons minds these terms describe specific anatomical abnormalities that need no further detailed explanations. They are used by the surgeon with the minimum or even no sensitivity. They don't have any unpleasant impact. The sad fact that these terms are strongly unpleasant and quite offensive to ordinary people especially when it comes to the pig snout expression. As they reach the patients, these terms have quite negative impact on them. In addition to the state of dissatisfaction from their nasal condition, they become severely disturbed and unhappy to hear these terms. "**It is best to be sensitive when describing peoples' physical appearance**" (Elizabeth Pope). Surgeons must be careful in using more acceptable descriptive words to their patients. With the clear advancement in anatomical knowledge these deformities could be described using more appropriate phrases. **These terms are totally avoided in this text and hopefully from all future textbooks.**

5. Innovative Approach to Rhinoplasty Photography

It is of great value to take multiple photographs in different specific views of the nose. The standard views are not sufficient to make clear detailed and scientific assessment of the different anatomical parts of the nose and face. They had to be modified and expanded to become of better value for the surgeon. The surgeon consequently is able to provide his patients with better assessment and clearer proposal for the surgery.

There are now more **editions to the standard views** that provide better assessment for the nasofacial relation, the effects of smiling and the angles around the nose.

Each anatomical area in the nose is studied by the newly introduced **specialized views**. These photographic views provide a wealth of tools for assessment planning. Each specific area of the nose is viewed better by the camera lens.

Multiplicity of the photographs are only of great value and advantage if they are **well displayed**.

As a three dimensional structure the nose can be seen from countless number of angles and views. A holistic view of the nose is important. A video recording of the nose and face from all directions seems like an ideal method to cover all of these angles and views. Nevertheless, a specific, well defined angle of photography captured by a fixed picture will give a solid document to each anatomical area targeted by this view.

6. The Standard and the Specialized Views

6.1. *The Importance of the Standard Views*

There are four well known **standard views** for the nose and face i.e. the **Frontal**, **Oblique**, **Lateral** and **Basal** views. These are excellent views in showing the **overall appearance of the nose in relation to the face** from the defined different angles.

6.2. *The Necessity for Specialized Views*

Advances in the surgical techniques of Rhinoplasty have lead the surgeons into further detailed procedures in the different anatomical areas of the nose. Highlighting the detailed anatomy of each of these areas by more **specialized photographic views** becomes a necessity. New views from different angles are therefore introduced. These views are:

1. The **Direct Dorsal Views**—non smiling and smiling
2. The **Backward Tilting Views** in two or three steps as the head is tilted backwards.
3. **Nasal Aperture Views**, right and left
4. **Rim-sill tests** in Nasal Aperture Views
5. The **Overhead Views** non smiling and smiling

6.3. *Upgrading the Standard Views*

More benefit is gained from the standard views by adding more views that demonstrate the effects of **smiling** as well as the **middle third** for the frontal, oblique and lateral views.

6.4. *The Advantages of photographic Anatomy*

Studying of the photographs must include the detailed description of the anatomical findings in each views. The correlation between the specific **photographic areas** of the nose and its corresponding **anatomical structures** creates a complete picture of **photographic anatomy** in the surgeon's mind. The normal and the abnormal anatomical areas are recognized, described, hence accurate diagnosis and decisions are greatly helped.

6.5. *Aesthetic photography of the Nose*

The plan to take photographs of the patient must clearly focus on the following two important facts;

(a) The main target is the nose
(b) The main objective is aesthetics

Aesthetic views for the nose must aim at taking photographs to the area of interest **at a direct angle** to have the complete view at the true maximal size of this area. Examples of these are:

- In the nasal aperture views the camera directly faces each **nasal aperture** separately in their naturally different angulation in order to see the natural size and appearance of the aperture shape size and margins.
- The **nasal dorsum** is best seen by a direct dorsal view where the camera directly faces the nasal dorsum.
- In the oblique views the camera faces directly the **lateral nasal wall**.

7. **The Four Areas of Rhinoplasty**

Aesthetic Rhinoplasty is not a single operation. Rhinoplasty is four **different operations;** one in each of the four anatomical areas of the nose.

Each one of the four surgeries is **a totally different procedure** that has different guidelines and techniques. The outcome of all **four surgeries must** produce a harmonized, **aesthetically attractive nose**. These four surgeries are:

i. **Anterior and Lateral wall surgery** for the Nasal tip and lateral crurae
ii. **Medial Wall Surgery** for the Nasal septum, the medial crurae and columella
iii. **Surgery of the Bony Pyramid** and **Mid Vault**
iv. **Alar Base Surgery** for Rim-sill folds, vestibular floors, flat triangles (also known as soft triangles) and **alae nasi**.

8. **Clinical Varieties of Noses Presenting for Rhinoplasty**

Patients seeking Rhinoplasty present with various nasal shapes and conditions. Each of these conditions required **combined regional surgeries** in one or more of the four areas of the nose. The common clinical presentations are:

(1) **The Large Nose**
(2) **The Bulky Nose**
(3) **The Crooked Nose**
(4) **The Deviated Nose and The Oblique Nose**
(5) **The Fractured Nose**
(6) **Finesse Rhinoplasty**
(7) **Secondary Rhinoplasty**
(8) **Ethnic Nose**
(9) **Child Rhinoplasty**
(10) **Special clinical conditions**:
 i. Developmental and Congenital anomalies e.g. dermoid cyst, Waadenburg syndrome, hypertelorism
 ii. Large Alae Nasi
 iii. Sliding tip

In each of these conditions, the same basic surgical techniques are pursued. Special attention is paid for each special case. Each of the major groups will be studied in further details.

9. **The Multiple Distinctive Views**

For accurate and comprehensive pre-operative photographic assessment, each patient needs multiple distinctive number of photographs. At least thirty photographs are needed. As well as the **standard views**, there are newly introduced **editions** to them, which added extra clinical significances. In addition the **Specialized views** are useful in scrutinizing each specific area of the nose.

9.1. ***The Standard Views***

The four standard views are:

- Frontal view: one photo
- Oblique views, right and left: two photos
- Lateral views, right and left: two photos
- Basal view: one photo

9.1.1. *New Editions to the Standard Views*
- The smiling full face, frontal view: one photo
- The smiling full face right and left lateral views: 2 photos
- The oblique midcheek and cheek marginal views: 2 photos
- The middle third views: These are specially important in large faces and small noses, as commonly seen in Asian noses.
  - Frontal View:1 photo
  - Oblique views, right and left midcheek and cheek marginal views: 4 photos
  - Lateral views right and left: 2 photos
- Smiling Basal View:1 photo

9.2. ***Specialized Views***
- Overhead views: 2 photos non-smiling and smiling
- Direct Dorsal views: 2 photos non-smiling and smiling

- Backward Tilting views: 2–3 photos in 2–3 backward steps
- Nasal Aperture views, right and left: 2 photos
- Rim-sill Tests, right and left: 2 photos

Thirteen new photographic editions are added to the six standard views. The newly suggested specialized views are 10–11 views.

The total number of photographs needed for pre-operative assessment is 29–30 photographs. Additional views are improvised in some individual cases.

9.3. *The Advantages of Multiple Views of the Nose*

It is of great advantage to have the general appearance of the **nose and face** as well as the detailed study of every anatomical component of the four anatomical areas of the nose.

The introduced new method of **photographic display** makes it easy for the surgeon to see all these details in an organized systematic way.

The display of two photographs beside each other to compare the pre-operative with the post-operative views is good enough to show one specific angle of the nose and face, but it is not good enough for displaying a group of four or more photographs at the same time. The display of only two photographs is insufficient to study all areas of the nose that are involved in the surgery. Having multiple new views means that we have to display groups of at least four photographs or more at the same time e.g. the pre and post operative smiling and non-smiling, right and left lateral and right and left oblique views. The pre and post operative photographs should be displayed above each other. Example of this; if we display the pre operative two or three steps of the Backward Tilting views beside each other, and the same post operative views are placed exactly below them, it will be easy for the eyes to immediately and quickly see and compare the six photographs at a glance i.e. seen at a glance.

Arrangement of the photographs should make it easy for the eyes of the surgeon to directly study and compare, not only between the preoperative and the postoperative photographs, but also to study many other anatomical facts that help in the preoperative assessment and post operative analysis. The following must be easily and clearly seen on displaying the photographs:

- Easy recognition of the **abnormal anatomical areas** versus the **normal areas**
- Direct comparison between the **right** and **left sides** of the face and nose.
- The **effect of smiling** on the nose, face, nasal base, cheeks and eyes. Comparison is made before and after surgeries.
- Observations of the **immediate, long term** and **post traumatic** changes on the nose and face.

10. The Value of Correct Display of the Multiple Views

Displaying photographs is made for many purposes:

- **Pre-operative** assessment.
  Thirty photos or more are displayed
- **Post-operative** Analysis.
  The overall number of the pre and post operative photographs may reach up to 60 photographs or more.
- **Tertiary study** as in cases of multiple surgeries, long term changes or trauma. More than 70 photos are displayed

10.1. *Displaying the Pre-operative Photographs*

For clear and direct display of **pre-operative** photographs many of the **comparative** or **sequential** anatomical areas of the nose and face must be seen closely **beside each other**. This is especially true in the following views:

- The **non-smiling** and **smiling** views are placed beside each other in order to give the direct visual impression of the anatomical changes that take place on smiling. This is seen in the **Frontal, Direct Dorsal**, **Overhead Basal and Lateral views**.
  The right and left smiling lateral views are especially good example to see the extent of nasal tip animation.
- The **right** and **left oblique views** must be seen side by side facing each other in the display. This is the best demonstration for comparison between the right and left sides of **nasal dorsum**. Nasal **hump** is more prominent on one side in cases of maxillary asymmetry.
- The **right** and **left lateral views** must be seen side by side facing each other to directly compare profiles, paranasal and nasal angles as well as alar grooves and columella.

- The two or three steps of the **backward tilting views** are placed beside each other for direct observation.
- The right and left **Nasal aperture views** are beside each other.
- The right and left **rim sill tests** must seen beside each other.

10.2. *Displaying the Post-operative and Tertiary Photos*

The post-operative photographs, one or more sets, are arranged in exactly the same pattern as the pre-operative ones. The two comparative and sequential photographs are placed **beside each other**. Each **post-operative** photographs is then placed **below** the corresponding pre-operative photograph.

The final presentation of the display is that the two comparative pre-operative photos are beside each other and the corresponding two post-operative photos are below them. **All four photos** are clearly and easily **seen in one place at a glance**. In cases of a third set of photographs i.e. second post-operative condition, photos are placed in a **third row below the previous two rows of photographs**.

Examples of this is having the pre-operative full face Frontal non-smiling and smiling photos above their equivalent post-operative non-smiling and smiling photos. It is therefore possible to see the effect of smiling on the nose and face pre-operatively and the outcome of surgery post operatively, all at the same time.

Another example is the pre-operative right and left rim-sill tests beside each other while their post-operative post-resection photos below them.

10.3. *The Order of Photographic Display*

Photographs are displayed in the order of their clinical significance which in turn reflects the extent of benefits.

Arrangement of the views is made in the following order:

- The Frontal Views full face (non-smiling and smiling) and mid third.
- The Overhead Views (non-smiling and smiling).
- The Direct Dorsal Views (non-smiling and smiling).
- The Backward Tilting Views (2–3 steps backwards).
- The Basal Views (non-smiling and smiling).
- The Nasal Aperture views (Right and left).
- The Rim-Sill tests (right and left).
- The Oblique Views full face and middle third; mid cheek and cheek margins.
- The Lateral views full face (non-smiling and smiling) and middle third.

11. **The Display of the Text**

The easy stereotyped display of photographs is associated with an equally easy stereotyped display of text. Each case is studied in exactly the same systematic pattern. In this way **photographs are seen at a glance** and the **texts are read at a glance**. The following items are discussed and the written before each case:

- Pre-operative Assessment
- Aims of Surgery
- Surgical plan
- Surgical procedure
- Post-Operative Analysis
- Commentary

In each case pre operative assessment, surgical plan, surgical procedure and post operative analysis are discussing the **four areas of the nose** and the corresponding **four Rhinoplasty surgical procedures**.

The four areas and their corresponding four surgeries of the nose are:

1. The **Frontolateral Walls** including the nasal tip
2. The **Medial Wall**, including the **Columella** and **Nasal Septum**
3. The **Bony Pyramid** and **MidVault**
4. **The Nasal Base** including the **Alar base**, the **Vestibular Floors** and the **Flat Triangles**.

P.S. Surgical **Delivery** of the lower lateral cartilages, **Defatting** and **Dome** weakening is indicated in the Atlas as D.D.D.

12. **Conclusion**

The simple stereotyped pattern of the display of the photographs and the text makes them easy to **see** and **read at a glance**.

SAG—Seen at A Glance

RAG—Read at A Glance

Display of photos

Frontal View (F.V.)	Frontal View Smiling (F.V.S.)	Frontal View Middle Third (F.V.MT.)	
Direct Dorsal View (D.D.V.)	Direct Dorsal View Smiling (D.D.V.S.)	Over Head View (O.H.V.)	Over Head View Smiling (O.H.V.S.)
Backward Tilting View (B.T.V.)	Steeper Backward Tilting View (S.B.T.V.)	Basal View (B.V.)	Basal View Smiling (B.V.S.)
Right Nasal Aperture View (R.N.A.V.)	Right Nasal Aperture View Rim Sill Test (R.N.A.V.R.S.T.)	Left Nasal Aperture View Rim Sill test (L.N.A.V.R.S.T.)	Left Nasal Aperture View (L.N.A.V.)
Oblique View Full Face Mid-Cheek Right (O.V.FF.MC.Rt.)	Oblique View Mid-Cheek Left (O.V.MC.Lt.)	Oblique View Middle Third Mid-Cheek Right (O.V.MT.MC.Rt.)	Oblique View Middle Third Mid-Cheek Left (O.V.MT.MC.Lt.)
Oblique View Cheek Margin Right (O.V.CM.Rt.)	Oblique View Cheek Margin Left (O.V.CM.Lt.)	Oblique View Middle Third Cheek Margin Right (O.V.MT.CM.Rt.)	Oblique View Middle Third Cheek Margin Left (O.V.MT.CM.Lt.)
Right Lateral View Right (Rt.L.V.)	Left Lateral View (Lt.L.V.)	Right Lateral View Smiling (Rt.L.V.S.)	Left Lateral View Smiling (Lt.L.V.S.)
Right Lateral View Middle Third (Rt.L.V.MT.)	Left Lateral View Middle Third Left (Lt.L.V.MT.)		

2 A Guide for Photographic Assessment and Analysis

The main objective of this guide is the critical **assessment** of the **pre-operative** photographs, followed by the comprehensive **analysis** of the **post-operative** photographs.

A large number of photographs and texts are displayed in this Atlas in an easy way that could be seen and read fairly quickly. SAG and RAG i.e. Seen at A Glance and Read at A Glance.

This guide meant to give an **in depth study** of the photographs. People may go to an art, science or history museum. Only those who have the informed knowledge, from the guiding notes, books or personnel, have the best benefit out of their visit.

The following guide is by no means a comprehensive one. More detailed study is made in the section of photography in the book of "Innovation in Rhinoplasty". Nevertheless the guide is a well informed foundation. From this start more information may be seen in each photograph, before and after surgery, for the best interest of the patients.

1. **The Contribution of Photography to Successful Rhinoplasty**
   Rhinoplasty photography is a major contributor to the seven Gold Standard Steps for Successful Rhinoplasty (see Introduction to Atlas) so that:

1.1. **Photographic Documentation and Photographic Display**
These two steps are solely made by successful photography. A wide range of highly professional, accurately standardized photographs of the nose and face are lucidly displayed.

1.2. **Pre-operative Assessment and Surgical Planning**
Critical assessment of the pre-operative photographs is of great help for better diagnosis, planning and consequently simple, short and correct surgical procedure with consistently better results.

1.3. **Post-operative Analysis**
Analysis of the short and long term results of surgery can only be achieved by taking photographs of the various views to the nose and face at different intervals. This is an excellent feedback for the surgeon to evaluate the different techniques in the different areas of the nose. Research work, future modifications and upgrading of many techniques can take place.

1.4. **Conclusion**
Assessment of the **pre-operative photographs** is invaluable for best planning and execution of surgery in the shortest time with best results.
Analysis of the **post-operative photographs** is invaluable for the best surgical evaluation, future advancement and avoiding mistakes.
The importance of individual history:
Unlike other types of surgeries, aesthetic or non-aesthetic, Rhinoplasty is not the same stereotyped operation. The nose is like a fingerprint every nose in this planet is different. Even the two sides of the same nose are different so that:
(a) Each nose has its own individualized surgery.
(b) The same nose may have different operation in different individuals according to their height, body built, social background, ethnicity and gender.
(c) Personal references; every individual prefers a certain look to the nose, some are quite conservatives and others would like to have radical changes in their noses.
(d) Rhinoplasty is associated with strong emotions and psychology. Candidates for Rhinoplasty are full of fear, hopes and dreams. Each candidate goes through five intensive psychological stages (see chapter of psychology of Rhinoplasy in Innovations of Rhinoplasty book).
(e) Rhinoplasty is combined professional, artistic and emotional endeavor. Not every competent surgeon is readily prepared to perform Rhinoplasty, and not every person with a deformed nose is readily prepared to have Rhinopasty.

M. H. A. Shafy, *Atlas of Clinical Cases in Rhinoplasty*,
https://doi.org/10.1007/978-3-031-07504-9_2

Benefits of individual history:

(a) Understanding the reason behind the shape of each nose i.e. the cause of deformity, depression, enlargement or otherwise.

(b) The personalized history puts life and humanize every individual case. Without this, it becomes too mechanical and too dry.

(c) The medical history alone is insufficient, the general, build of the body, psychological and emotional state,personal overall preferences, gender, type of personality, social status, social life, individual hobbies and activities, all these are factors that help in making decisions of the type of surgery that suits this individual and to proceed for surgery or avoid it altogether.

Important Note:

In this Atlas the individual relevant history is omitted in all cases. Some may contain detailed personal information that is not suitable for publication.

2. **Pre-operative Photographic Assessment**

   Not all information could be seen at the time of clinical examination of patients. Photographs highlight specific anatomical areas that could not be seen by the clinicians eyes. Pre-operative photographic assessment proved of great value in surgical planning and decisions. Each of the four areas of Rhinoplasty is critically assessed.

2.1. **Photographic Assessment of Frontolateral Walls**

Frontolateral walls study is mainly concerned about the nasal tip. Photographically the nasal tip is studied in its **shape**, **position** and **size**. The **shape** of the tip photographically expressed as **tip definition** while **position** of the tip is expressed as **tip projection**.

2.1.1. **Tip Definition**

Tip definition means that the nasal tip, made by the two middle crurae, is **small** and **prominently well identified** from the surrounding alae nasi. This is to be distinguished from the **flat ill defined**, **large** and **bulky nasal tips**.

A thick skinned nasal tip is usually large and bulky. It **overshadows the alae nasi** on both sides. The alae nasi may hardly be seen or not seen at all. The superior alar grooves, (see Anatomy section) are filled with the subdermal fat. They become short, flat and ill recognized.

The subdermal fat of the **middle** and **lateral crurae** makes the tip amorphously continuous with the alae nasi on both sides. The tip is unrecognized and is ill defined.

Defatting of the middle and lateral crurae results in a **slim and small nasal tip** without the need to directly stitch the domes. The **superior alar grooves**, being uncovered of all the fat, they become **deep**, **long** and **visible**. The **alae nasi** come into view, and share in nasal aesthetics with the nasal tip.

How does defatting works

i. **The superior alar groove** anatomically consists of two components:
   - **Alar muscular groove** i.e. between the ala nasi and the muscular triangle posteriorly
   - **Alar crural groove** i.e. between the ala nasi and the lateral crus anteriorly.

     Defatting the **lateral crurae** clears the fat off the junction between the lateral crurae and the alae nasi. The superior alar grooves become more apparently deeper and consequently longer.
ii. **The alae nasi** becomes more apparent after defatting its junctional area with the lateral crurae. The bounderies of their bodies become clearer. As they are pulled medially, they became better seen and look smaller and well defined. Aesthetics of the alae nasi generally improve.
iii. **The nasal tip** becomes smaller by defatting the **middle crurae**. Nasal tip definition is further enhanced by defatting the **lateral crurae**. The overlying skin becomes thinner.

Tip definition is best seen in the following views:

- Frontal Views.
- Over Head Views.
- Direct Dorsal Views
- Backward Tilting Views.
- Basal Views.
- Nasal Aperture Views.

The **superior alar grooves** are best seen in:

- Direct Dorsal Views
- Oblique Views
- Lateral Views

2.1.2. **Tip Projection**

This term is used to express the **height** and the **shape of the tip** at the end of the nasal dorsum. For aesthetically pleasing projection, the nasal tip should be **at the same level** or **slightly higher** than the nasal dorsum. In the **lateral views** the angle of the tip should be near to 90 degrees. This is best coupled with a 90 degrees nasolabial angle.

Nasal tip projection is best seen in the **lateral views** and to lesser extend in the **oblique views**.

2.1.3. **Tip Size**

Tip size is aesthetically significant. Too small ill defined or too large and bulky are two unaesthetic tips. It is directly related to the **skin thickness** and the **sizes of the middle and lateral crurae**. Bifidity or grooving of the middle crurae are unaesthetic. The size of nasal tip is seen in all views but predominantly better seen in the **Frontal, Direct Dorsal, Backward Tilting** and **Basal views**.

2.1.4. **The Light Reflex**

The light reflex is looked for at the domes of the nasal tip. **Bifid nasal tip** reflects **two spots** of light reflex. An **aesthetically pleasing nasal tip** reflects **one spot of light reflex**.

The light reflex of the nasal tip is better seen in the Frontal and Backward Tilting views.

2.2. **Photographic Assessment of the Medial Wall**

The medial wall is made of **the columella, the medial crurae** and **the caudal cartilagenous septum**. The three subcutenous structures of the medial wall that are photographically significant are:

1. The columella
2. The caudal cartilagenous septum including the anterior septal angle at the end of the nasal dorsum.
3. The Inferior Vestibular Bands (I.V.B.), including the nasal sill bands that go, abutting the posterior then the superior margins of the medial crurae on both sides (see the chapter of Histological Studies)
   - The columella has two component
     - The anterior firm part made by the medial crurae
     - The posterior soft fold between the medial crurae and the filtrium of the upper lip.

All views except the Direct Dorsal and Overhead Views are important in studying the medial wall.

The **Backward Tilting**, **Basal** and the **Nasal Aperture** views are the specialized views for the medial wall photography. These are followed by the Oblique and Lateral views.

2.2.1. **Assessement of the Deviated and/or Elongated Caudal Septum**

Aesthetic effects of caudal septal deviation and/or elongation may take place, **laterally, inferiorly** or **anteriorly**. Photographically the medial wall is looked for in the following areas:

a. **Laterally**
   - The deviated caudal septum pushes the **medial crus** including the I.V.B. (Inferior Vestibular Band) laterally distorting the **shape** of **nasal aperture** and produces unequal nasal openings in **size** and shape. This is best seen in the **Backward Tilting, Basal** and **Nasal Aperture Views**.

b. **Inferiorly**

   The caudal septum may be elongated inferiorly:
   - Pushing the two components of the columella, the firm crurae and the soft fold, producing a **protruded columella**. This is best seen in the Frontal, Oblique and Lateral views.
   - The long caudal septum pushes the **ipsilateral nasal sill band inferiorly** to become at a lower level than the contralateral nasal sill band. This is best to seen in the Frontal and Backward Tilting views.
   - The severely deviated caudal margin of the cartilaginous septum may be **seen through** the nasal aperture cavity.

     The inferior changes are best seen in the **Frontal, Oblique** and **Lateral view**. Other specialized views demonstrates these changes to lesser extent.

c. **Anteriorly**
   - The **height** of the anterior septal angles is shown in the **supratip area** i.e. the weak triangle as **supra tip depression** or **supratip elevation** in cases of low and high anterior septal angle consequently.

     Unilateral bulge of middle or **lateral crurae** may be caused by a high severely deviated cartilagenous septum.

     These changes are best seen in the **Lateral, Oblique, Backward Tilting** and **Nasal Aperture Views**.

2.2.2. **Assessment of the Columella**

- The **protruding** and **hanging** columella are best seen in the Lateral and Oblique views.
- **Thickness, bifidity** and **lateral columellar protrusions** are best seen in the Basal and Nasal Aperture views.

2.2.3. **The Light Reflex**

The light reflex of the columella is observed normally as one spot or two spots in cases of grooving and bifidity. This is best seen in the Backward Tilting and Basal Views.

2.3. **Photographic Assessment of the Bony Pyramid**

The bony pyramid is assessed photographically for:

2.3.1. **Height**

- Depression: supratip, midvault, saddle deformities or skislope depression. Depressions may be post traumatic or development.
- Elevation: osteocartilagenous humps and supratip elevation.
- Irregularities following trauma, accidental or surgical.

2.3.2. **Deviation**

The bony pyramid may be deviated off the midline in the **sagital plane**. Deviation is best seen in the Frontal, Direct Dorsal and Overhead Views.

Deviated bony pyramid is commonly seen in developmental bilateral maxillary asymmetry.

2.3.3. **Obliquity**

The bony pyramid may be oblique to one side in the **axial plane**. Oblique bony pyramid is best seem in the Backward Tilting Views.

Oblique bony pyramid is commonly seen following **traumatic** fracture or surgery.

Combined **deviation** and **obliquity** of the bony pyramid is seen in bilateral **maxillary asymmetry** i.e. the developmentally oblique bony pyramid is always associated with deviation of the nose to one side, while traumatically oblique bony pyramid is not associated with deviation of the nose.

The maxillary bone is larger in one side than the other. The oblique bony pyramid and bilateral maxillary asymmetry are best seen in Backward Tilting Views where one cheek is high and narrow while the opposite cheek is low and wide.

2.3.4. **Dorsum**

The dorsum of the bony pyramid, from the nasion at the nasofrontal angle to the anterior septal angle, is best seen in the **Lateral** and **Oblique views**.

Other views demonstrates the dorsum and sidewalls in different and useful angles i.e. the nasal aperture views.

2.3.5. **Side Walls**

Wide base, unequal or **irregular sidewalls** are unaesthetic. The sidewalls are seen in **all views** except Basal Views. Each of the views has a special angle to the side wall. The unequal sidewalls and wide base of the body pyramid are best seen in the Backward Tilting views. Irregularities of the sidewalls are best seen in the Frontal and Oblique views.

2.3.6. **The Light Reflex**

The Light Reflex of the nasal dorsum of special aesthetic and photographic importance. It is best seen in the Direct Dorsal Views.

2.4. **Photographic Assessment of the Alar Base**

The nasal base includes the **alar base, flat triangles** (also known as the **soft triangles**), the **vestibular floors** and the **nasal sill bands**. The nasal openings are no more than two gaps that separate the vestibular floors posteriorly from the flat triangles anteriorly.

2.4.1. **Why the Alar Base and not the Nasal Base?**

The alar base is the most significant surgically of all of the three structures of the nasal base.

The **Alar Base** is therefore referred to as the fourth area of Rhinoplasty rather than the nasal base.

2.4.2. **The Alae Nasi**

The alae nasi are photographically significant in its structural body as well as its relations and attachments to the upper lip.

2.4.2.1. **The Alar Bodies**

Alar bodies are best seen in the lateral and oblique views. They are observed for:

- The **alar size** and **shape**; **columello alar relationship**:
  Too **small** alae nasi expose the lateral columellar walls and vice versa, too **large** alae nasi may become at a lower level than the columella which might be completely hidden. This is mostly seen in Asian noses.
- **Alar-Tip Relationship**
  The alae nasi should appear anteriorly as two gentle protrusion on the sides of the nasal tip. This is best seen in the **Frontal, Direct Dorsal** and **Overhead views**. Different angles of viewing the alae nasi are the **Backward Tilting** and **Basal Views**.
  Smiling and Alar Flare
  Smiling views demonstrates the extent of **alar flare**. It is not uncommon to have **asymmetrical sizes** of alae nasi and **asymmetrical alar flare** on smiling. Asymmetrical smile is associated with different sizes and shapes of cheek balls, levels and shapes of the nasolabial folds as well as different lateral angles of the lips.

2.4.2.2. **The Alar Grooves**

The **superior** and **posterior alar grooves** are compared on their **length** and **depth** before and after surgeries.

- The **superior alar groove** is an alar nasal groove i.e. between the superior margin of the ala nasi and the lateral crus and the muscular triangle from before backwards (see anatomy section in anatomy section of Innovations in Rhinoplasty). It is mainly affected by the subdermal **fatty layer** that covers the lateral crurae.

The **superior alar grooves** are best seen in the **Direct Dorsal, Overhead, Oblique and Lateral Views**.

- The **posterior alar groove** is an alar lip groove i.e. between the posterior margin of the ala nasi and the upper lip (see anatomy section of Innovations in Rhinoplasty). It is mainly affected by the size and thickness of the **posterior segments of the rim-sill folds**.

The **posterior alar grooves** are seen in the **Basal, Backward Tilting** and **Nasal Aperture Views**.

2.4.2.3. **The Alar Margins**

- The **inferior alar margins** i.e. **alar rims** are best seen in the Backward Tilting, Basal and Nasal Aperture Views.
  The length, shape and light reflexes are observed.
- The **Rim Sill Test** to demonstrates the posterior and inferior segments of the rim-sill folds.
  - A **long inferior segment** produces **wide nasal aperture** while **thick posterior segment** produces **bulky alar base** and bulky lower third of the nose.
  - Bulky posterior segment has an acute angle with the upper lip giving a **flat tire appearance**.
  - The posterior and inferior **excisional segment scars** are looked for and seen in post-operative photographs.
  - **Light Reflexes** are observed off the inferior margins (Basal and Nasal Aperture Views).

2.4.3. **The Flat Triangles and the Vestibular Floors**

The **Flat Triangles** (also known as the **soft triangles**) and the **Vestibular Floors** Including the **Nasal Sill Bands** are best seen in the Backward Tilting, Basal and Nasal Aperture Views. **Light Reflexes** are observed at the margins of the flat triangles. (Nasal Aperture Views).

2.5. **The Light Reflex**

The hairless glistening surfaces and margins of the nasal skin reflects lines and spots of light (refer to the main text):

a. **Surface light reflex**:
   i. Dorsal light reflex: a line of light is reflected off the skin of the nasal dorsum (Direct Dorsal Views).
   ii. Tip light reflex: one or more spots of light is reflected off the glistening skin cover of the domes of the nasal tip. (Frontal and Backward Tilting Views).
b. **Marginal light reflex:**

Light is reflected from the following margins:

i. Inferior alar margins (Nasal Aperture and Basal Views).
ii. Nasal sill bands (Nasal Aperture and Oblique Views).
iii. Lateral columellar margins (Lateral Views).
iv. Inferior margins of the flat triangles (Nasal Aperture Views).

Absent Light Reflex

The light reflex is absent in:

a. The weak and soft areas e.g. rim-sill folds and posterior columellar fold.
b. Anatomically disturbed areas e.g. caudal dislocation or irregular dorsal anatomy.

The presence or absence of light reflex is of aesthetic and surgical significances. Distorted preoperative light reflexes improve after surgery to become one regular line, in cases of dorsal and marginal light reflexes, and one spot in cases of the nasal tip light reflex. This is an additional method of assessing better postoperative surgical results.

3. **Post-operative Analysis and Comments**

The post operative comprehensive analysis of aesthetics of each of four areas of Rhinoplasty is beneficial for the **patients** and the **surgeons** alike.

Patients understand in more details the changes after surgery. Some patients surprisingly may forget what their noses looked like.

Any residual deformity or misshapen area could be seen and discussed with the surgeon.

Surgeons benefit from the feedback of successes, mistakes and failures. Long term results are significantly useful in all cases.

Many lessons are learned so that surgeons are continuously improving, correcting and developing new techniques.

In the post-operative analysis, **the post-operative photographs** are examined after going through the pre-operative photographic assessment, aims of surgery, surgical plan and the surgical procedure. Better aesthetic results in each of the four areas of Rhinoplasty are described in the different photographic views as follows:

3.1. **Antrolateral Wall**

- **Tip Definition**: nasal tip is smaller with thinner and smoother overlying skin. It is more prominent and well identified from the alae nasi on both sides. The alae nasi come into view to become clearly visible and share in nasal aesthetics (Frontal, Direct Dorsal, Overhead, Backward Tilting and Basal Views).
- **Tip projection**: The nasal tip at the same level of the nasal dorsum with good aesthetic angle. This is coupled with good aesthetic nasolabial angle (lateral and oblique views).
- The **light reflex** is clear and appear as one or two spots off the nasal tip.

3.2. **The Medial Wall**

- Correction of septal deviation leads to:
  - Nasal apertures: Nasal openings are closer in size and shape to each other.
  - Unilateral bulge of medial crus overcome.
  - Unilateral inferior displacement of nasal sill band is amended. Both bands become at the same horizontal level.
  - The protrusion of the caudal cartilagenous margin is no longer seen.
  - Unilateral bulge of the middle or lateral crus have leveled.
- Hanging columella or protrusion columella have gone.
- Supratip elevation/or depression become more level.
- Mobility of the tip is gone.
- The **light reflex** is observed (Basal and Backward Tilting Views).

3.3. **Bony Pyramid**

- **Bony pyramid aesthetics**: the nasal dorsum is straight and the sidewalls are smooth and narrow (all views except the Basal Views).
- **The light reflex** is seen as an uninterrupted line off the nasal dorsum (Direct Dorsal Views).

3.4. **Alar Base**

- **Superior alar groove aesthetics** improved by defatting. The grooves become longer and deeper (Oblique, Lateral and Direct Dorsal grooves).
- **Posterior alar groove aesthetics** improved:
  - By defatting alone: After defatting the lateral crurae the alae nasi are pulled medially and the angles of the posterior alar grooves become wider. Aesthetics of the alae nasi improve as they become clearly seen. (Backward Tilting and Nasal Aperture Views).
  - By defatting as well as excising the posterior segments of the rim-sill folds. The flat tire appearance is no longer present. (Backward Tilting, Basal and Nasal Aperture Views).
- **Alae nasi aesthetics improve** by defatting alone or together with rim-sill fold excision. The alae nasi are pulled medially widening the posterior alar grooves. They become more visible and smaller in size. (Backward Tilting, Basal and Nasal Aperture Views).
- **Nasal aperture aesthetics:**
  - **The size** of the nasal openings are reduced:
    - i By **defatting alone**, in some, but not in all cases.
    - ii By **Defatting** as well as **excising the inferior segments of the rim-sill folds**. (Backward Tilting, Basal and Nasal Aperture views).
  - **The shape** of nasal openings.
  - **Defatting alone** of the frontolateral walls enhances aesthetics of the nasal openings with or without affecting their size. They become more elegantly oval on shape. (Backward Tilting, Basal and Nasal Aperture views).
  - **Defatting** and **excision of the rim-sill folds** transforms the nasal apertures from **thick walled wide** and **rounded** openings with **transverse long axes** to **thin walled, small oval** openings with **anterior long axes**. (Backward Tilting, Basal and Nasal Aperture views).
- The marginal **light reflexes** are observed off the inferior alar margins, nasal sill bands, margins of the flat triangle and the lateral columellar margins (Basal, Nasal Aperture, Oblique and Lateral views).

Part II

Large Nose Rhinoplasty

Part II: Clinical Case 1

3

Preoperative Assessment

1. **Frontolateral walls**
   Large and bulky frontolateral walls overshadowing the alae nasi. The nasal tip was flat and ill defined. (Frontal, Direct Dorsal and Backward Tilting Views).
2. **Medial Wall**
   Mobile tip (lateral smiling views).
3. **Bony pyramid**
   a. Wide base of the bony pyramid (Frontal, Direct Dorsal and Backward Tilting Views).
   b. Diffuse dorsal light reflex (Direct Dorsal Views).
4. **Alar base**
   a. Wide alar base, due to long inferior segments, and bulky, due to thick posterior segments of Rim Sill folds (Backward Tilting, Basal and Nasal Aperture Views).
   b. There is natural asymmetrical alae nasi. They are different in size and shape, the left ala nasi being slightly larger (Frontal direct your soul and overhead views).
   c. The nasal sill band is flat i.e. it is not elevated from the level of lip skin (Backward Tilting, Basal, and Nasal Aperture Views).

Aims of Surgery

1. Overall reduction of the nasal size.
2. Reduce the bulk of the lower third of the nose.
3. Reduce the width and bulk of the alar base.

Surgical Plan

1. **Frontolateral walls**
   a. D.D.D. including weak triangle to reduce the bulk of nasal tip and supra tip area. Rasping of the fibrous dermal layer of the frontolateral walls to further reduce the thickness of the skin.
   b. Bilateral cephalic trim of the lateral crurae.
2. **Medial Wall**
   Division of depressor septi muscles.
3. **Bony pyramid**
   Osteotomies and medialization of the lateral bony walls to reduce the width of the bony pyramid.
4. **Alar base**
   Resection of both components of the Rim Sill folds, i.e. the posterior thick segments, to reduce the alar bulk, and the inferior long segments, to reduce the size of Nasal openings.

Surgical Procedure

As per Surgical Plan.

Post-Operative Analysis

1. **Frontolateral**
   a. Tip definition: nasal tip is smaller with thinner and smoother overlying skin. It is more prominent and well identified from the alae nasi on both sides. The alae nasi come into view to become clearly visible and share in nasal aesthetics (Frontal, Direct Dorsal, Overhead, Backward Tilting and Basal Views).
   b. Tip projection: The nasal tip at the same level of the nasal dorsum with good aesthetic angle. This is coupled with good aesthetic nasolabial angle (lateral and oblique views).
   c. Tip light reflex is seen as one spot off the nasal tip. (Frontal and Backward Tilting Views).
2. **Medial Wall**
   Tip mobility was not completely overcome.
3. **Bony Pyramid**
   a. Bony pyramid aesthetics: the nasal dorsum is straight and the sidewalls are smooth and narrow (all views except the Basal Views).
   b. Dorsal light reflex is seen as an uninterrupted line off the nasal dorsum (Direct Dorsal Views).

M. H. A. Shafy, *Atlas of Clinical Cases in Rhinoplasty*,
https://doi.org/10.1007/978-3-031-07504-9_3

4. **Alar Base**
   a. Superior alar groove aesthetics improved by defatting. The grooves become longer and deeper (Oblique, Lateral and Direct Dorsal grooves).
   b. Posterior alar groove angles and aesthetics of the alae nasi are improved. The alae nasi are pulled medially widening the posterior groove angles. The alae nasi are better seen and look smaller in size (Nasal Aperture and Oblique Views).
   c. Nasal Aperture Aesthetics: The flat nasal sill bands have made it difficult to produce rounded lateral alar angles post-operatively. Nevertheless nasal apertures are smaller and aesthetically more acceptable.
   d. Marginal light reflexes are seen off the inferior alar margins.

Commentary

a. Removing the two hypodermal fatty layers were not sufficient to reduce thickness of nasal tip skin. The dermal layer was further thinned out by rasping. This step is better avoided in open Rhinoplasty due to division of the two columellar arteries and lack of tip blood supply.
b. In these cases, of flat nasal sill bands, only the **posterior** segments of the rim sill folds are excised. The **inferior** segments are better preserved to maintain the lateral rounded shapes of the nasal apertures.

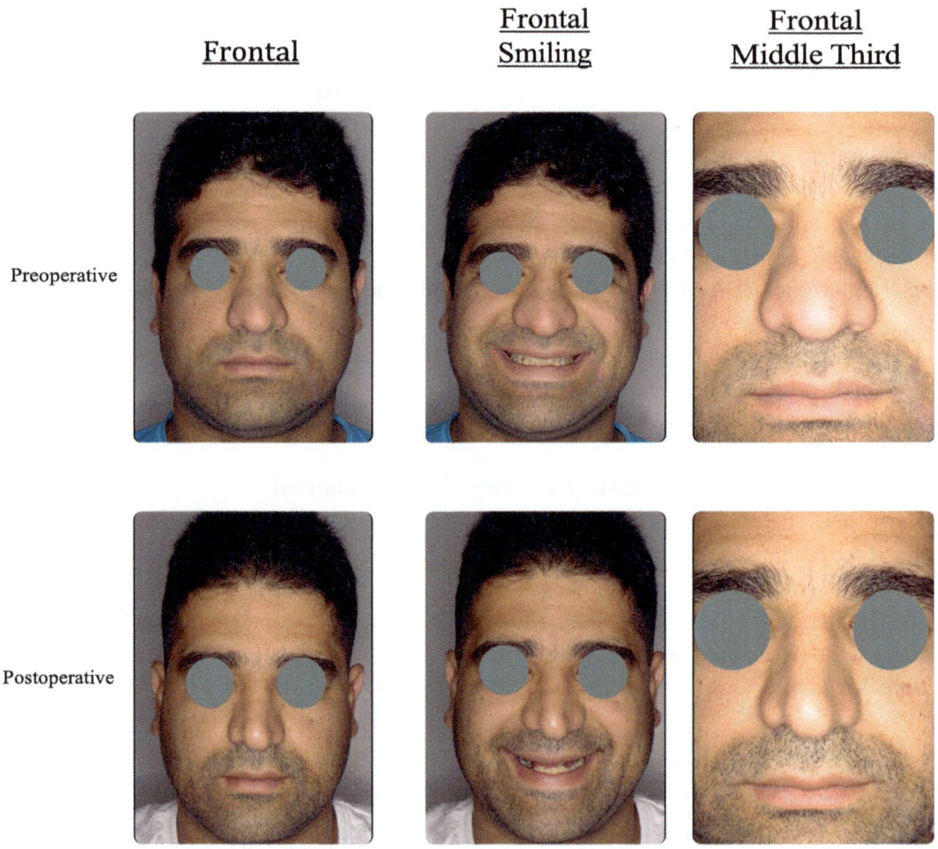

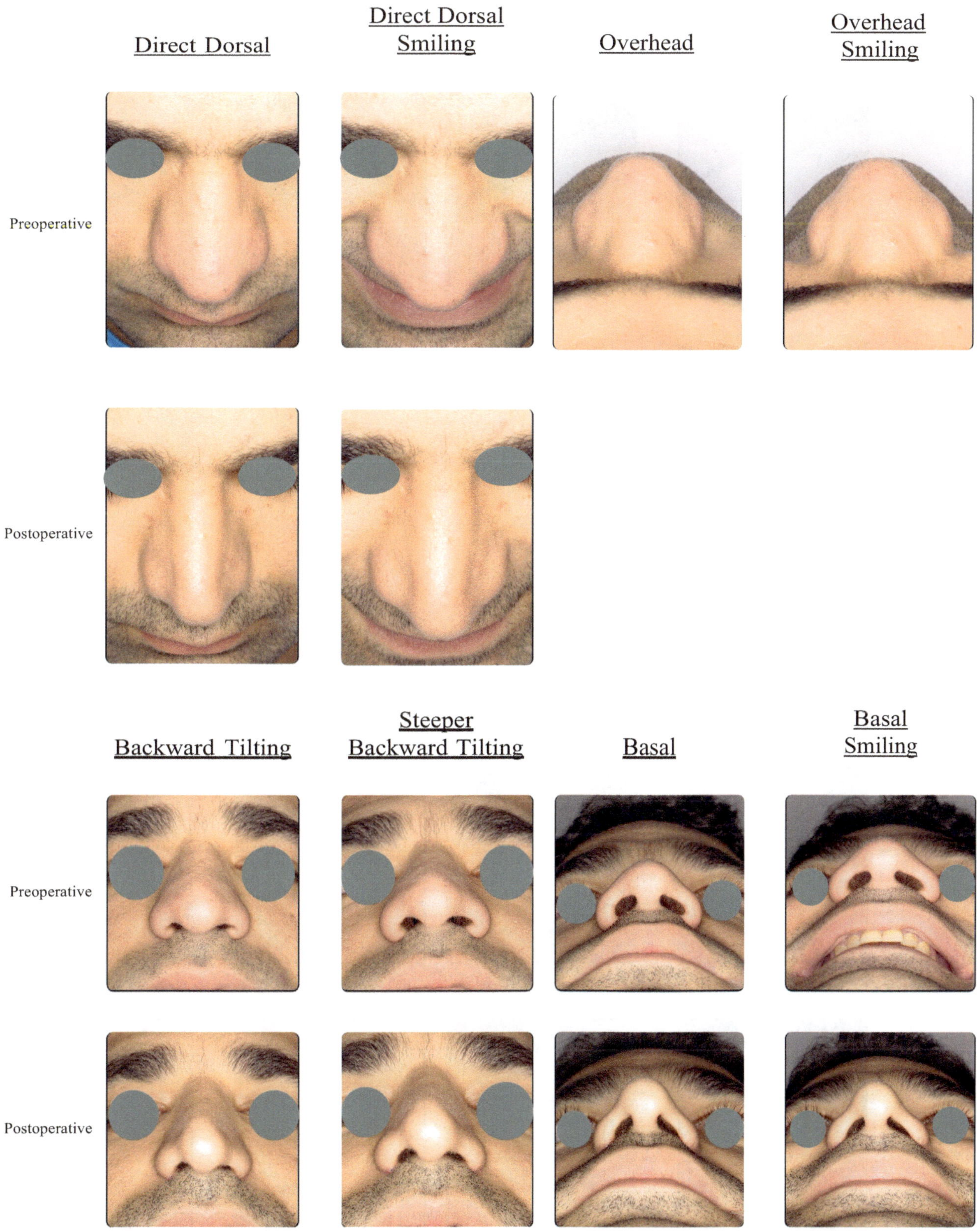
Direct Dorsal
Direct Dorsal Smiling
Overhead
Overhead Smiling
Preoperative
Postoperative
Backward Tilting
Steeper Backward Tilting
Basal
Basal Smiling
Preoperative
Postoperative

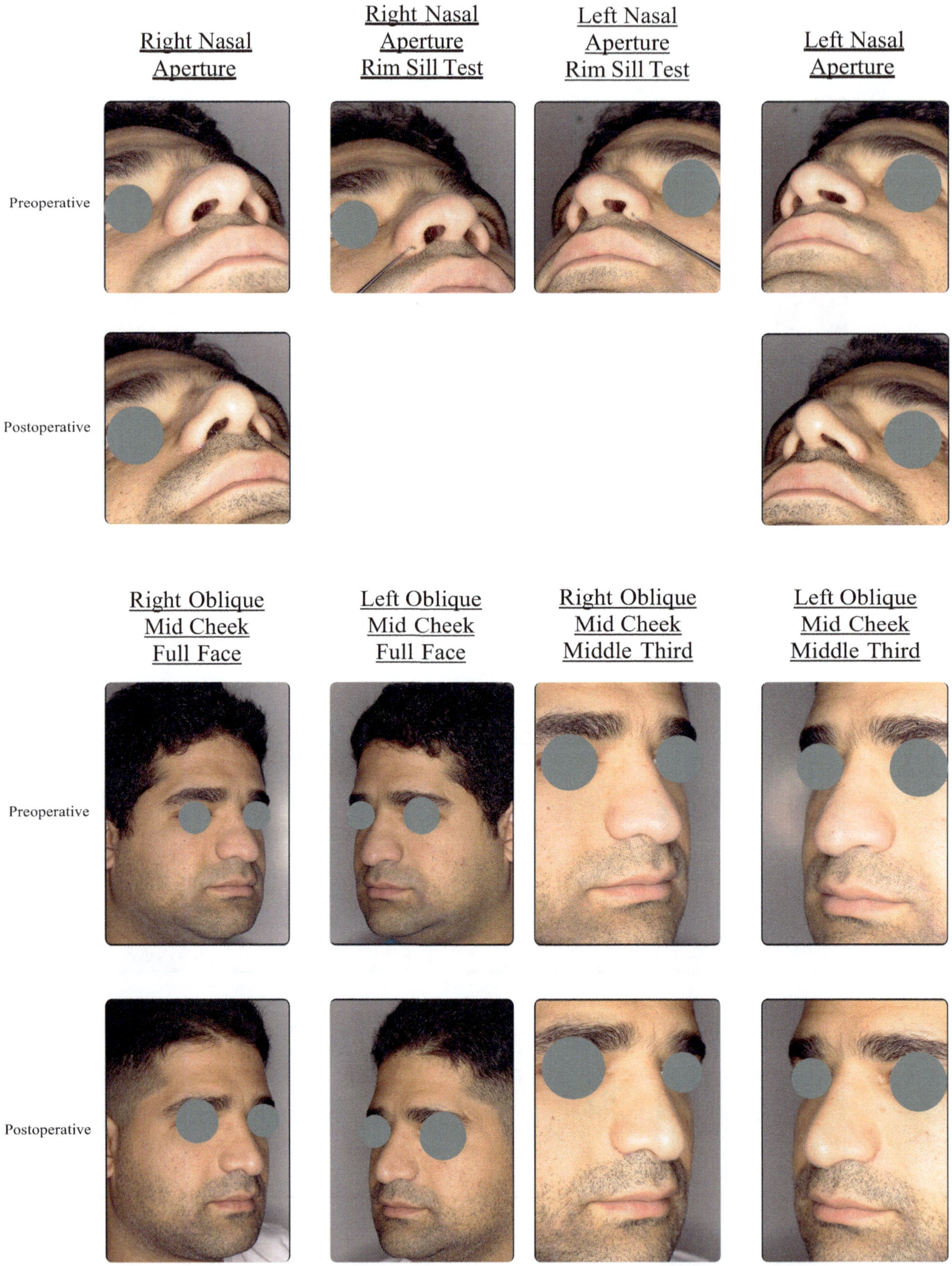
Right Nasal Aperture
Right Nasal Aperture Rim Sill Test
Left Nasal Aperture Rim Sill Test
Left Nasal Aperture
Preoperative
Postoperative
Right Oblique Mid Cheek Full Face
Left Oblique Mid Cheek Full Face
Right Oblique Mid Cheek Middle Third
Left Oblique Mid Cheek Middle Third
Preoperative
Postoperative

Right Oblique Cheek Margin Full Face | Left Oblique Cheek Margin Full Face | Right Oblique Cheek Margin Middle Third | Left Oblique Cheek Margin Middle Third

Preoperative

Postoperative

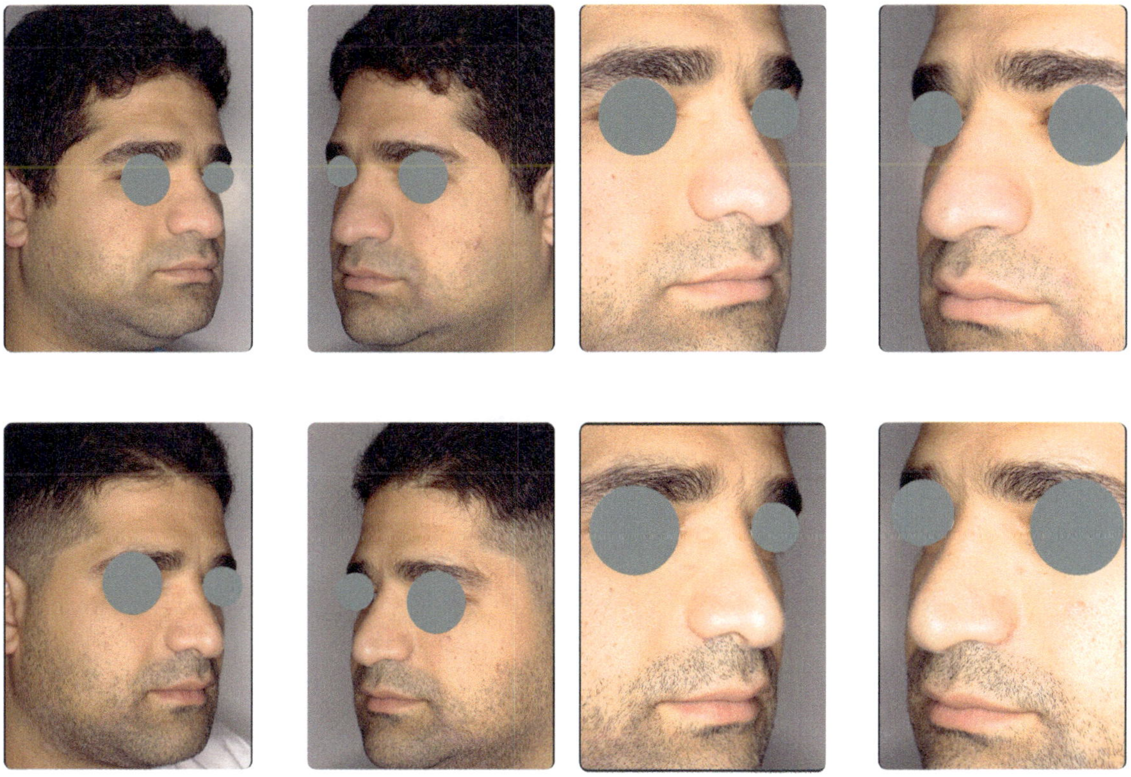

Right Lateral | Left Lateral | Right Lateral Smiling | Left Lateral Smiling

Preoperative

Postoperative

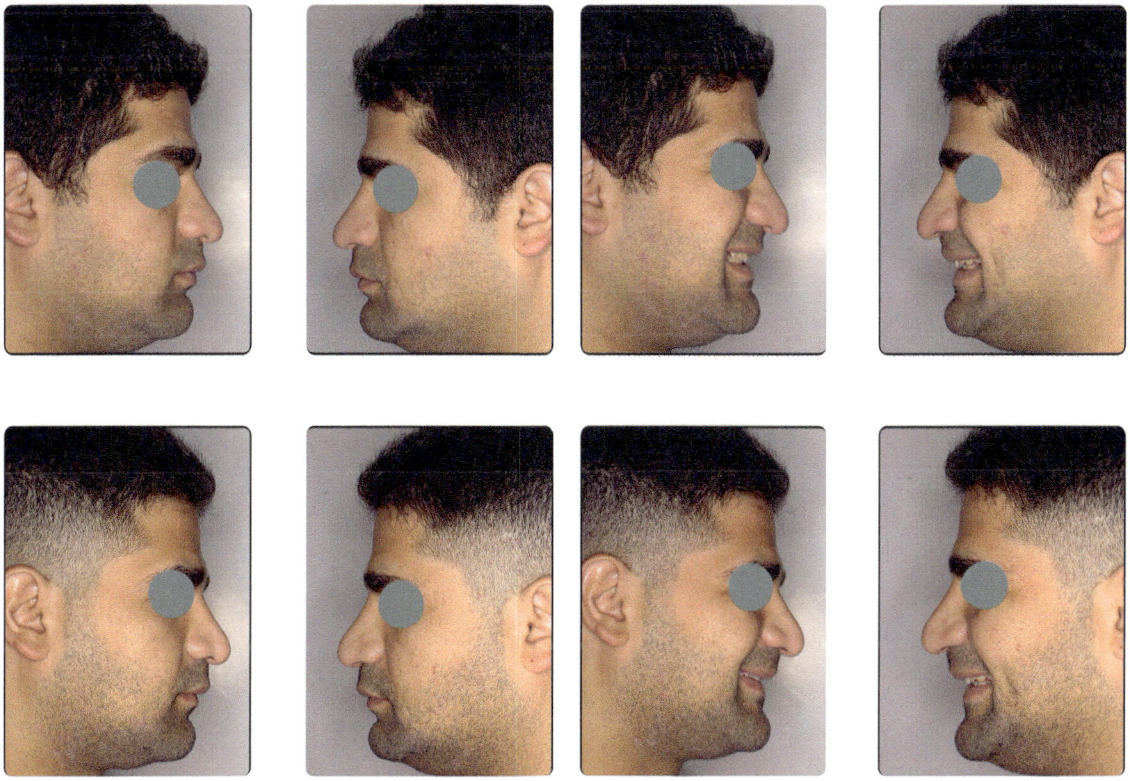

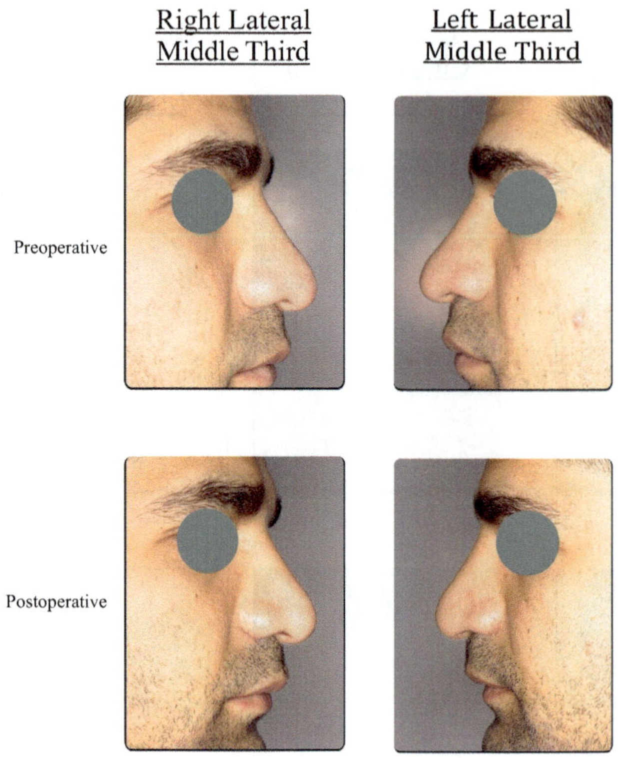
Right Lateral
Middle Third
Left Lateral
Middle Third
Preoperative
Postoperative

4 Part II: Clinical Case 2

Preoperative Assessment

1. **Frontolateral walls**
   Large, bulbous tip that overshadows the alae nasi (frontal, direct dorsal and overhead views).
2. **Medial Wall**
   Mobile tip (lateral smiling views).
3. **Bony pyramid**
   a. Osteocartilaginous hump (Lateral, and Oblique Views).
   b. Wide base of the bony pyramid (Direct Dorsal, Overhead and Backward Tilting Views).
   c. The boney pyramid is oblique, but not deviated, to the right due to bilateral maxiliary asymmetry. The right cheek is wide and low and the left cheek is high and narrow (Frontal and Backward Tilting Views).
   d. Abscent dorsal light reflex (preoperative Direct Dorsal Views).
4. **Alar base**
   Wide alar base, nasal apertures are thick walled wide and rounded. Acute posterior groove, angles with the upper lip, giving the impression of a flat tire appearance (Backward Tilting and Basal Views).

Aims of Surgery

1. Reduction of the overall size and bulk of the nose, including the nasal tip, boney pyramid and alar base.
2. Abolish the mobile tip.

Surgical Plan

1. **Frontolateral walls**
   a. DDD including the weak triangle to reduce the size and bulk of the nasal tip and supra tip area.
   b. Cephalic trim of the lateral crurae to reduce the size.
2. **Medial Wall**
   Division of the Depressor Septi muscles.
3. **Bony pyramid**
   a. Excision of the osteocartilaginous hump.
   b. Osteotomies and medialization of the lateral bony walls to reduce the width of the bony pyramid.
   c. Kasanjian maneuver to the left i.e. cross fracture of the bony pyramid after osteotomies (see Surgery of the Bony Pyramid in Text).
4. **Alar base**
   Resection of the posterior and inferior segments of the rim-sill folds.

Surgical Procedure

As per Surgical Plan.

Post-Operative Analysis

1. **Frontolateral**
   a. Tip definition: the nasal tip is smaller with thinner and smoother overlying skin. It is more prominent and well identified from the alae nasi on both sides. The alae nasi come into view to become clearly visible and share in nasal aesthetics (Frontal, Direct Dorsal, Overhead, Backward Tilting and Basal Views).
   b. Tip projection: The nasal tip at the same level of the nasal dorsum with good aesthetic angle. This is coupled with good aesthetic nasolabial angle (lateral and oblique views).
   c. Tip light reflex is seen as one spot off the nasal tip. (Frontal and Backward Tilting Views).
2. **Medial Wall**
   Tip mobility was not completely overcome.
3. **Bony Pyramid**
   a. Bony pyramid aesthetics: the nasal dorsum is straight and the sidewalls are smooth and narrow (all views except the Basal Views).
   b. Dorsal light reflex is seen as an uninterrupted line off the nasal dorsum (Direct Dorsal Views).

M. H. A. Shafy, *Atlas of Clinical Cases in Rhinoplasty*,
https://doi.org/10.1007/978-3-031-07504-9_4

4. **Alar Base**
   a. Superior alar groove aesthetics improved by defatting. The grooves become longer and deeper (Oblique, Lateral, Direct Dorsal and Overhead Views).
   b. Posterior alar groove aesthetics improved by defatting as well as excision of the inferior and posterior segments of the rim-sill folds. The flat tire appearance is no longer present. (Backward Tilting, Basal and Nasal Aperture Views).
   c. Alae nasi aesthetics improved. They are pulled medially become better seen, smaller and share in nasal aesthetics. (Nasal Aperture, Oblique and Lateral Views).
   d. Nasal Aperture Aesthetics improved:
      i. The size of the nasal openings are reduced by defatting as well as excising the inferior segments of the rim-sill folds. (Backward Tilting, Basal and Nasal Aperture views).
      ii. The shape of nasal openings improved. Defatting and excision of the rim-sill folds transformed the nasal apertures from thick heavy wide and round openings with transverse long axes to become thin delicate small oval openings with anterior long axes. (Backward Tilting, Basal and Nasal Aperture views).
   e. Marginal light reflexes are better seen at:
      i. The inferior alar and flat triangular margins. The light reflex is absent from the rim-sill folds. The latter were accurately excised (Nasal Aperture Views).
      ii. Nasal sill bands (Oblique Views).
      iii. Lateral crural prominences (Lateral Views).

Commentary

a. Photographs of the lateral views apparenly show a flat nasofrontal angle. The oblique views show a well formed nasofrontal angle. This was confirmed by palpation. The excess hairs of eyebrows have given the impression of the flat angle in the lateral view photographs. The surgeon must not rush into reducing the nasofrontal angle based on the photographic appearance.
b. Photographs were taken 10 days postoperatively (note the fresh alar scar in the postoperative frontal view). A more uniform reduction in the size of the bony pyramid, midvault and nasal tip will take place in the long term.
c. The overall size of the nose is smaller and proportionately suites his face better than before surgery. Patient's wish was fulfilled. Naso-facial relationships are best seen in the frontal, oblique and lateral views.

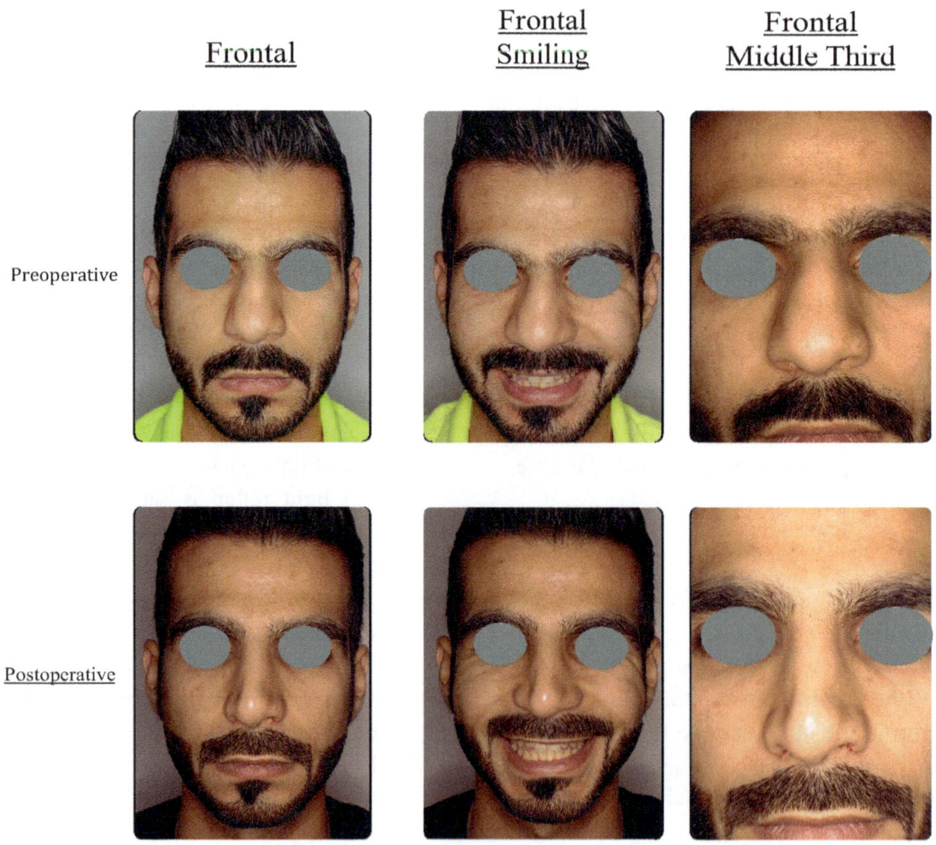

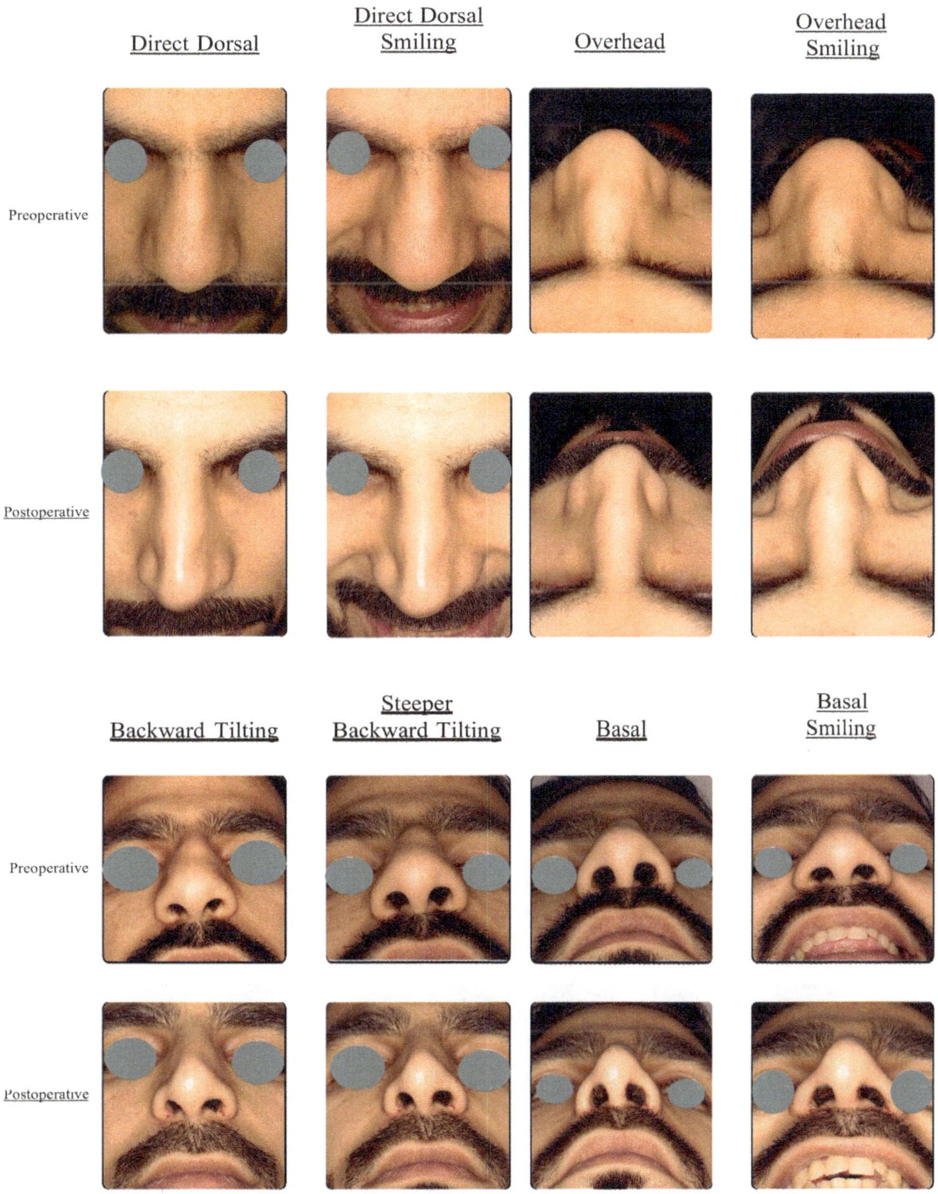
Direct Dorsal
Direct Dorsal Smiling
Overhead
Overhead Smiling
Preoperative
Postoperative
Backward Tilting
Steeper Backward Tilting
Basal
Basal Smiling
Preoperative
Postoperative

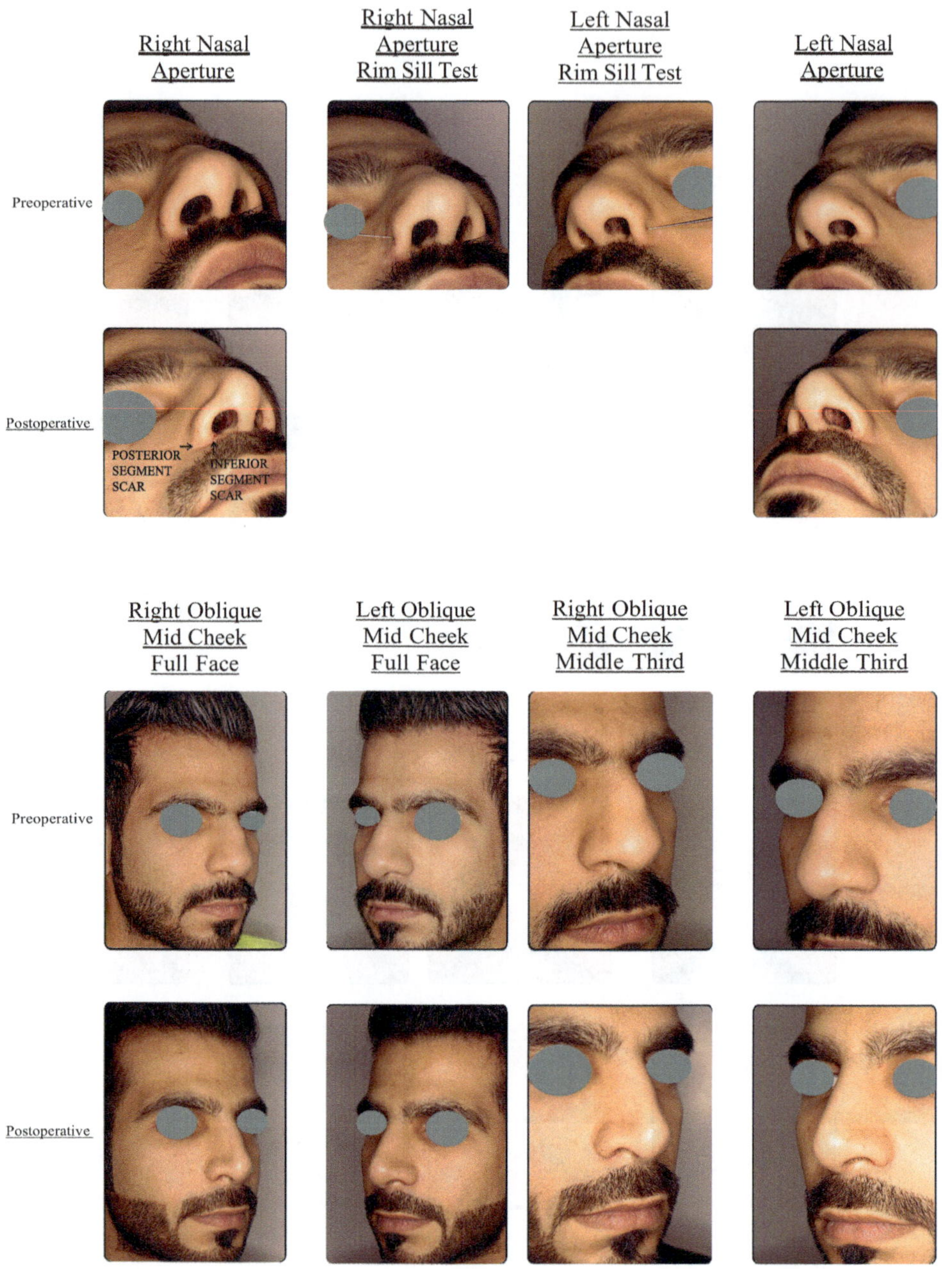
Right Nasal Aperture
Right Nasal Aperture Rim Sill Test
Left Nasal Aperture Rim Sill Test
Left Nasal Aperture
Preoperative
Postoperative
POSTERIOR SEGMENT SCAR
INFERIOR SEGMENT SCAR
Right Oblique Mid Cheek Full Face
Left Oblique Mid Cheek Full Face
Right Oblique Mid Cheek Middle Third
Left Oblique Mid Cheek Middle Third
Preoperative
Postoperative

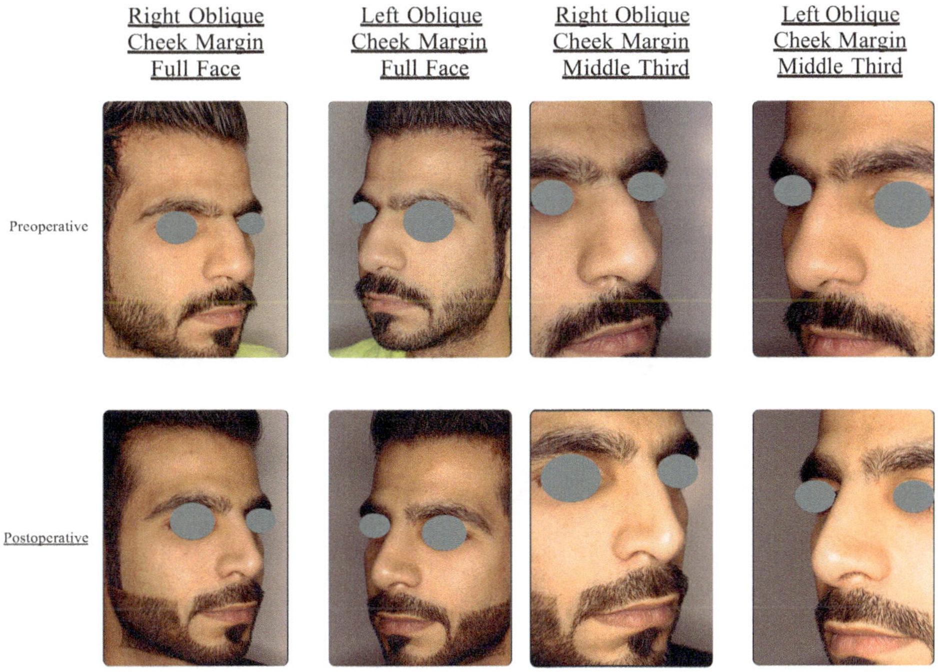
Right Oblique Cheek Margin Full Face
Left Oblique Cheek Margin Full Face
Right Oblique Cheek Margin Middle Third
Left Oblique Cheek Margin Middle Third
Preoperative
Postoperative

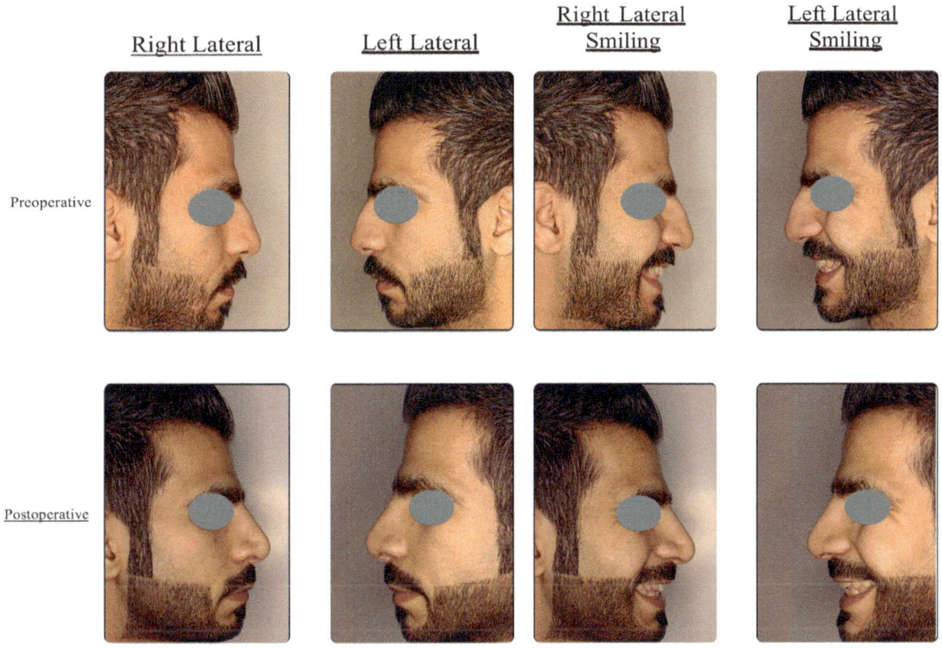
Right Lateral
Left Lateral
Right Lateral Smiling
Left Lateral Smiling
Preoperative
Postoperative

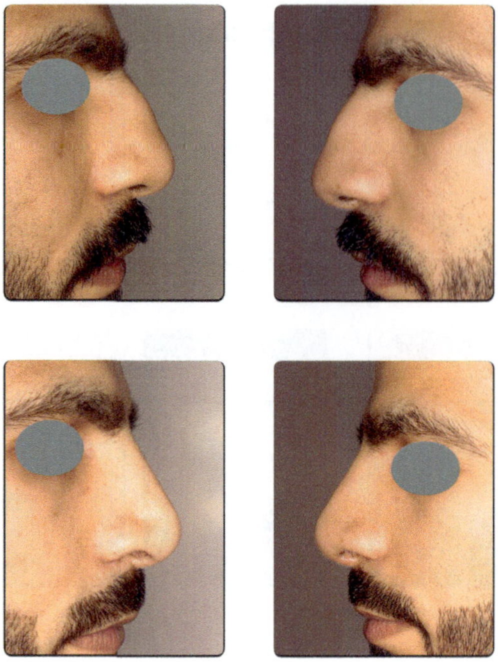
Right Lateral Middle Third
Left Lateral Middle Third
Preoperative
Postoperative

Part II: Clinical Case 3

5

Preoperative Assessment

1. **Frontolateral walls**
   Large Bulbous tip that overshowed the alae nasi (frontal and direct dorsal views).
2. **Medial Wall**
   Nil of note.
3. **Bony pyramid**
   a. Wide base of the boney pyramid (Direct Dorsal and Backward Tilting Views).
   b. Small osteocartilagenous hump (Oblique, Lateral, Backward Tilting and Nasal Aperture Views).
   c. The dorsal light reflex was defused (pre-operative Direct Dorsal Views).
4. **Alar base**
   Bilateral high alar arches (Lateral and Oblique Views).

Aims of Surgery

1. Smaller nasal tip.
2. Reduction of the size of the bony pyramid.
3. Lowering the alar margins.

Surgical Plan

1. **Frontolateral walls**
   a. DDD including the weak triangle to reduce the size and bulk of the nasal tip and supra tip area.
   b. Bilateral cephalic trim of lateral crurae to reduce the size.
2. **Medial Wall**
   Nil of note.
3. **Bony pyramid**
   a. Excision of the osteocartilaginous hump.
   b. Osteotomies and medialization of the lateral bony walls to reduce width of the bony pyramid.
4. **Alar base**
   Lowering inferior margins of the alae nasi using bony septal grafts.

Surgical Procedure

a. As per Surgical Plan.
b. Boney, septal grafts were used to reinforce the inferior margins of the alae nasi.

Post-Operative Analysis

1. **Frontolateral Walls**
   a. Tip definition improved i.e. the tip is slimmer and prominently well identified. The overlying skin is thinner. The alae nasi come into view to share in nasal aesthetics (Frontal, Direct Dorsal, Overhead, Backward Tilting and Basal Views).
   b. Tip projection: the nasal tip is at the same level of the nasal dorsum with good aesthetic angle. This is coupled with good aesthetic nasolabial angle (Lateral and Oblique Views).
   c. Tip light reflex is seen as one spot off the nasal tip. (Frontal and Backward Tilting Views).
2. **Medial Wall**
   Nil of Note.
3. **Bony Pyramid**
   a. Bony pyramid aesthetics: the nasal dorsum is straight and the sidewalls are smooth and narrow (all views except the Basal Views).
   b. Dorsal light reflex is seen as a regular one line off the nasal dorsum (Direct Dorsal Views).
4. **Alar Base**
   a. The superior alar grooves now clear off fat, become deeper, longer and visible (Direct Dorsal, Oblique and Lateral Views).
   b. Posterior alar groove aesthetics improved by defatting. Flat tire appearance is no longer present as the posterior alar groove angle with the upper lip became wider. (Backward Tilting, Basal and Nasal Aperture Views).
   c. Nasal aperture aesthetics aesthetics improved by defatting:

M. H. A. Shafy, *Atlas of Clinical Cases in Rhinoplasty*,
https://doi.org/10.1007/978-3-031-07504-9_5

   i. The size of the nasal openings are reduced, only by defatting.
   ii. The shapes of nasal openings become more elegantly oval. (Backward Tilting, Basal and Nasal Aperture views).
d. Aesthetics of the alae nasi improved:
   i. The alar margins become at a lower level with better relation with the columella.
   ii. The bodies of alae nasi are pulled medially after defatting, widening the posterior alar grooves. They are better seen and look smaller in size. (Nasal Apaerture, Basal and Oblique Views).
e. Marginal light reflexes are clearly seen at:
   i. Inferior alar margins (Nasal Aperture Views).
   ii. The nasal sills are too short to be seen in the oblique views.
   iii. Lateral crural prominences (Lateral Views).

Commentary

a. The post operative photographs were taken on the 10th post operative day.
b. The inferior alar margins are aesthetically in a better location with improved columello-alar relationship.

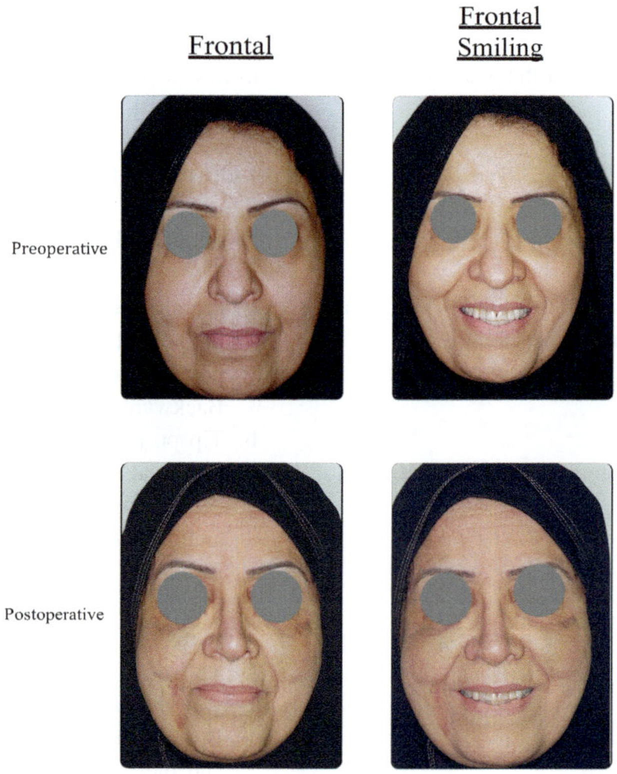

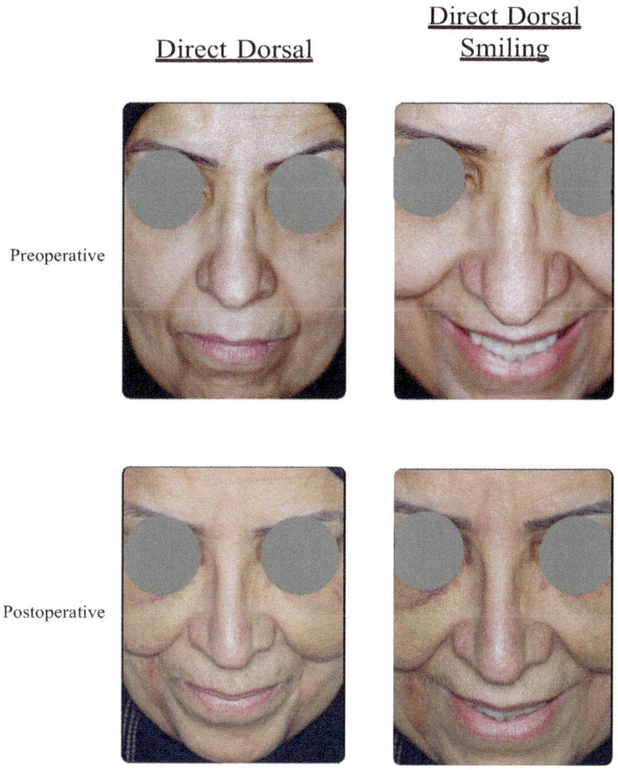
Direct Dorsal
Direct Dorsal Smiling
Preoperative
Postoperative

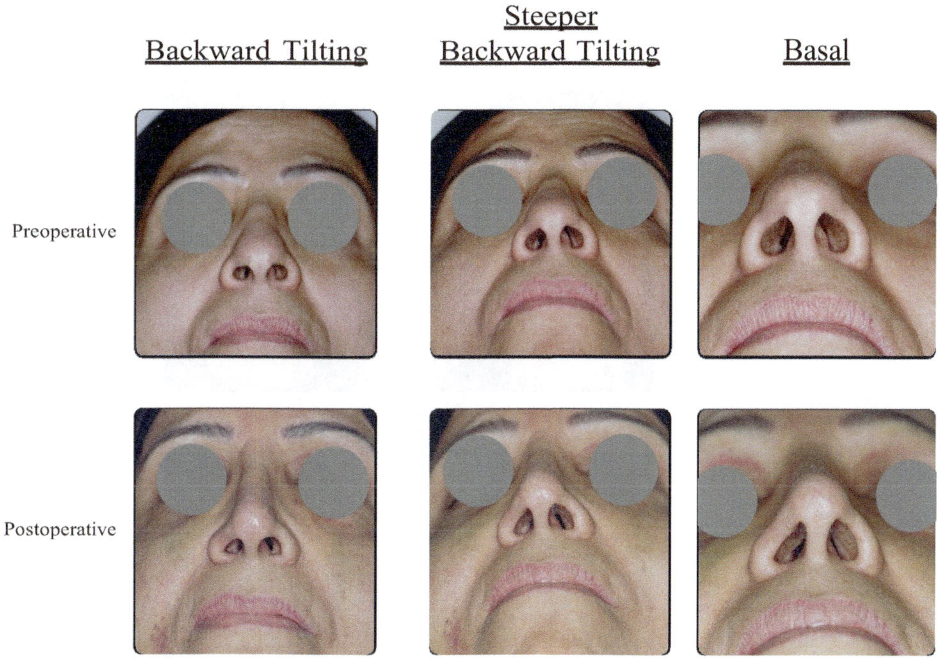
Backward Tilting
Steeper Backward Tilting
Basal
Preoperative
Postoperative

Right Nasal Aperture | Right Nasal Aperture Rim Sill Test | Left Nasal Aperture Rim Sill Test | Left Nasal Aperture

Preoperative

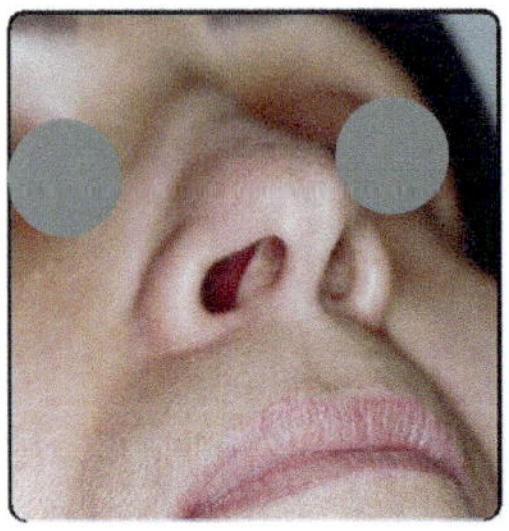

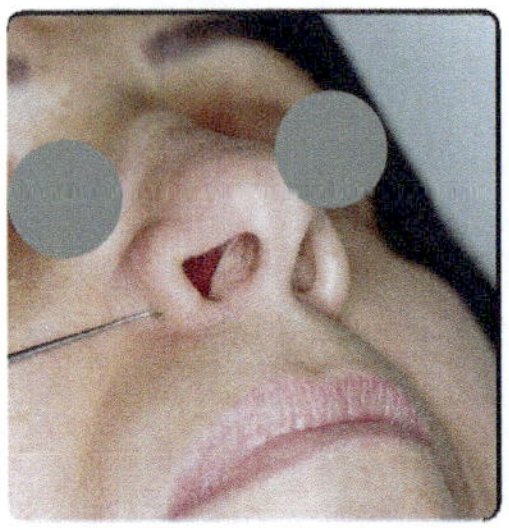

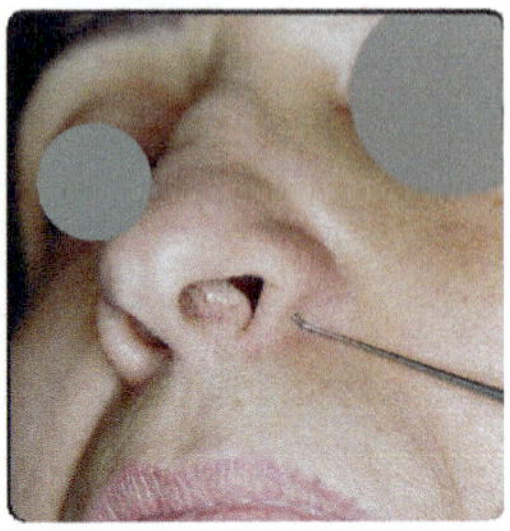

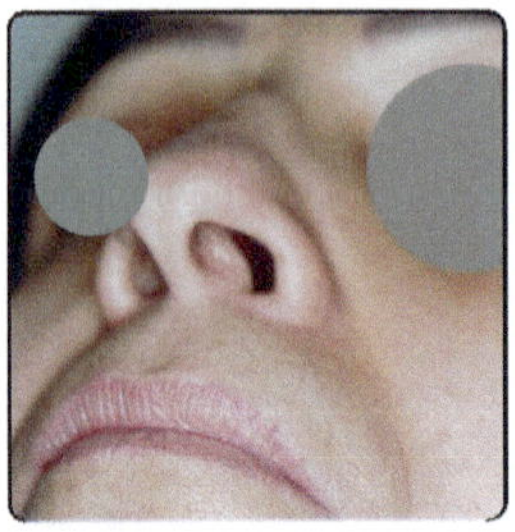

Postoperative

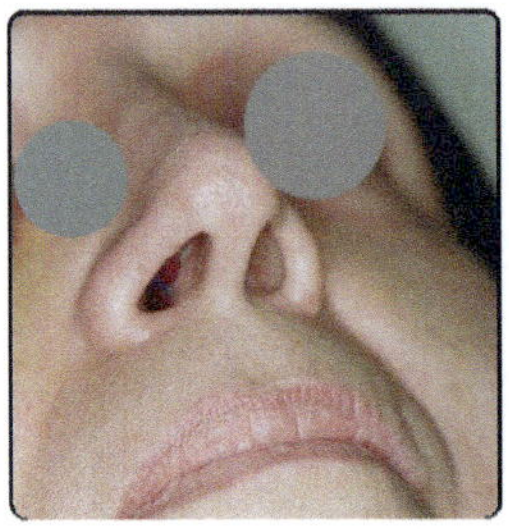

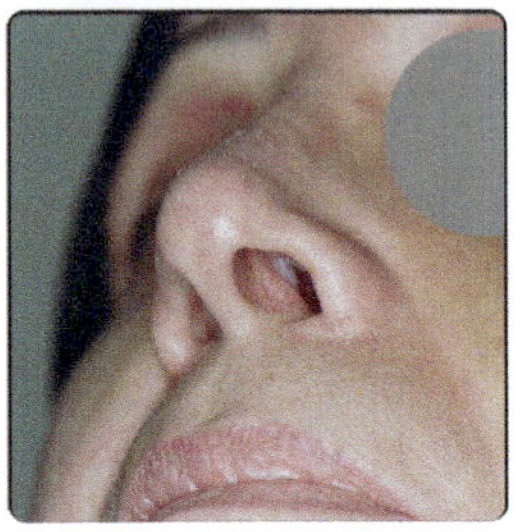

Right Oblique Mid Cheek Full Face | Left Oblique Mid Cheek Full Face

Preoperative

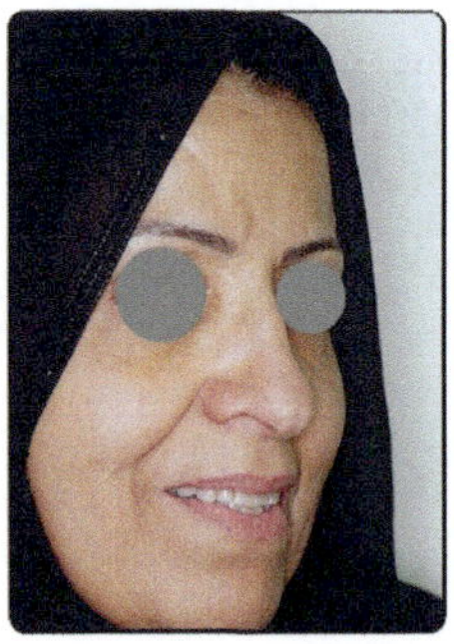

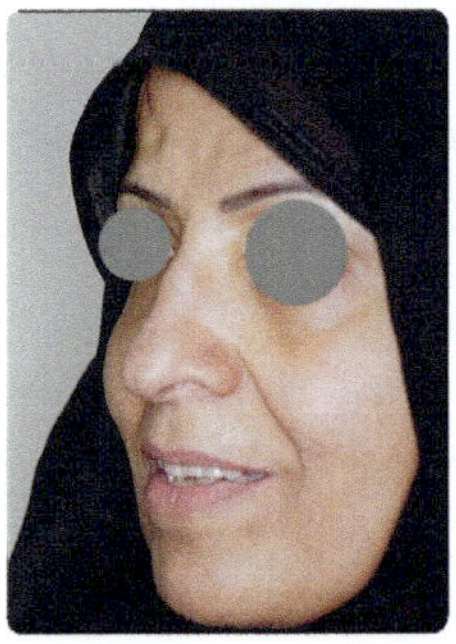

Postoperative

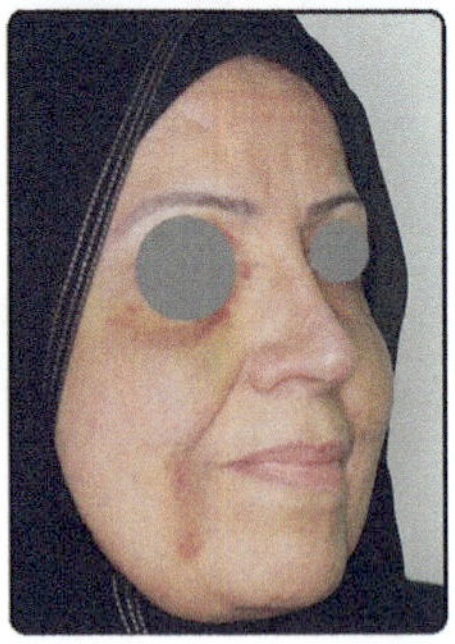

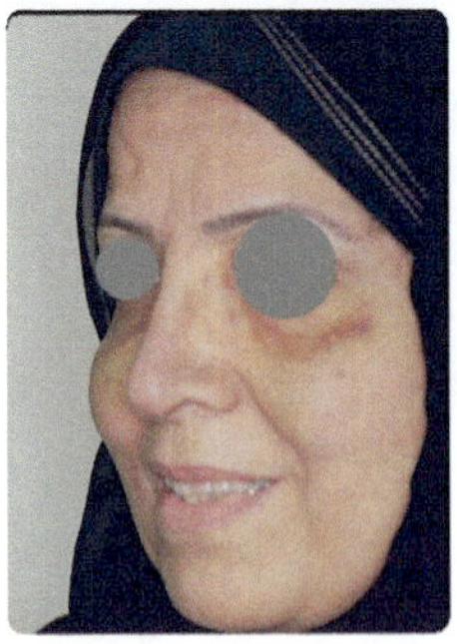

Right Oblique Cheek Margin Full Face	Left Oblique Cheek Margin Full Face

Preoperative

Postoperative

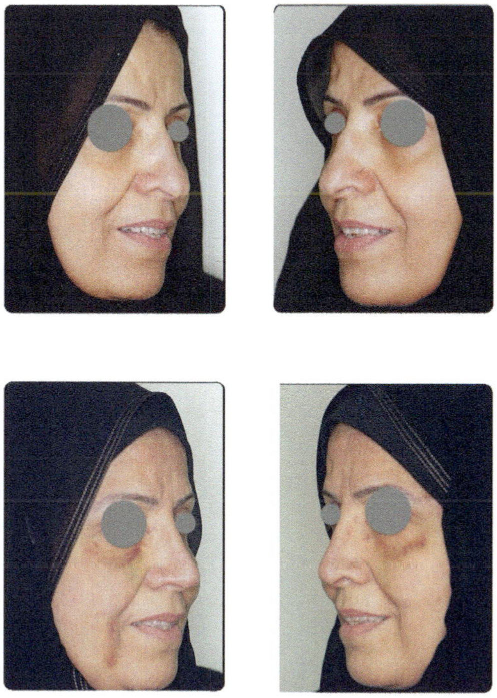

Right Lateral	Left Lateral	Right Lateral Smiling	Left Lateral Smiling

Preoperative

Postoperative

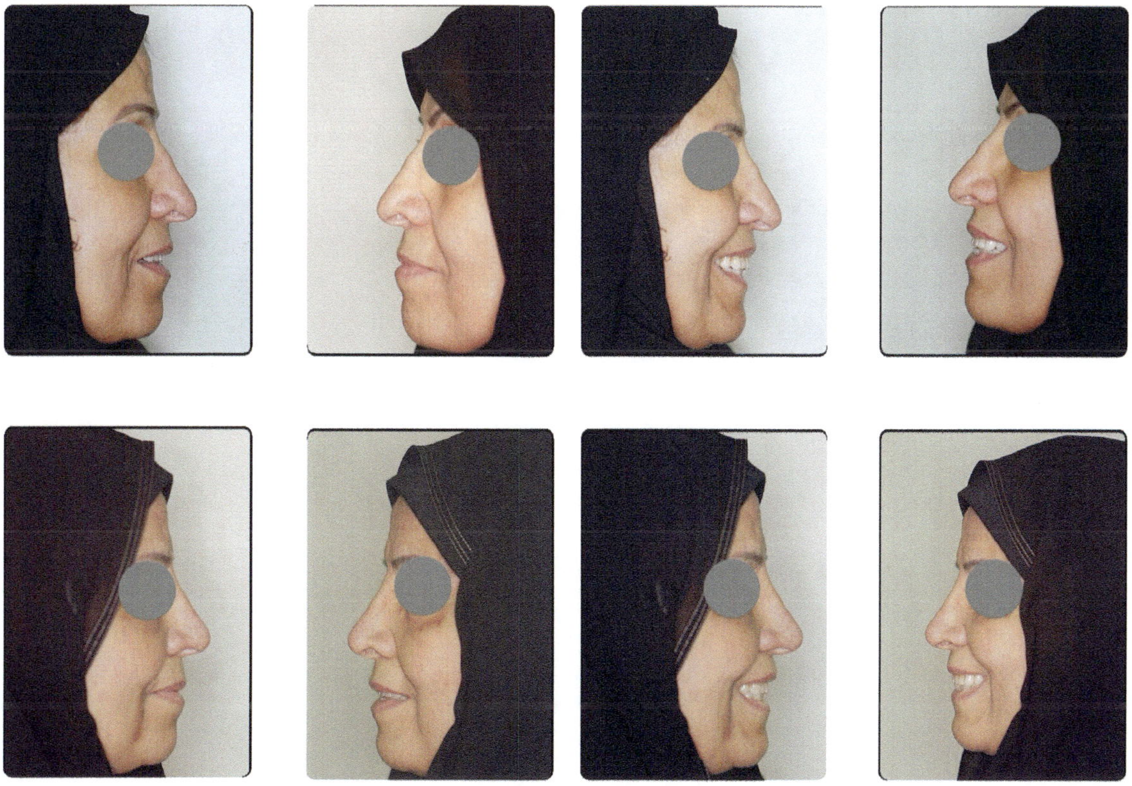

Part II: Clinical Case 4

6

Preoperative Analysis

1. **Frontolateral walls**
   Large bulbous tip that overshadows the alae nasi (Frontal and Direct Dorsal Views).
2. **Medial Wall**
   a. Plunging tip, i.e. drooping inferiorly with acute nasolabial angle. (Lateral Smiling Views).
   b. Mobile tip, the tip moves inferiorly on smiling (Lateral Smiling Views).
3. **Boney pyramid**
   a. Osteocartilaginous hump (Oblique, Lateral and Nasal Aperture Views).
   b. Wide base of the bony pyramid (Frontal, Direct Dorsal and Backward Tilting Views).
   c. Distorted dorsal light reflex (pre-operative, Direct Dorsal Views).
4. **Alar base**
   The nasal openings are thick, heavy and rounded. (Basal and Nasal Aperture Views).

Aims of Surgery

1. Reduce the size and bulk of the nasal tip.
2. Overcome the plunging and the mobile tip.
3. Reduce the overall size of the nose.

Surgical Plan

1. **Frontolateral walls**
   a. DDD including the weak triangle to reduce the size and bulk of frontolateral walls.
   b. Bilateral cephalic trim of the lateral crurae to reduce the size.
2. **Medial Wall**
   a. Septoplasty as well as trimming few millimeters off the caudal cartilaginous septum.
   b. Minimal trim of the membranous septum, i.e. the two sides of the loose vestibular skin.
   c. Division of the Depressor Septi muscles.
3. **Boney pyramid**
   a. Excision of the osteocartilaginous hump.
   b. Bilateral Osteotomies and medialization of the bony side walls.
4. **Alar base**
   Nil of note.

Surgical Procedure

As per Surgical Plan.

Post-Operative Analysis

1. **Frontolateral Wall**
   a. Tip definition improved i.e. the tip is slimmer and prominently well identified with thinner overlying skin. The alae nasi come into view to share in nasal aesthetics (Frontal, Direct Dorsal, Overhead, Backward Tilting and Basal Views).
   b. Tip projection: the nasal tip is at the same level of the nasal dorsum with good aesthetic angle. This is coupled with good aesthetic nasolabial angle (lateral and oblique views).
   c. Tip light reflex is seen as one spot off the nasal tip. (Frontal and Backward Tilting Views).
2. **Medial Walls**
   Plunging as well as mobility of the nasal tip were managed by:

i. Excision of the osteocartilaginous hump,
ii. Excision of the membranous septum, including its two loose skin layers, as well as trimming of few millimeters of the caudal (vestibular) septum,

M. H. A. Shafy, *Atlas of Clinical Cases in Rhinoplasty*,
https://doi.org/10.1007/978-3-031-07504-9_6

iii. Division of the Depressor Septi muscles. Mobile tip is totally abolished post-operatively (pre- and post-operative lateral views, smiling and non-smiling).

3. **Bony Pyramid**
   a. Bony pyramid aesthetics improved: the nasal dorsum is straight and the sidewalls are smooth and narrow (all views except the Basal Views).
   b. Dorsal light reflex is seen as a regular one line off the nasal dorsum (Direct Dorsal Views).
4. **Alar Base**
   a. The superior alar grooves now clear off fat, become deeper, longer and visible (Direct Dorsal, Oblique and Lateral Views).
   b. Posterior alar groove aesthetics improved by defatting. Flat tire appearance is no longer present, as the posterior alar groove angle with the upper lip became wider. (Backward Tilting, Basal and Nasal Aperture Views).
   c. Alae nasi aesthetics improved by defatting. They moved medially widening the posterior alar grooves, become better seen and look smaller in size (Nasal Aperture, Basal and Oblique Views).
   d. Nasal aperture aesthetics improved by defatting:
      i. The size of the nasal openings are the same.
      ii. The shape of nasal openings become more elegantly oval. (Backward Tilting, Basal and Nasal Aperture views).
   e. Marginal light reflexes are clearly seen at:
      i. Inferior alar margins (Nasal Aperture Views).
      ii. Nasal sill bands (Oblique Views).
      iii. Lateral crural prominences (Lateral Views).

Commentary

a. The overall size of the nose is smaller and proportionately suites his face better than before surgery. Patient's wish was fulfilled. Naso-facial relationships are best seen in the frontal, oblique and lateral views.
b. Enhanced aesthetic of the nose have had a dramatic effects on the overall appearance of the face. The beauty of each part of the face, namely, the eyes, the cheeks, the forehead, the chin and even the smile have all been enhanced.
c. The nasal openings looked relatively wide pre-operatively. After two steps defatting, there was release of tension of the ballooned frontolateral skin which draped the naturally small-size lower lateral cartilages. The alar margins are relaxed and consequently the nasal openings became smaller and triangular in shape. No alar resection was needed (pre- and post-operative Basal Views and Right and Left Nasal Aperture Views).
d. **The plunging mobile tip** was overcome by the combined work in the following areas of the nose:
   i. The fronto-lateral walls: defatting, and cephalic trim of the lateral crurae.
   ii. Median wall.: septoplasty, excision of the membranous septum, trimming of the caudal septum and devision of the depressor septi muscles.
   iii. The bony pyramid and mid volt: excision of the osteo-cartilaginous hump and medialisation of the sidewalls of the bony pyramid.

Frontal | Frontal Smiling | Frontal Middle Third

Preoperative

Postoperative

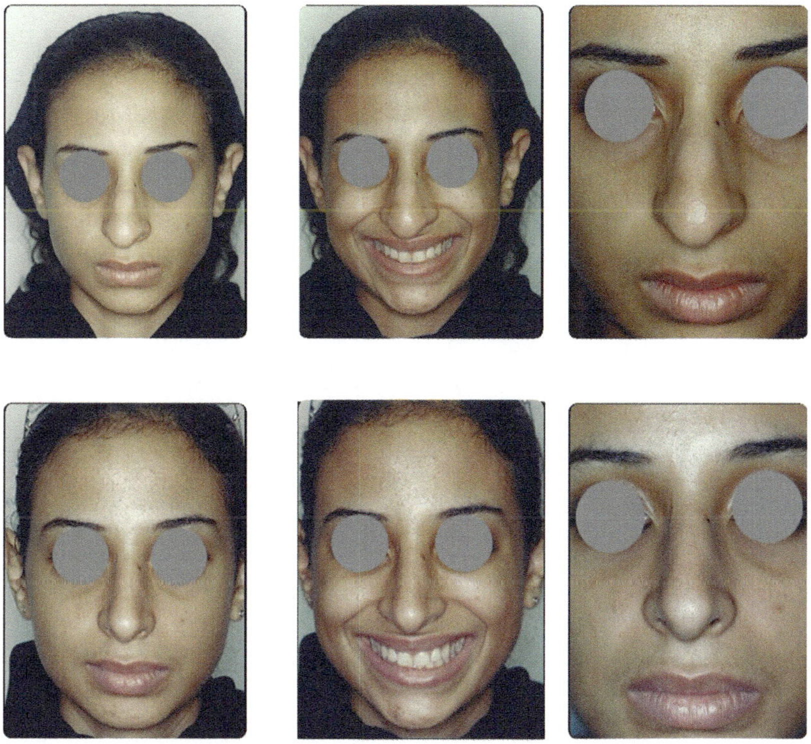

The nasofacial relationship is enhanced postoperatively as the width of the nose and tip have been reduced.

The aesthetics of the eyes, cheeks and upper lip are im-

Direct Dorsal | Direct Dorsal Smiling

Preoperative

Postoperative

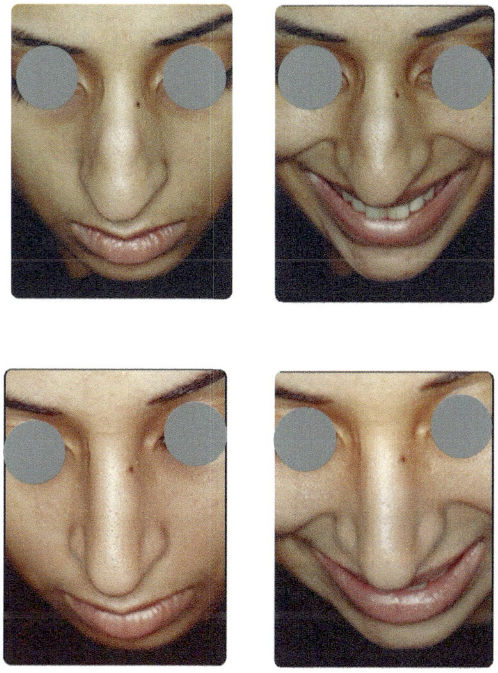

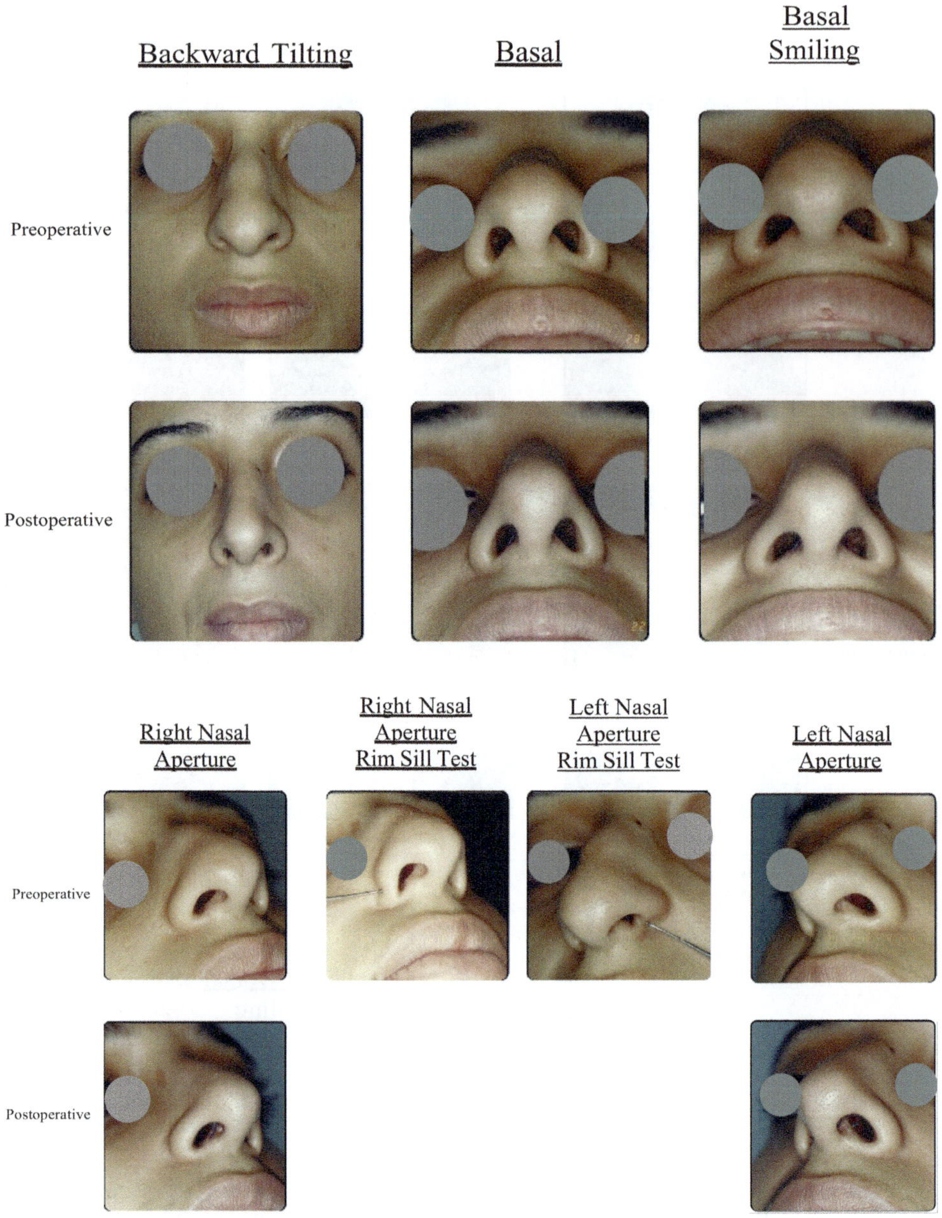
Backward Tilting
Basal
Basal Smiling
Preoperative
Postoperative
Right Nasal Aperture
Right Nasal Aperture Rim Sill Test
Left Nasal Aperture Rim Sill Test
Left Nasal Aperture
Preoperative
Postoperative

Right Oblique Mid Cheek Full Face	Left Oblique Mid Cheek Full Face	Right Oblique Mid Cheek Middle Third	Left Oblique Mid Cheek Middle Third

Preoperative

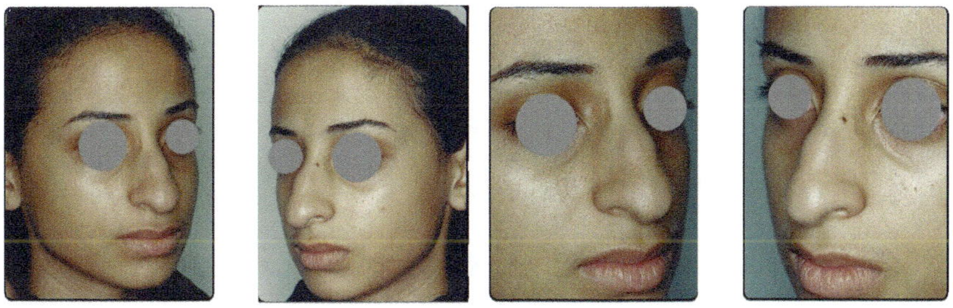

Postoperative

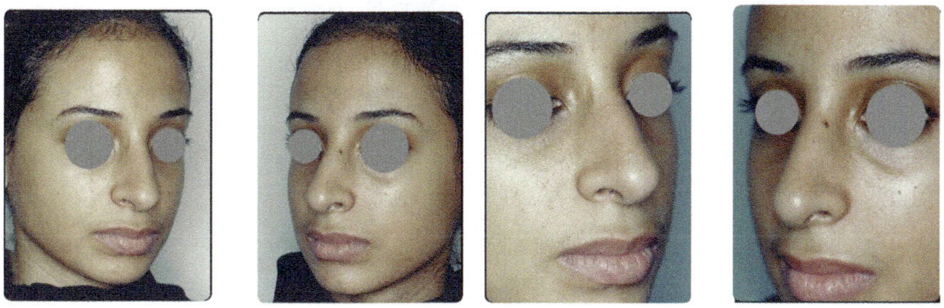

Right Oblique Cheek Margin Full Face	Left Oblique Cheek Margin Full Face	Right Oblique Cheek Margin Middle Third	Left Oblique Cheek Margin Middle Third

Preoperative

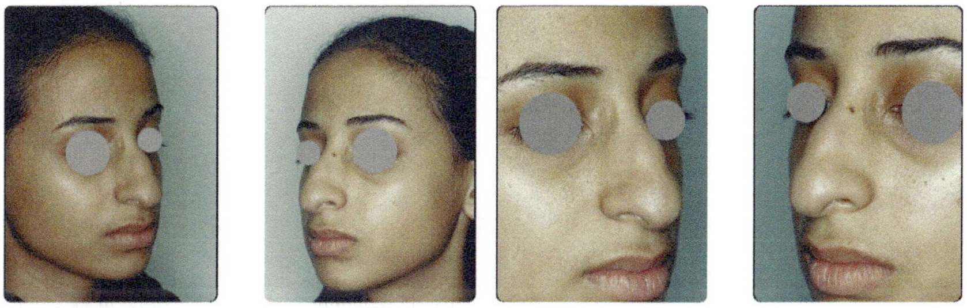

Postoperative

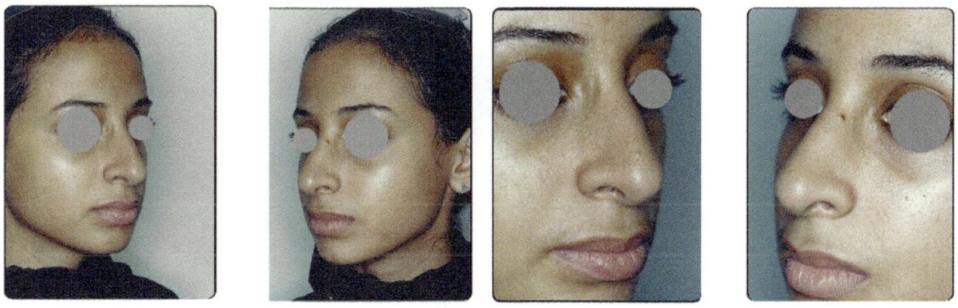

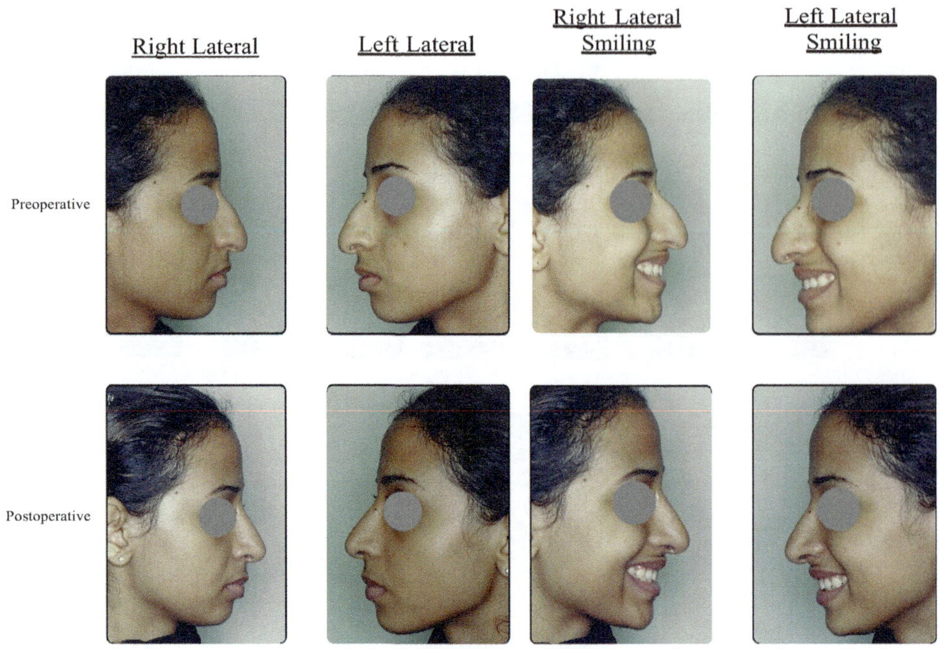
Right Lateral
Left Lateral
Right Lateral Smiling
Left Lateral Smiling
Preoperative
Postoperative

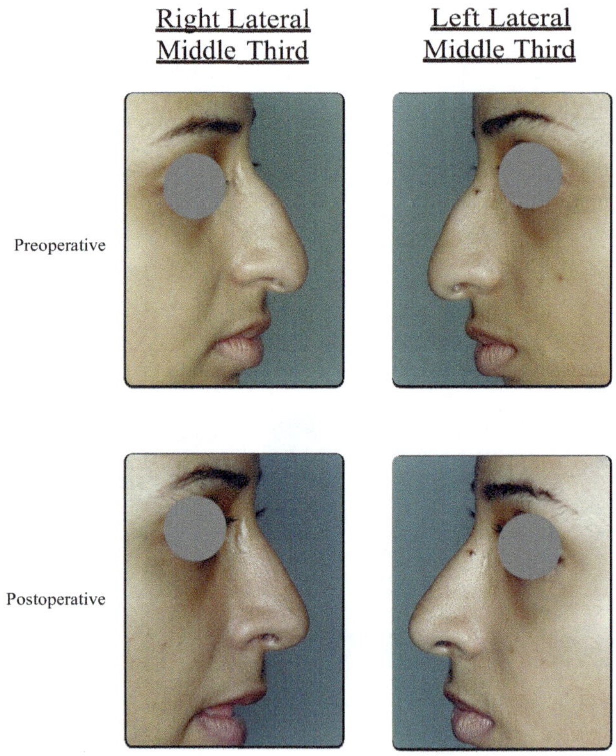
Right Lateral Middle Third
Left Lateral Middle Third
Preoperative
Postoperative

7 Part II: Clinical Case 5

Preoperative Assessment

1. **Frontolateral walls**
   Large and bulky frontolateral walls that overshadow the alae nasi (Frontal, Direct Dorsal and Overhead Views).
2. **Medial Wall**
   a. Mobile tip (Lateral Smiling View).
   b. Pluning tip i.e. drooping inferiorly with acute nasolabial angle (pre-operative Lateral Smiling View).
3. **Bony pyramid**
   a. Wide base of the boney pyramid (Frontal, Direct Dorsal, Overhead and Backward Tilting Views).
   b. Osteocartilaginous hump which is oblique, but not deviated, to the right side due to bilateral maxillary asymmetry. The right cheek is wide and low while the left cheek is high and narrow. (Frontal and Backward Tilting Views).
4. **Alar base**
   Wide alar flare on smiling despite the acceptable width of the alar base (Frontal pre-operative smiling views).

Aims of Surgery

1. Overall reduction of the size and bulk of the nose.
2. Centralization of the nasal obliquity.
3. Abolish the mobile plunging tip.
4. Reduction of the size of the alar base and the wide alar flare on smiling.

Surgical Plan

1. **Frontolateral walls**
   a. DDD including the weak triangle to reduce the bulk of nasal tip and supra tip area.
   b. Cephalic trim of the lateral crurae to reduce the size of the nasal tip.
2. **Medial Wall**
   a. Division of the depressor septi muscles.
   b. Trim of few mm. of the caudal cartilaginous and membranous septum.
3. **Bony pyramid**
   a. Excision of the osteocartiligenous hump.
   b. Osteotomies with Kasanjian maneuver to the left i.e. cross fracture of the bony pyramid after osteotomies. (see Surgery of the Bony Pyramid in Text).
4. **Alar base**
   Excision of the inferior segments of the rim-sill folds to reduce the alar flare on smiling.

Surgical Procedure

a. As per Surgical Plan.
b. Resection of the rim sill segments was not necessary.

Post-Operative Analysis

1. **Frontolateral Walls**
   a. Tip definition improved i.e. slimmer and prominently well identified with thinner overlying skin. The alae nasi come into view to share in nasal aesthetics (Frontal, Direct Dorsal, Overhead, Backward Tilting and Basal Views).
   b. Tip projection: The nasal tip at the same level of the nasal dorsum with good aesthetic angle. This is coupled with good aesthetic nasolabial angle (lateral and oblique views).
   c. Tip light reflex is seen as one spots off the nasal tip. (Frontal and Backward Tilting Views).
2. **Medial Wall**
   The mobile and plunging nasal tip was managed by (pre- and post-operative lateral views, smiling and non-smiling):

M. H. A. Shafy, *Atlas of Clinical Cases in Rhinoplasty*,
https://doi.org/10.1007/978-3-031-07504-9_7

   a. Excision of the osteocartilaginous hump,
   b. Trimming of a few millimeters of the caudal cartilaginous and membranous septum,
   c. Division of the Depressor Septi muscles.
3. **Bony Pyramid**
   a. Bony pyramid aesthetics improved: the nasal dorsum is straight and the sidewalls are smooth and narrow (all views except the Basal Views).
   b. Dorsal light reflex is seen as a regular one line off the nasal dorsum (Direct Dorsal Views).
4. **Alar Base**
   a. The superior alar grooves now clear off fat, become deeper, longer and visible (Direct Dorsal, Oblique and Lateral Views).
   b. Posterior alar groove aesthetics improved by defatting. Flat tire appearance is no longer present. (Backward Tilting, Basal and Nasal Aperture Views).
   c. Alae nasi aesthetics improved. Defatting pulled the alar bodies medially widening the posterior alar grooves. The alae nasi are better seen and look smaller in size. (Nasal Aperture and Oblique Views).
   d. Nasal aperture aesthetics improved: after the defatting procedure the lateral walls were propped up, the alar base was sufficiently narrowed and did not need further surgical reduction. The nasal openings look smaller, thin walled and nicely oval in shape.
   e. Alar flare, on smiling, surprisingly reduced after defatting only. No alar resection was needed.
   f. Marginal light reflexes are clearly seen at:
      i. Inferior alar margins (Nasal Aperture Views).
      ii. Nasal sill bands (Oblique Views).
      iii. Lateral crural prominences (Lateral Views).

Commentary

a. Care must be taken to avoid dramatic changes in these types of extremely shy individuals. This might have an unpredictable psychological impact on bashful personalities.
b. The skin surface irregularities became smoother following defatting.

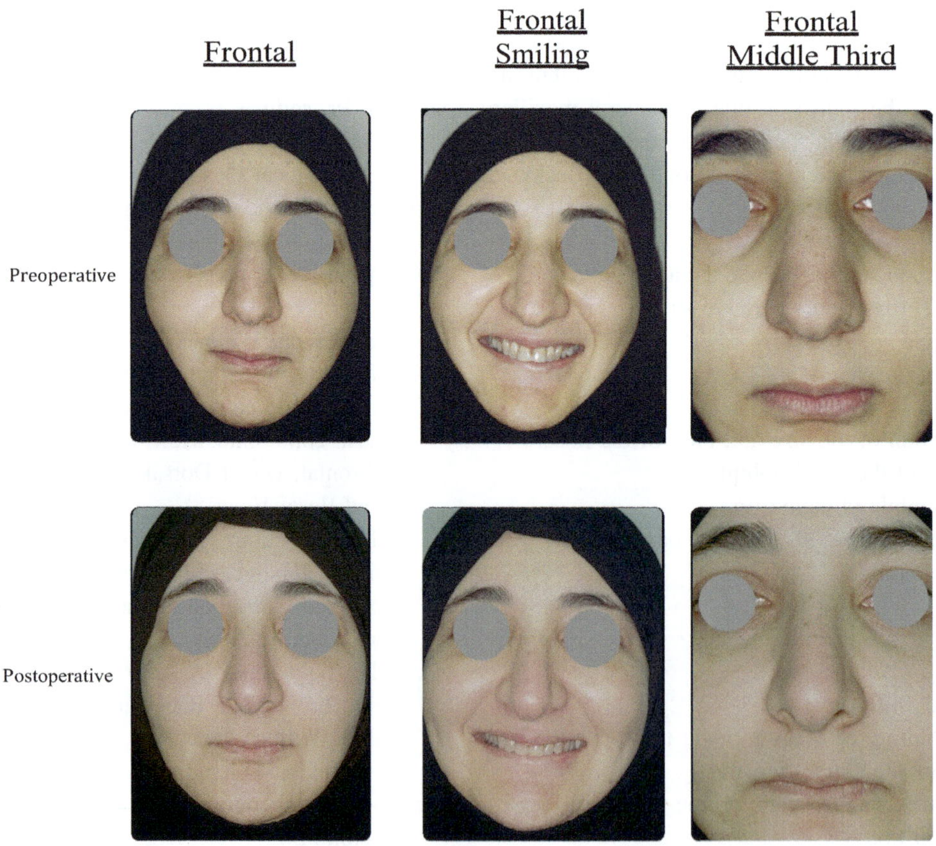

Direct Dorsal | Direct Dorsal Smiling | Overhead | Overhead Smiling

Preoperative

Postoperative

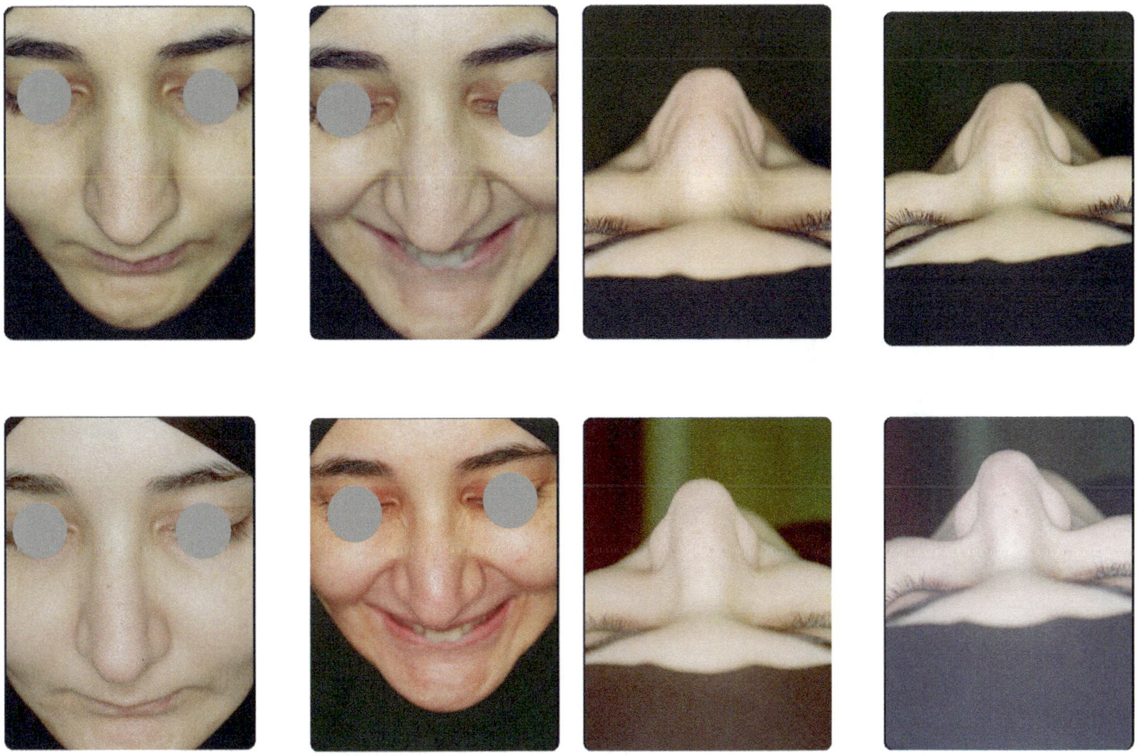

Backward Tilting | Steeper Backward Tilting | Basal

Preoperative

Postoperative

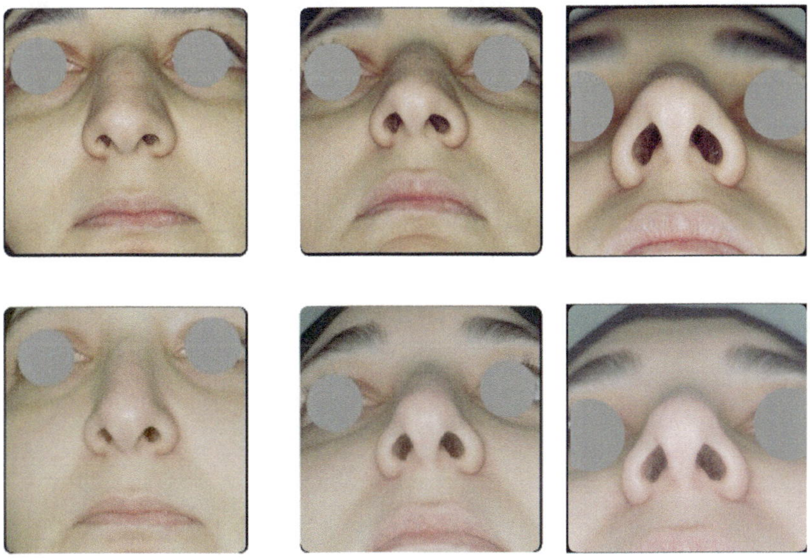

Right Nasal Aperture | Right Nasal Aperture Rim Sill Test | Left Nasal Aperture Rim Sill Test | Left Nasal Aperture

Preoperative

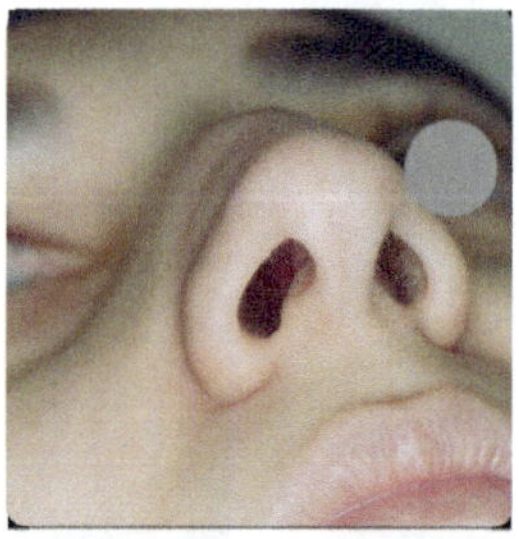
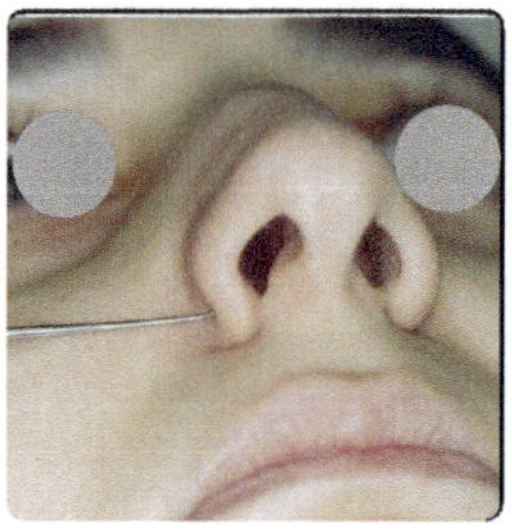
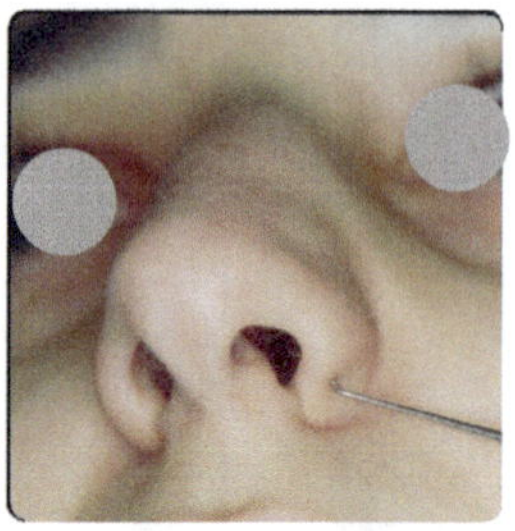
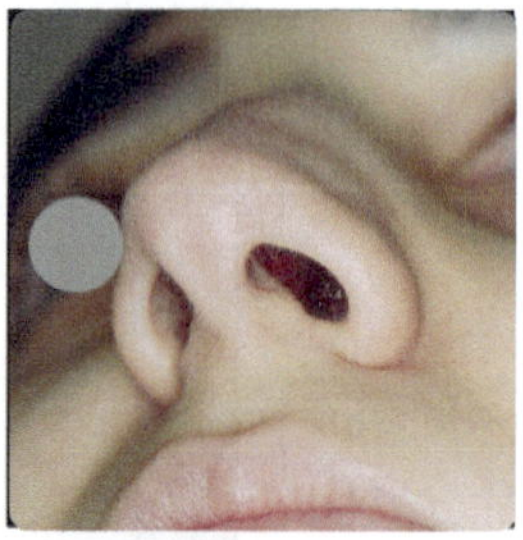

Postoperative

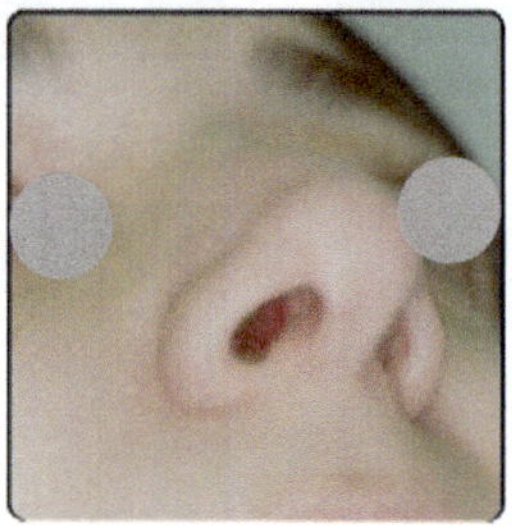
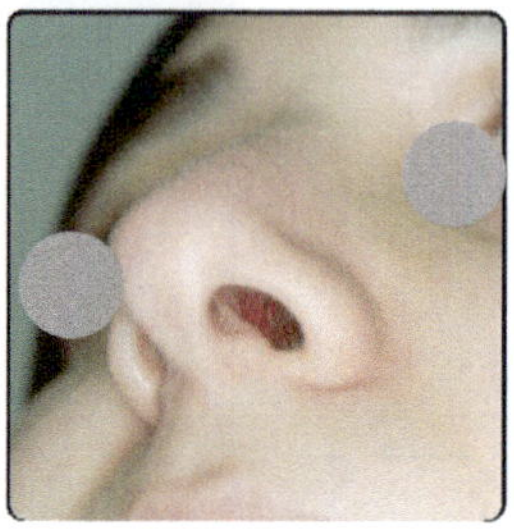

Right Oblique Mid Cheek Full Face | Left Oblique Mid Cheek Full Face | Right Oblique Mid Cheek Middle Third | Left Oblique Mid Cheek Middle Third

Preoperative

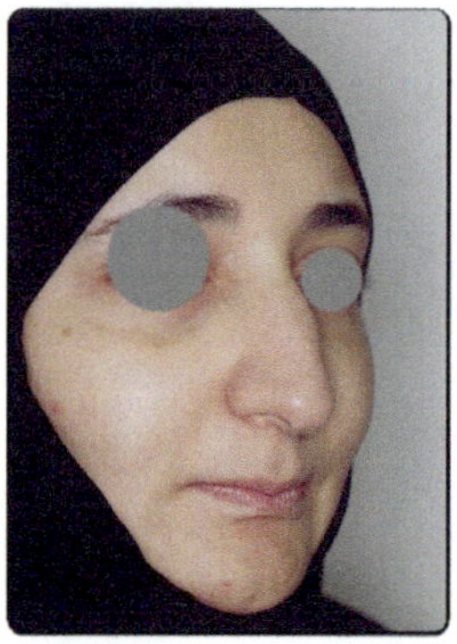
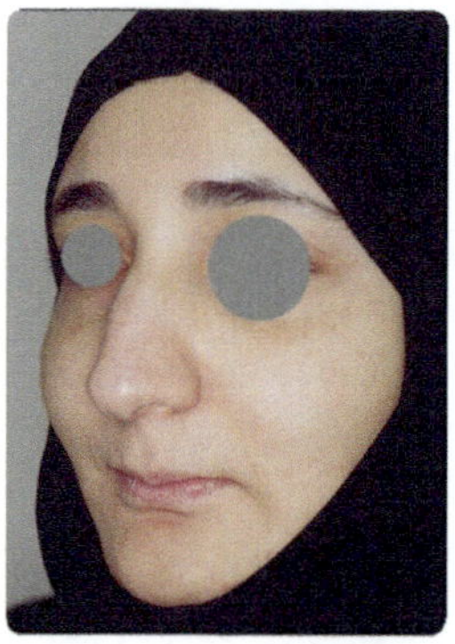
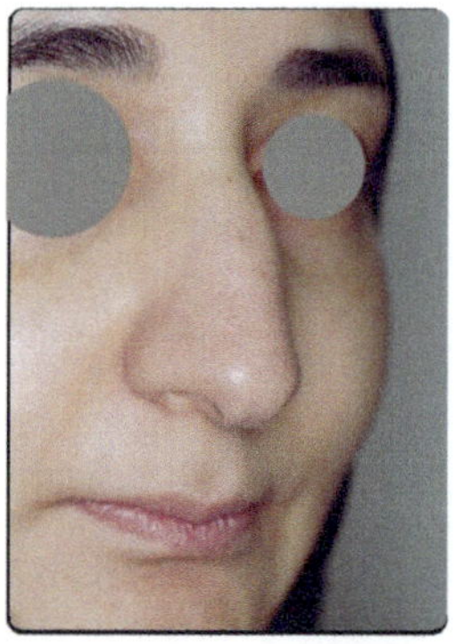
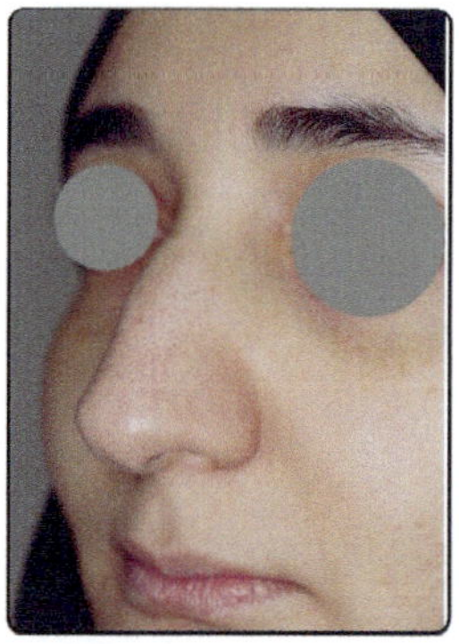

Postoperative

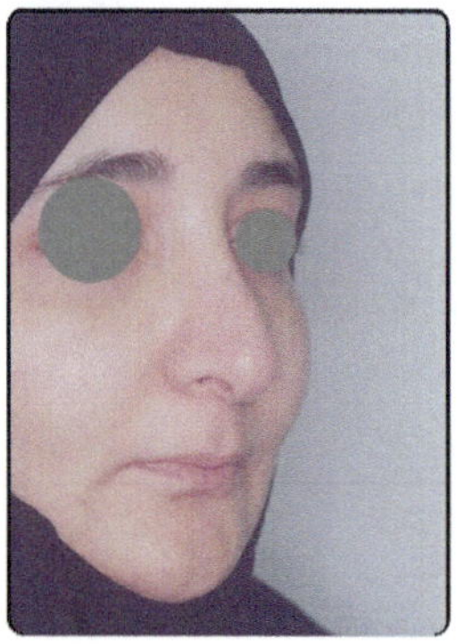
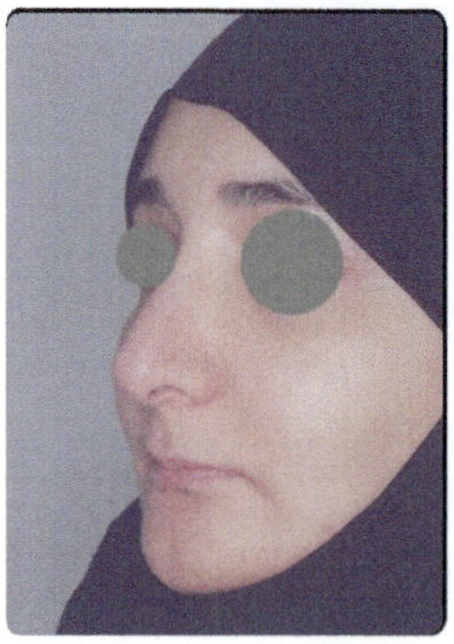
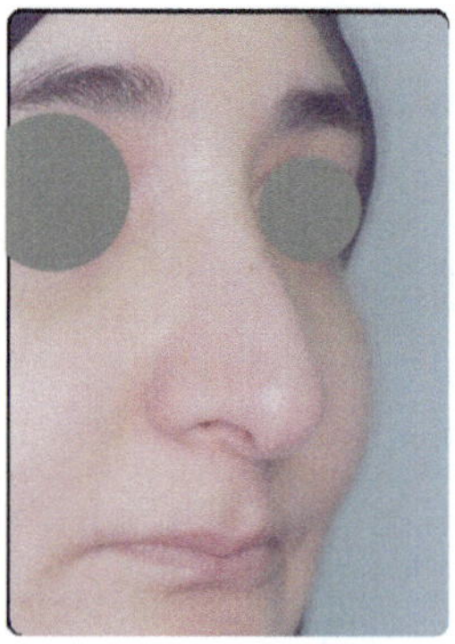
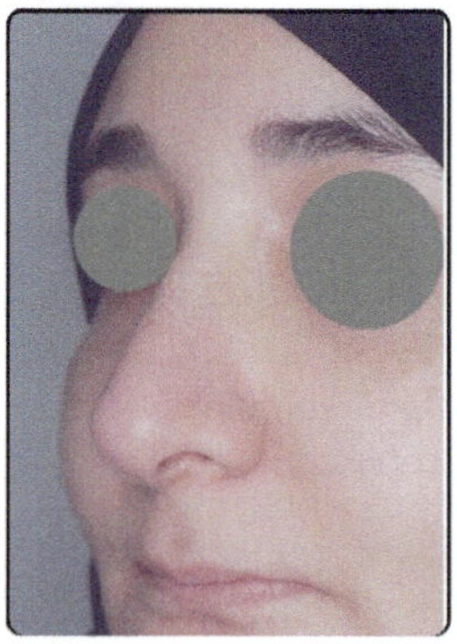

Right Oblique Cheek Margin Full Face	Left Oblique Cheek Margin Full Face	Right Oblique Cheek Margin Middle Third	Left Oblique Cheek Margin Middle Third

Preoperative

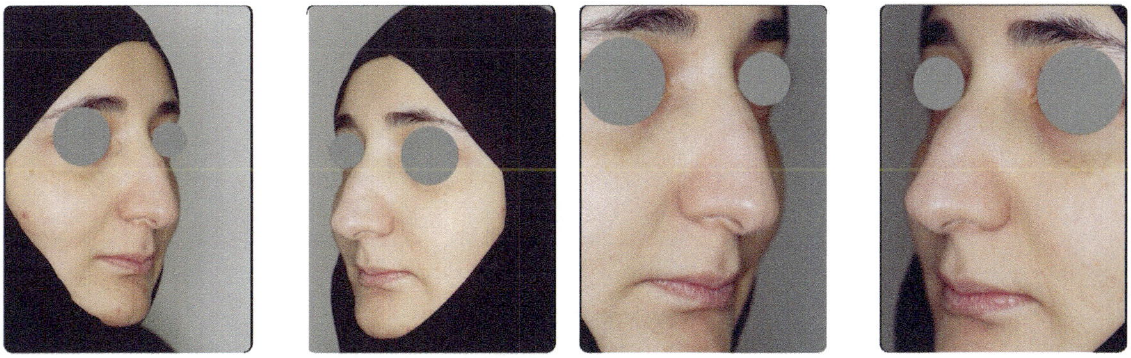

Postoperative

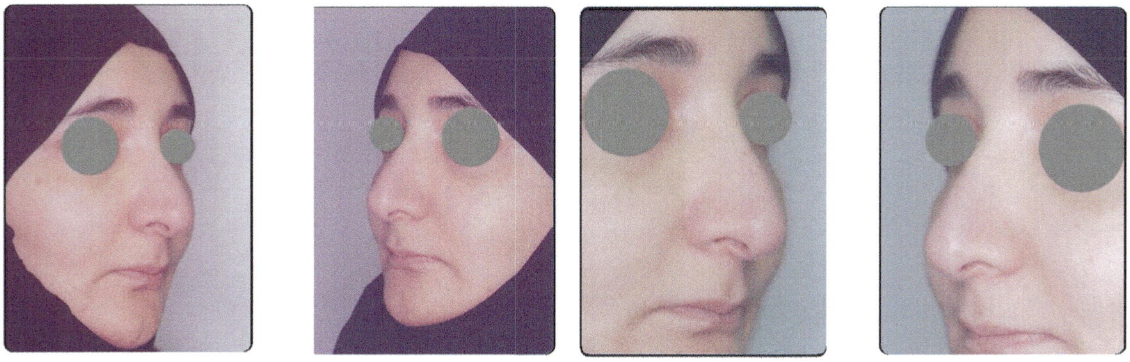

Right Lateral	Left Lateral	Right Lateral Smiling	Left Lateral Smiling

Preoperative

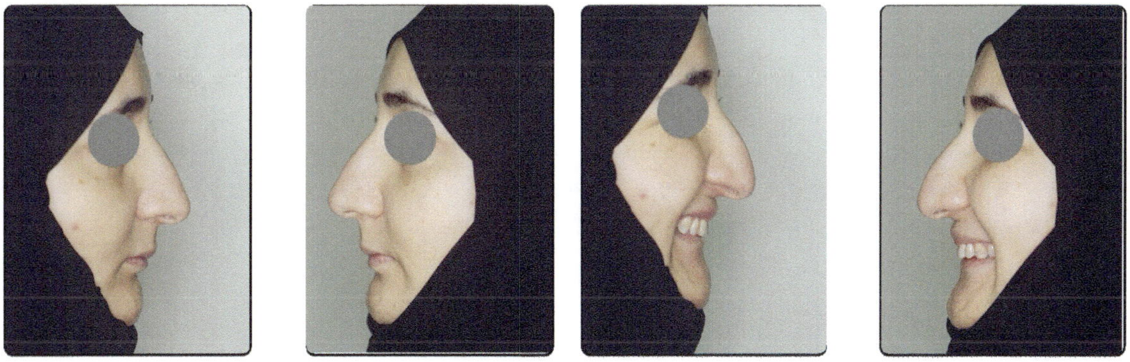

Postoperative

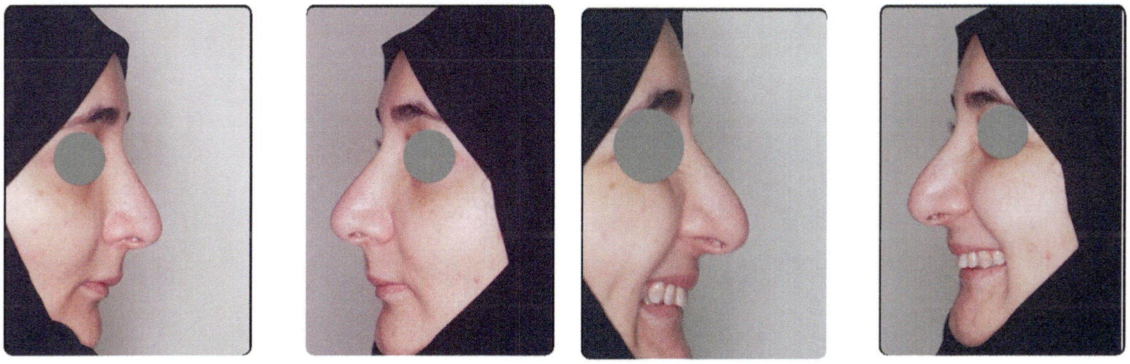

Right Lateral Middle Third | Left Lateral Middle Third

Preoperative

Postoperative

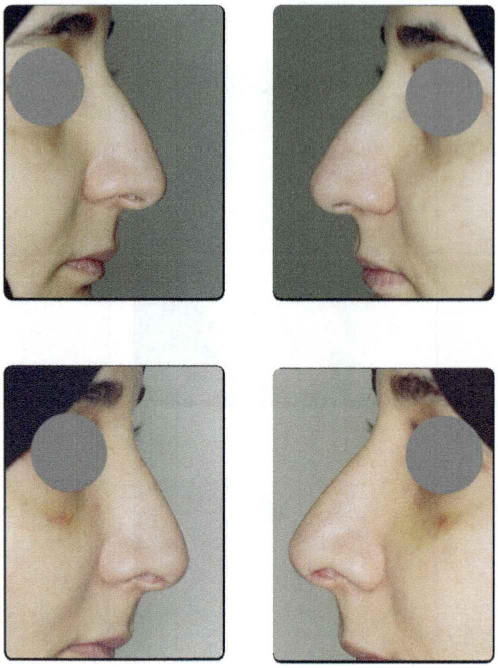

Part II: Clinical Case 6

8

Preoperative Assessment

1. **Frontolateral walls**
   a. Large frontolateral walls. The nasal tip is of reasonable size but pointing inferiorly (Pre-operative Frontal View).
   b. The nasal tip was counter deviated to the right side while the bony pyramid deviation was to the left. A crooked nose is a nose with a bend or twist in its body (preoperative Frontal, and Backward Tilting Views).
   c. The lateral crurae together with the alae nasi are displaced forward by the long rim still folds. They both make a wide flat interior wall. Their normal lateral location is taken away and replaced by the long rim-sill folds (Frontal, and Backward Tilting Views).

2. **Medial Wall**
   Nil of note.

3. **Boney pyramid**
   a. Wide base of the bony pyramid (Frontal and Backward Tilting Views).
   b. Osteocartilaginous hump predominantly to the left due to bilateral maxillary asymmetry. The right cheek is wide and low while the left cheek id narrow and high. (Backward Tilting Views).
   c. The bony pyramid was both deviated (Frontal View) and oblique (Backward Tilting View) to the left. The lower third of the nose is counter deviated to the right.

4. **Alar base**
   a. The rim sill folds are very long, thick and laterally angulated. They created fourth lateral walls to nasal apertures, in addition to the columella, the nasal sill bands and the alae nasi.
   b. The alae nasi are located anteriorly instead of laterally, together with the lateral crurae. The nasal apertures are rectangular in shape look apparently wide (Backward, Tilting, and Basal Views).

Aims of Surgery

1. Correct the crookedness of the nose.
2. Reduce the size of the nose.
3. Improve the aesthetics of the nasal apertures.
4. Readjust the positions of the lateral crurae and alae nasi back to their natural normal location in the lateral nasal walls.

Surgical Plan

1. **Frontolateral walls**
   DDD including the weak triangle to reduce the bulk of frontolateral walls.
2. **Medial Wall**
   Nile of Note.
3. **Boney pyramid**
   a. Excision of the osteocartilaginous hump.
   b. Osteotomies and Kasanjian maneuver to the right i.e. cross fracture of the bony pyramid after osteotomies to centralize it.
4. **Alar base**
   Excision of the long and bulky inferior and posterior segments of the rim sill folds.

Surgical Procedure

As per Surgical Plan.

Post-Operative Analysis

1. **Frontolateral Walls**
   a. The nasal tip becames small, round and no longer pointing inferiorly.
   b. Tip projection: the nasal tip is at the same level of the nasal dorsum with good aesthetic angle. This is

M. H. A. Shafy, *Atlas of Clinical Cases in Rhinoplasty*,
https://doi.org/10.1007/978-3-031-07504-9_8

coupled with good aesthetic nasolabial angle (lateral and oblique views).
   c. Tip light reflex is seen as one spot off the nasal tip (Frontal Views).
   d. The lateral crurae and alae nasi came back to their normal location at the lateral nasal in walls.
2. **Medial Wall**
   The inferior alar and lateral columellar margins regained the normal anatomical relations as the alae nasi came came dawn from the anterior to natural lateral location.
3. **Bony Pyramid**
   a. Bony pyramid aesthetics improved: the nasal dorsum is straight and the sidewalls are smooth and narrow (all views except the Basal Views).
   b. Dorsal light reflex is a straight line post-operatively as compared to the interrupted reflex pre-operatively. (Frontal Views).
4. **Alar Base**
   a. Following the excision of the rim-sill folds, the alae nasi were pulled downwards and medially in order to be attached to nasal sill bands. This resulted in the following positive aesthetic effects:
      a. Three walled nasal openings instead of four.
      b. The nasal apertures are not only smaller sized, but they became thin walled due to the removal of the thick long rim-sill folds.
      c. The margins of the alae nasi have moved downwards losing their unpleasant v-shaped appearance (Frontal views).
      d. Together with excision of the nasal hump and osteotomies the whole nose had became smaller, shorter and straight.
   b. Marginal light reflexes are clearly seen at:
      a. Inferior alar margins (Nasal Aperture Views).
      b. Nasal sill bands (Oblique Views).
      c. Lateral crural prominences (Lateral Views).

Commentary

a. Visually the nose looked long and pointing down simulating a plunging tip. The nasolabial angle was approximately 90 degrees preoperatively and is the same postoperatively. Therefore it is not a plunging tip. The visual effect is due to the unusually long and thick rim sill folds. This resulted in the unaesthetically displaced alae nasi upwards and laterally (Backward Tilting and Lateral Views). The alar margins on both sides give a V-shaped appearance that looks like a plunging tip (Oblique and Lateral Views).
b. The alar margins and the nasal sill bands are quite short in this patient's nose as compared to the long and thick rim sill folds.
c. The long and thick rim-sill folds had the following negative effects on nasal aesthetics:
   i. Large size of the lower third of the nose.
   ii. Wide rectangular shaped nasal apertures.
   iii. The lateral walls, including the lateral crurae and alae nasi, were displaced forwards and upwards, producing a broad anterior nasal wall that has v-shaped inferior margins. Simple excision of these very large rim sill folds was sufficient to reverse all these changes. The nose looks remarkably smaller with small triangular shaped apertures. The alae nasi and lateral crurae are more naturally placed back to the lateral walls.

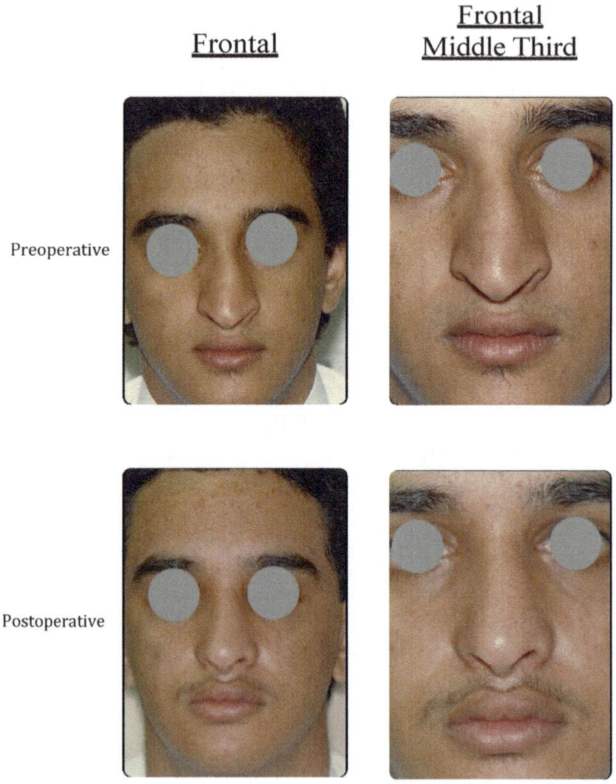

Backward Tilting | Steeper Backward Tilting

Preoperative

Postoperative

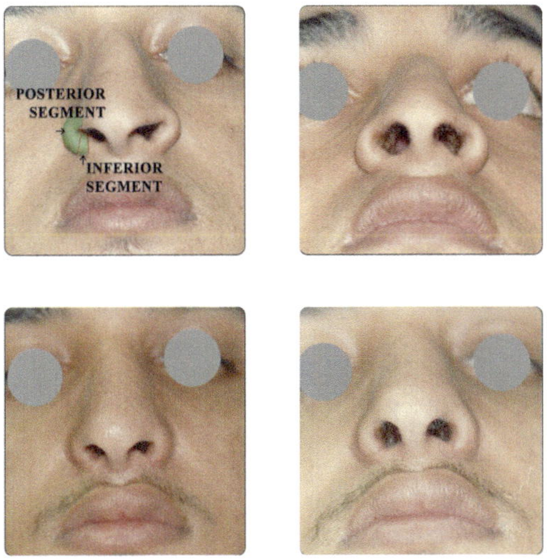

Right Nasal Aperture Rim Sill Test | Left Nasal Aperture Rim Sill Test

Preoperative

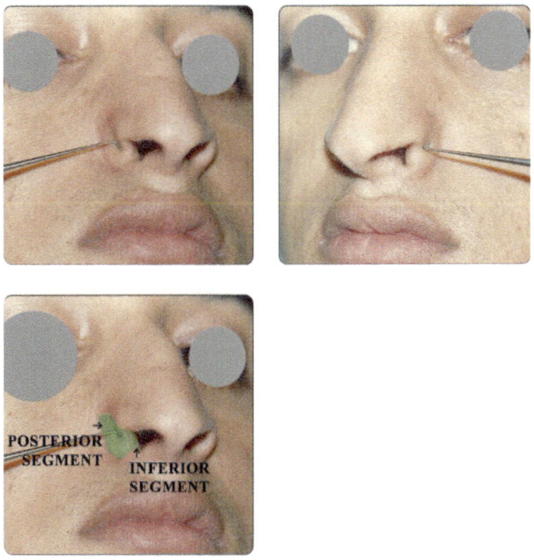

Right Oblique Cheek Margin Full Face | Left Oblique Cheek Margin Full Face | Right Oblique Cheek Margin Middle Third | Left Oblique Cheek Margin Middle Third

Preoperative

Postoperative

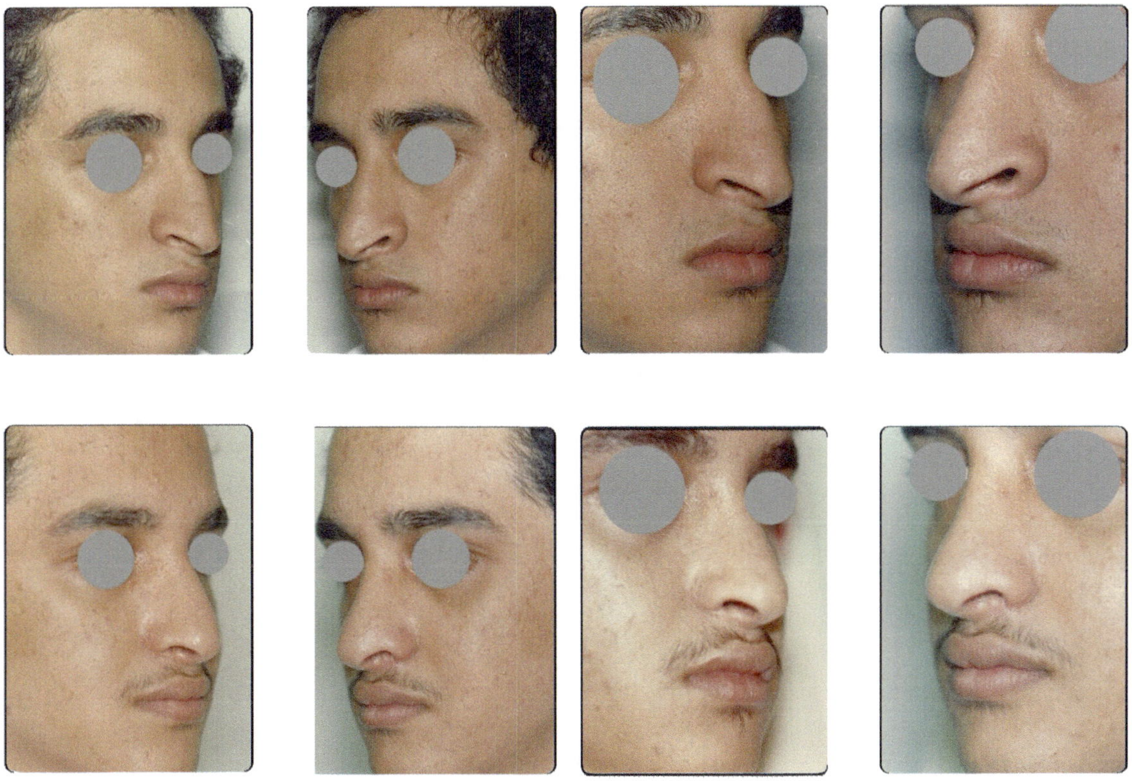

Right Lateral

Left Lateral

Preoperative

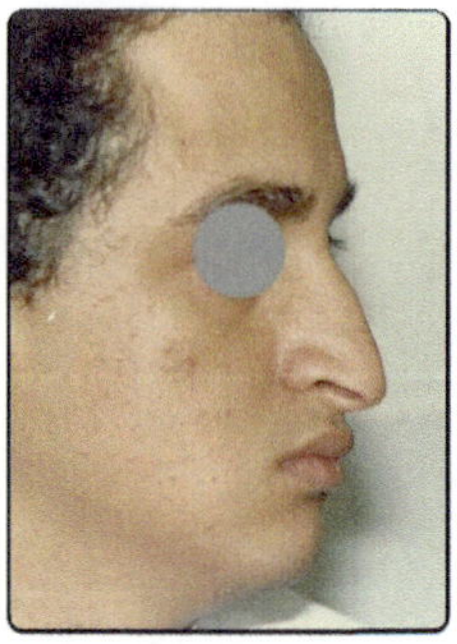

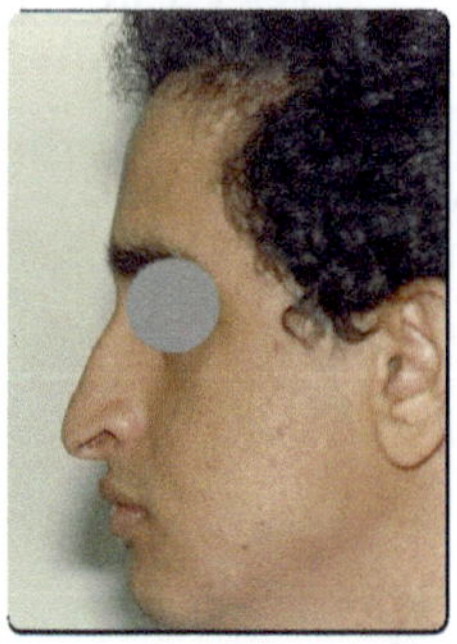

Postoperative

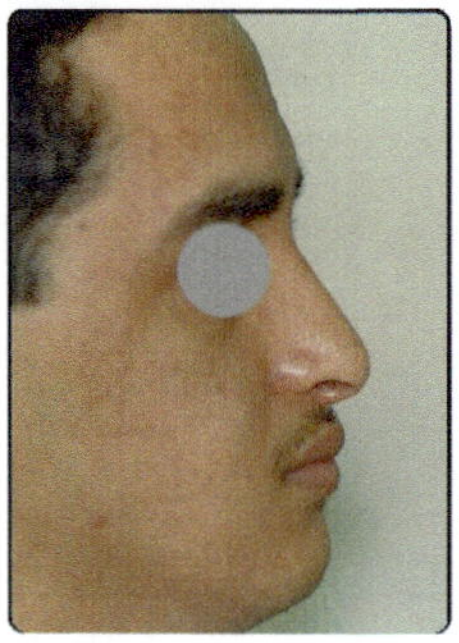

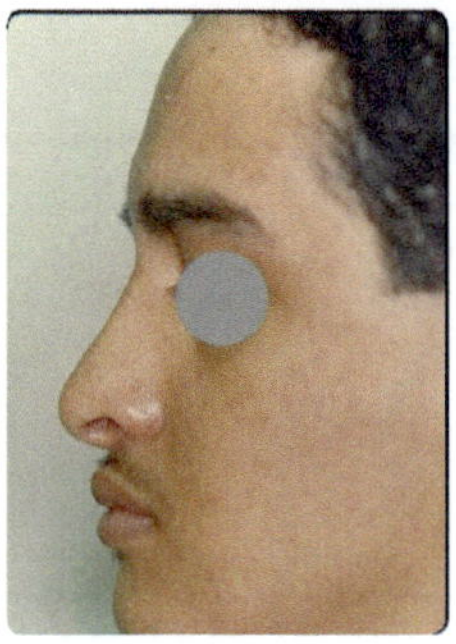

Right Lateral
Middle Third

Left Lateral
Middle Third

Preoperative

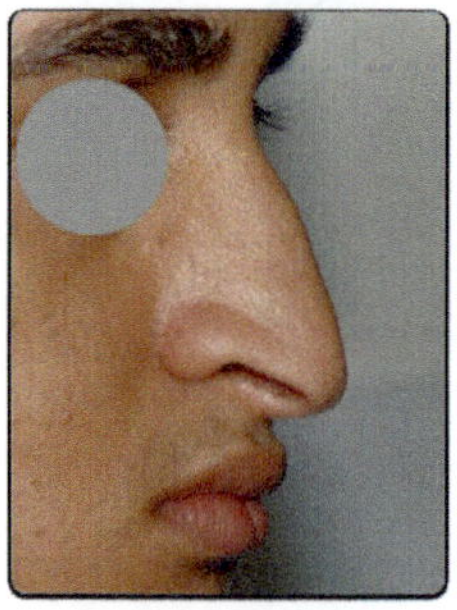

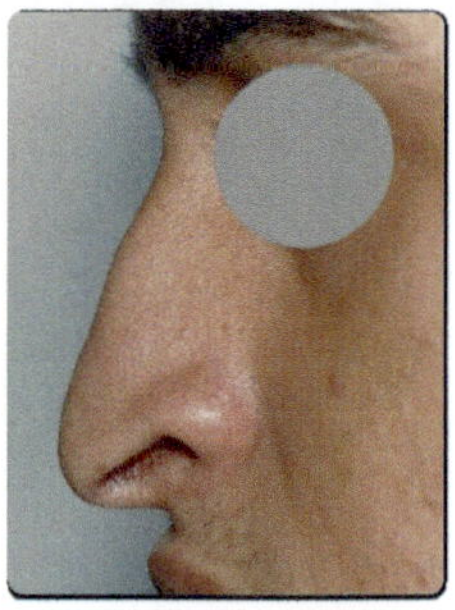

Postoperative

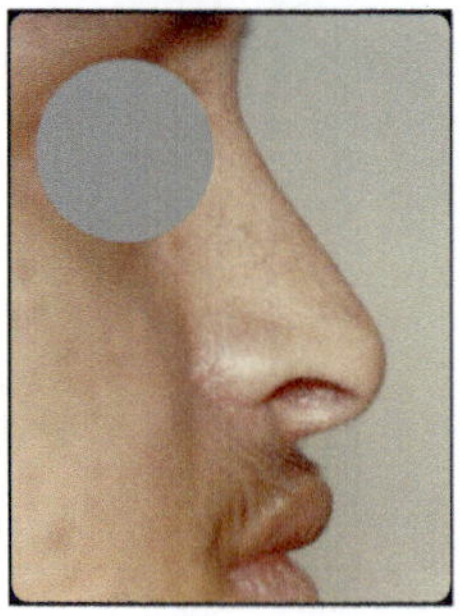

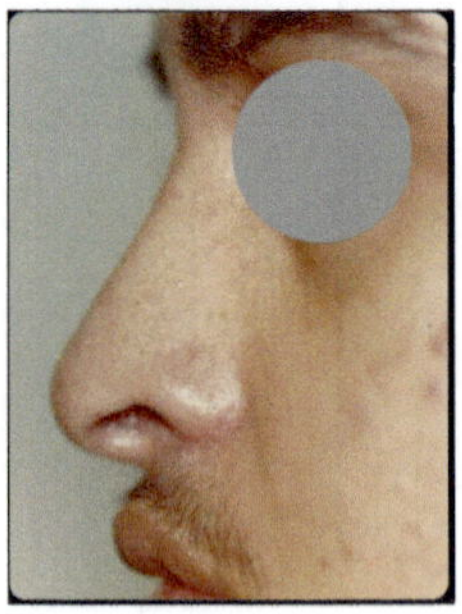

Part II: Clinical Case 7

9

Preoperative Assessment

1. **Frontolateral walls**
   Small but bulky tip partly overshadowing the alae nasi (Frontal Views).
2. **Medial Wall**
   a. Full nasolabial angle due to bulky anterior nasal spine (Lateral Views).
   b. Tight upper lip (pre-operative Lateral Views).
   c. Lateral prominence of the medial crurae (Basal Views).
   d. Mobile tip (Lateral Smiling Views).
3. **Boney pyramid**
   a. Osteocartilaginous hump (Oblique, Lateral, Backward Tilting and Nasal Aperture Views).
   b. Wide base of the bony pyramid (Frontal, Direct Dorsal, Overhead and Backward Tilting Views).
   c. Irregular dorsal light reflex.
4. **Alar base**
   a. Tight upper lip (Lateral smiling, and non-smiling views).
   b. The left ala nasi is naturally larger than the right. This gives the impression of asymmetrical smile. (Frontal Non-Smiling and Smiling Views).

Aims of Surgery

1. Reduce the bulk of the nasal tip.
2. Reduce the size and length of the nose.
3. Abolish the mobility of the tip and the tight upper lip.

Surgical Plan

1. **Frontolateral walls**
   a. DDD including the weak triangle to reduce the bulky nasal tip and supra tip area.
   b. Cephalic trim of lateral crurae to reduce the size.
2. **Medial Wall**
   a. Septoplasty: reducing the length and the height of the cartilaginous septum.
   b. Division of the depressor septi muscles, to overcome the mobile tip, and division of the frenulum transorally to abolish the tight upper lip.
3. **Boney pyramid**
   a. Excision of the osteocartilaginous hump down to the level of the anterior septal angle.
   b. Osteotomies and medialization of the lateral bony walls reduce the width of the bony pyramid.
4. **Alar base**
   Nil of note.

Surgical Procedure

a. As per Surgical Plan.
b. Septoplasty. right caudal dislocation (out of the maxillary groove) was found and corrected. The caudal margin was reduced by 2 mm. Part of the dorsal cartilaginous septum was removed with the cartilaginous hump. The anterior angle of the septum was slightly reduced as it was filling and elevating the supra tip area i.e. the weak triangle.
c. Having finished the operation the two domes were found to be of unequal height. Small pieces of crushed septal cartilage were placed over the tip to balance its shape and produce the final projecting appearance.
d. Transcolumellar nylone stitch across the posterior margins of the medial crurae and the inferior vestibular bands. This helped to overcome the lateral prominences of the medial crurae. Nylon stitch was used and removed after 6–8 weeks.

M. H. A. Shafy, *Atlas of Clinical Cases in Rhinoplasty*,
https://doi.org/10.1007/978-3-031-07504-9_9

Post-Operative Analysis

1. **Frontolateral Walls**
   a. Tip definition: the nasal tip is smaller with thinner and smoother overlying skin. It is more prominent and well identified from the alae nasi on both sides. The alae nasi come into view to become clearly visible and share in nasal aesthetics (Frontal, Direct Dorsal, Overhead, Backward Tilting and Basal Views).
   b. Tip projection: The nasal tip at the same level of the nasal dorsum with good aesthetic angle. This is coupled with good aesthetic nasolabial angle (lateral and oblique views).
   c. Tip light reflex is seen as one spot off the nasal tip. (Frontal and Backward Tilting Views).
2. **Medial Wall**
   a. The fullness in the nasolabial angle is gone (Lateral views).
   b. The tightness in the upper lip is released (Lateral Smiling views).
   c. The lateral crural prominences disappeared (Basal and Nasal Aperture Views).
3. **Bony Pyramid**
   a. Bony pyramid aesthetics: the nasal dorsum is straight and the sidewalls are smooth and narrow (all views except the Basal Views).
   b. Dorsal light reflex is a straight line post-operatively (Direct Dorsal Views).
4. **Alar Base**
   a. The superior alar grooves now clear off fat, become deeper, longer and visible (Direct Dorsal, Oblique and Lateral Views).
   b. Aesthetics of the alae nasi improved. They are no longer stretched by the long nose and better seen after defatting (Nasal, Aperture, Oblique and Lateral Views).
   c. Nasal aperture aesthetics improved:
      a. The size of nasal apertures equalized after correction of septal deviation (basal Views).
      b. The shapes of nasal apertures became nicely oval rather than long slit like openings (Backward Tilting and Basal views).
   d. Marginal light reflexes are clearly seen at:
      a. Inferior alar margins (Nasal Aperture Views).
      b. Nasal sill bands (Oblique Views).
      c. Lateral crural prominences (Lateral Views).

Commentary

a. It is not enough to only reduce the nasal hump, the whole size of the nose must be reduced as well. A long nose without a hump is just as bad as a long nose with a hump.
b. The new, smaller size of the nose is in proportion to the other facial features, namely the lips, chin, cheeks and eyes.

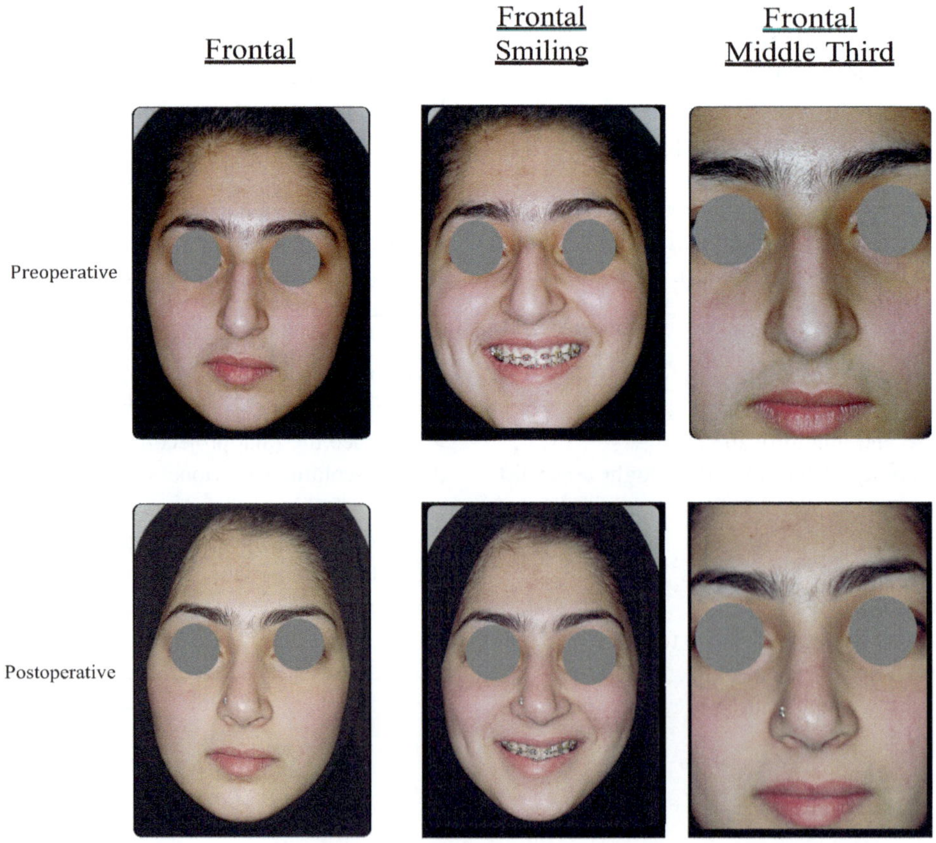

Direct Dorsal | Direct Dorsal Smiling | Overhead

Preoperative

Postoperative

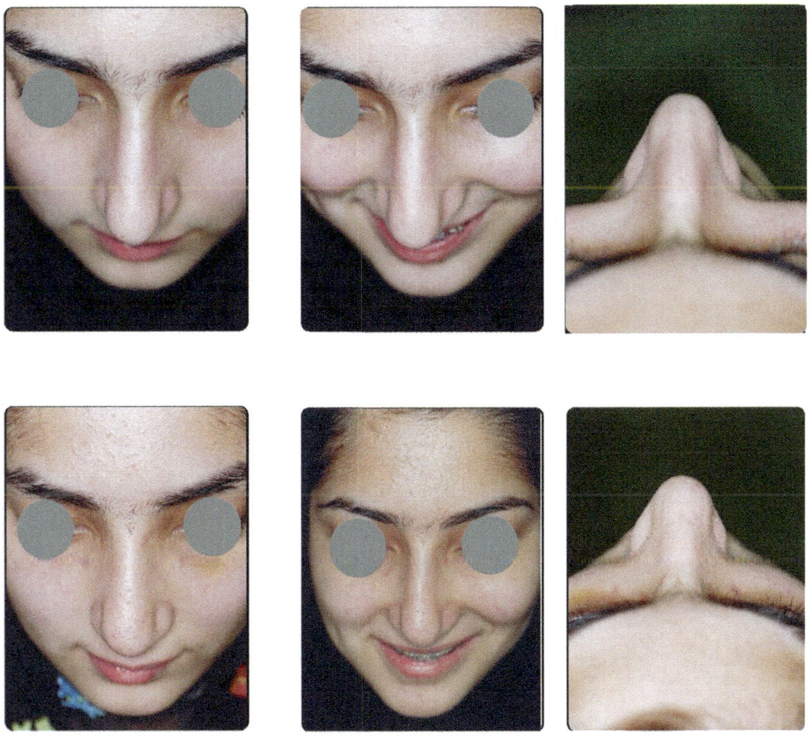

Backward Tilting | Steeper Backward Tilting | Basal | Basal Smiling

Preoperative

Postoperative

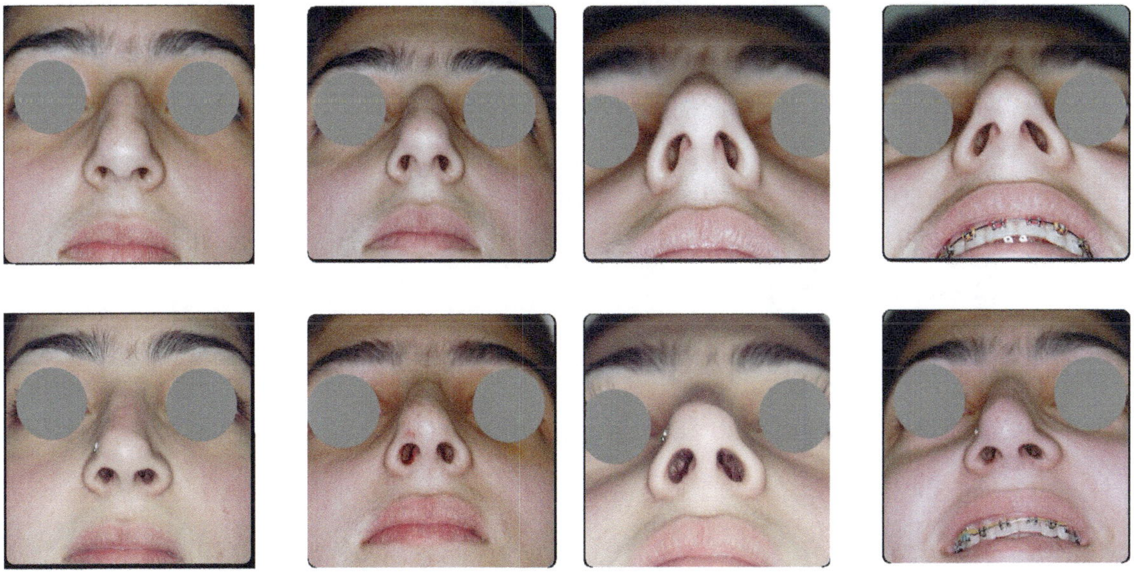

Right Nasal Aperture | Left Nasal Aperture

Preoperative

Postoperative

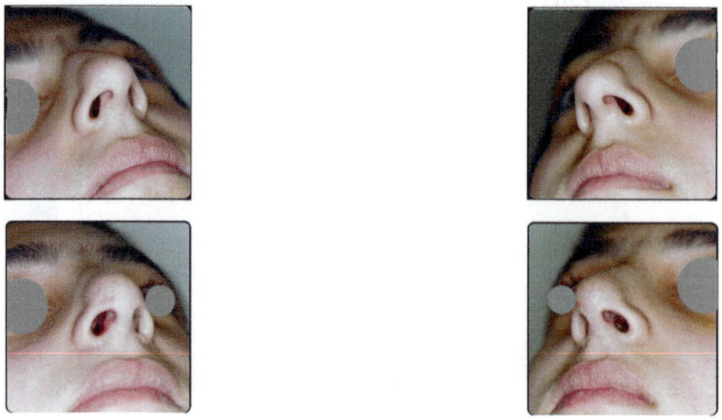

Right Oblique Mid Cheek Full Face | Left Oblique Mid Cheek Full Face | Right Oblique Mid Cheek Middle Third | Left Oblique Mid Cheek Middle Third

Preoperative

Postoperative

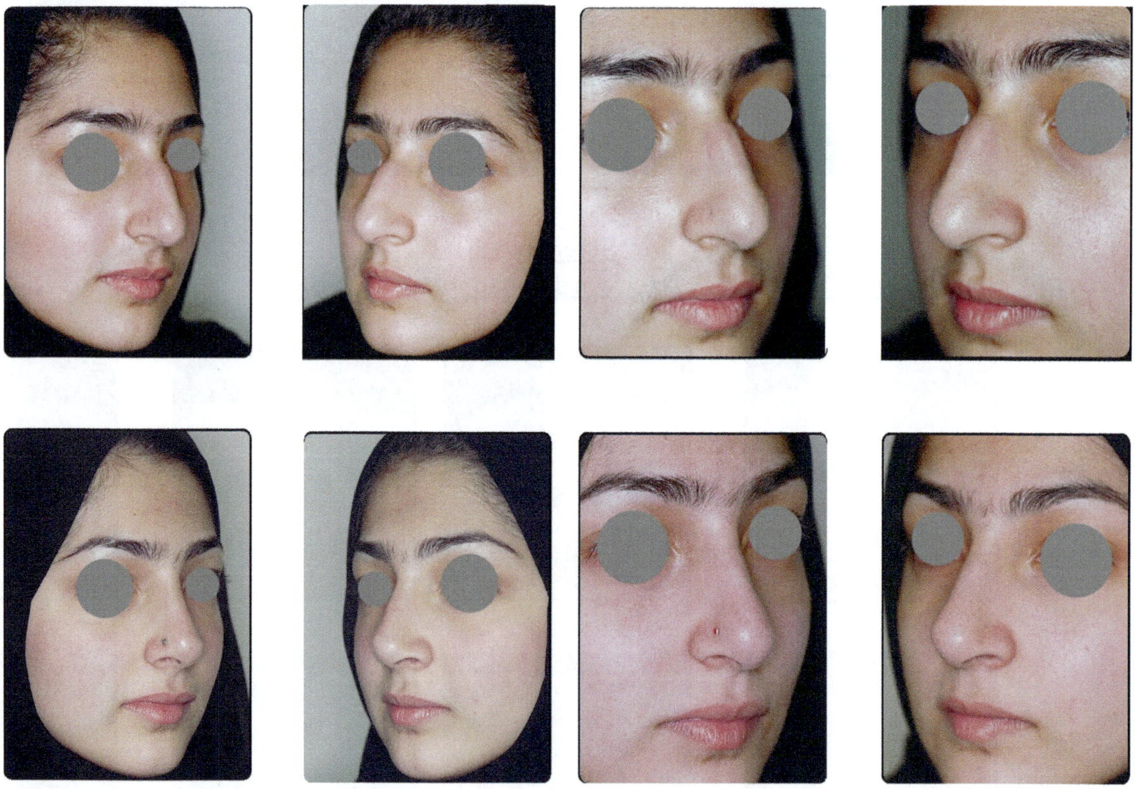

Right Oblique Cheek Margin Full Face | Left Oblique Cheek Margin Full Face | Right Oblique Cheek Margin Middle Third | Left Oblique Cheek Margin Middle Third

Preoperative

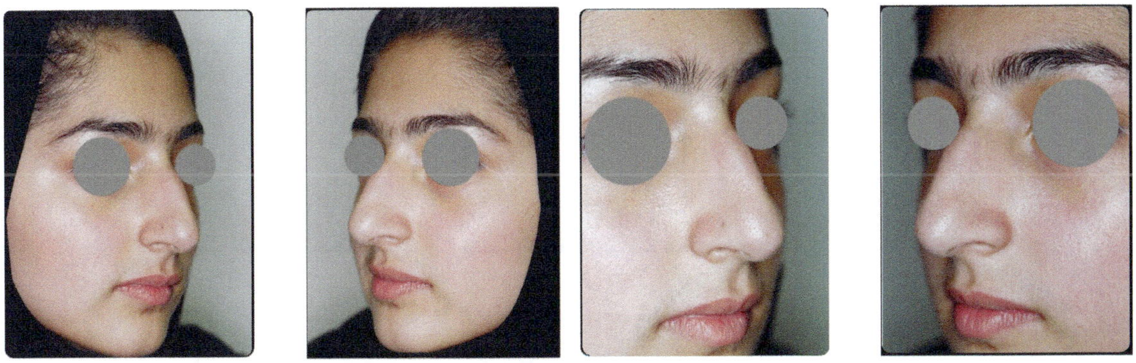

Postoperative

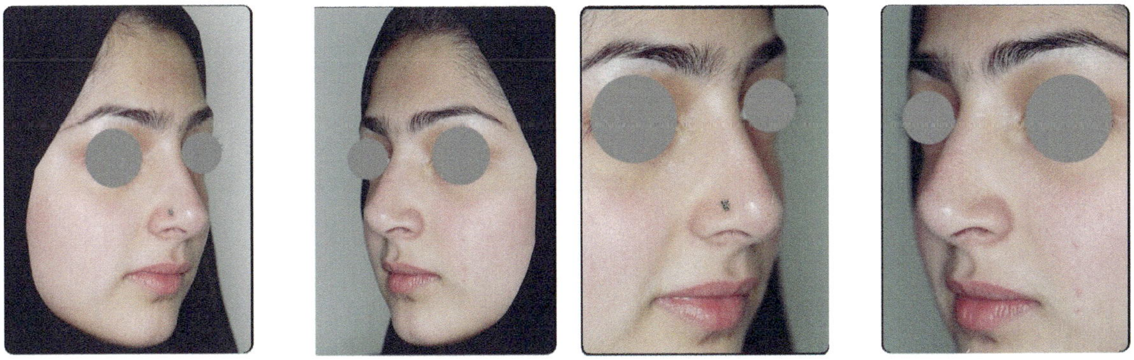

Right Lateral | Left Lateral | Right Lateral Smiling | Left Lateral Smiling

Preoperative

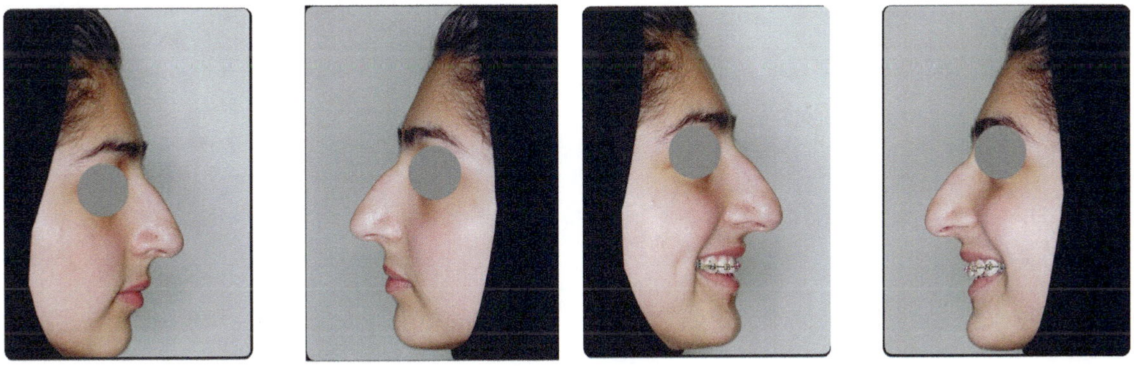

Postoperative

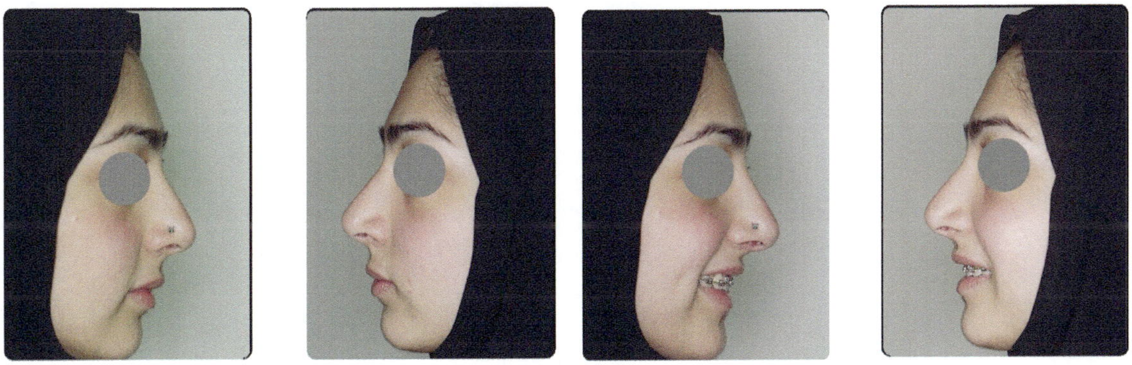

Right Lateral Middle Third | Left Lateral Middle Third

Preoperative

Postoperative

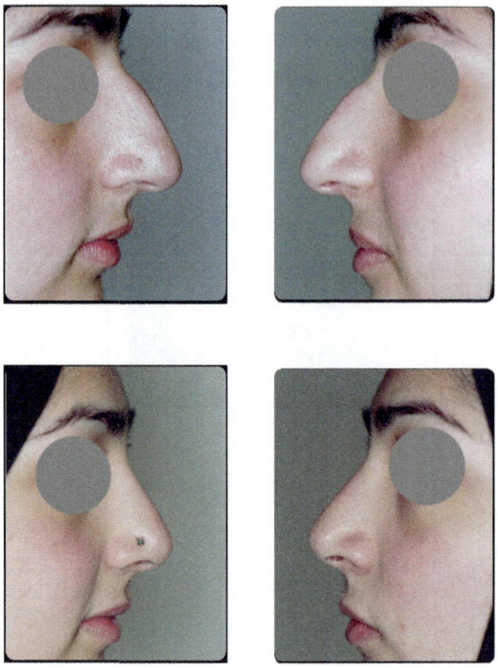

10 Part II: Clinical Case 8

Preoperative Assessment

1. **Frontolateral Walls**
   Large, bulky and ill defined nasal tip (Frontal and Basal Views) despite of the good projection (lateral views).
2. **Nasal Septum**
   Nil of note.
3. **Boney pyramid**
   a. Wide base of the boney pyramid (Frontal, Direct Dorsal and Backward Tilting Views).
   b. Small osteocartilagenous hump (Backward Tilting, Oblique and Lateral Views). This is rather the normal anatomical concavoconvex bodies of the nasal bones (see Anatomy Section in Text).
4. **Alar base**
   Wide alar base due to **long inferior segments** of rim-sill folds. Bulky alar base due to **thick posterior segments** of the rim sill folds (Basal and Nasal Aperture Views). Note the inferior and posterior segments of the left rim-sill test appearance are a pale area.

Aims of Surgery

Reduction of the overall size and bulk of the nose.

Surgical Plan

1. **Frontolateral walls**
   a. DDD including the weak triangle to reduce the bulk of frontolateral walls and supra tip area.
   b. Cephalic trim of the lateral crurae to reduce the size of frontolateral walls.
2. **Medial Walls**
   Nil of note
3. **Boney pyramid**
   a. Excision of the osteocartilagenous hump.
   b. Osteotomies and medialization of the lateral bony walls to reduce the width of the bony pyramid.
4. **Alar base**
   Bilateral resection of the inferior and posterior segments of the rim sill folds.

Surgical Procedure

As per Surgical Plan

Post-Operative Analysis

1. **Frontolateral Walls**
   a. Tip definition improved: the tip is slimmer and prominently well identified with thinner overlying skin. The alae nasi come into view to share in nasal aesthetics (Frontal, Direct Dorsal, Overhead, Backward Tilting and Basal Views).
   b. Tip projection: the nasal tip is at the same level of the nasal dorsum with good aesthetic angle. This is coupled with good aesthetic nasolabial angle (lateral and oblique views).
   c. Tip light reflex is seen as one spot off the nasal tip. (Frontal and Backward Tilting Views).
2. **Medial Walls**
   Nil of Note.
3. **Bony Pyramid**
   a. Bony pyramid aesthetics improved: the nasal dorsum is straight and the sidewalls are smooth and narrow (all views except the Basal Views).
   b. Dorsal light reflex is seen as an uninterrupted line off the nasal dorsum (Direct Dorsal Views).
4. **Alar Base**
   a. The superior alar grooves now clear off fat, become deeper, longer and visible (Direct Dorsal, Oblique and Lateral Views).
   b. Posterior alar groove aesthetics improved by defatting as well as excising the posterior segments of the rim-sill folds. The impression of the flat tire appearance is no longer present. (Backward Tilting, Basal and Nasal Aperture Views).

M. H. A. Shafy, *Atlas of Clinical Cases in Rhinoplasty*,
https://doi.org/10.1007/978-3-031-07504-9_10

c. Alae nasi aesthetics improved: they are pulled medially become better seen, smaller in size and share in nasal aesthetics. (Nasal Aperture, Oblique and Lateral Views).
d. Nasal aperture aesthetics:
   a. The wide lateral bowing of alae nasi and thick base of the rim-sill folds have dramatically improved (Backward Tilting, Basal and Nasal Aperture Views).
   b. The sizes of the nasal apertures are smaller and the shapes become more elegantly oval (Backward, Tilting, Basal and Nasal Aperture Views).
e. Marginal light reflexes are clearly seen at:
   i. The inferior alar and flat triangular margins. Reflex is absent from the rim-sill folds which were accurately excised. This is better seen in the left than the right aperture views. The left has more direct angle of photography.
   ii. Nasal sill bands (Oblique Views).
   iii. Lateral crural prominences (Lateral Views).

Commentary

Post-operative photographs were taken on the seventh postoperative day immediately after removing the plaster cast and the stitches. Further uniform reduction in the size and bulk is expected in the following months and years.

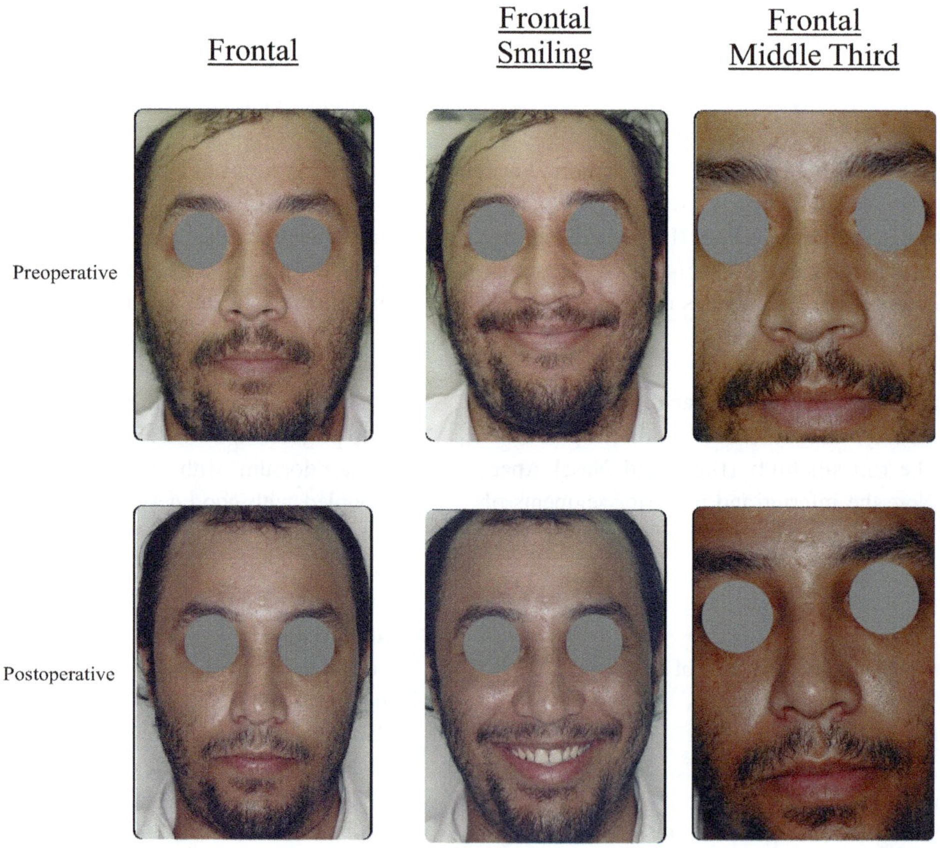

Direct Dorsal

Preoperative

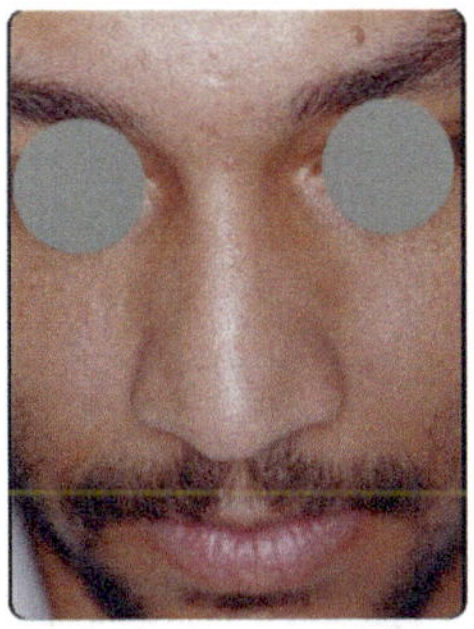

Postoperative

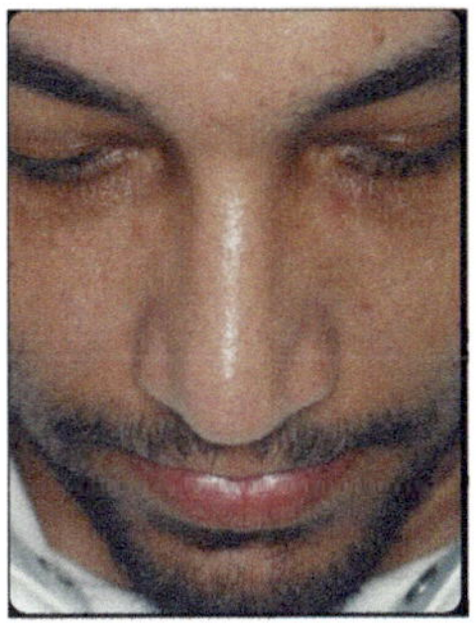

Backward Tilting | **Steeper Backward Tilting** | **Basal**

Preoperative

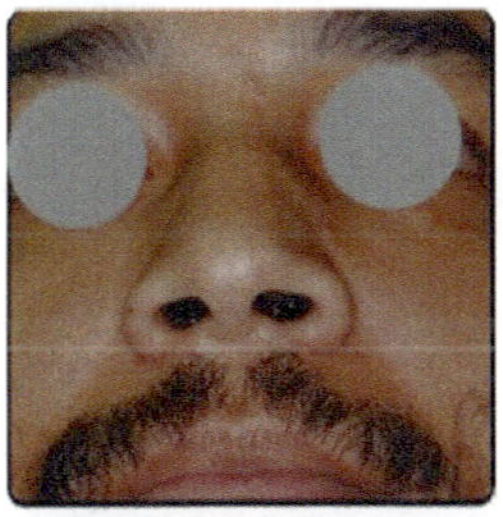

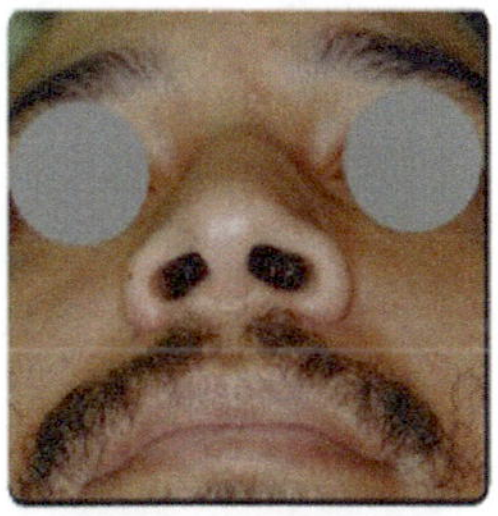

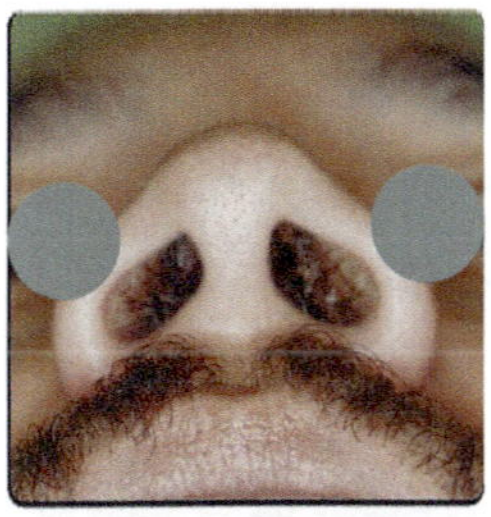

Postoperative

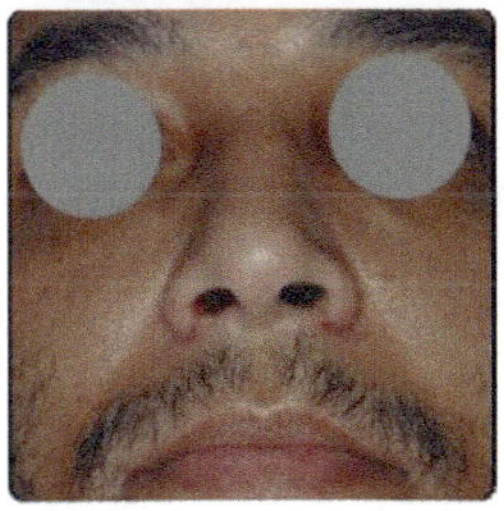

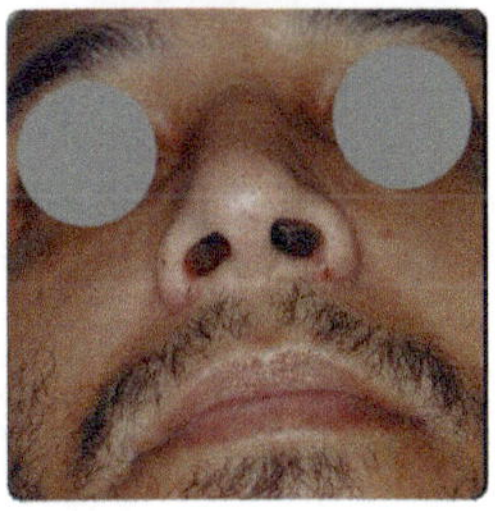

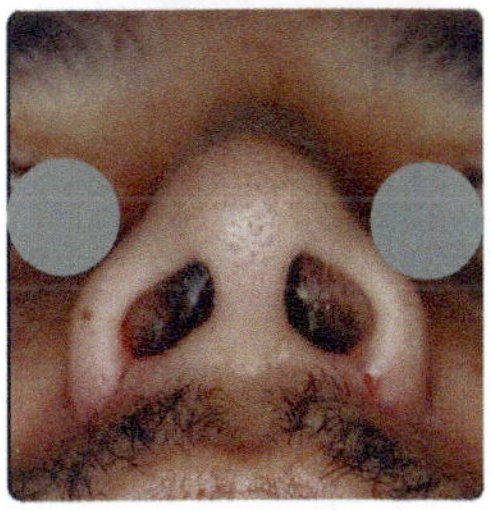

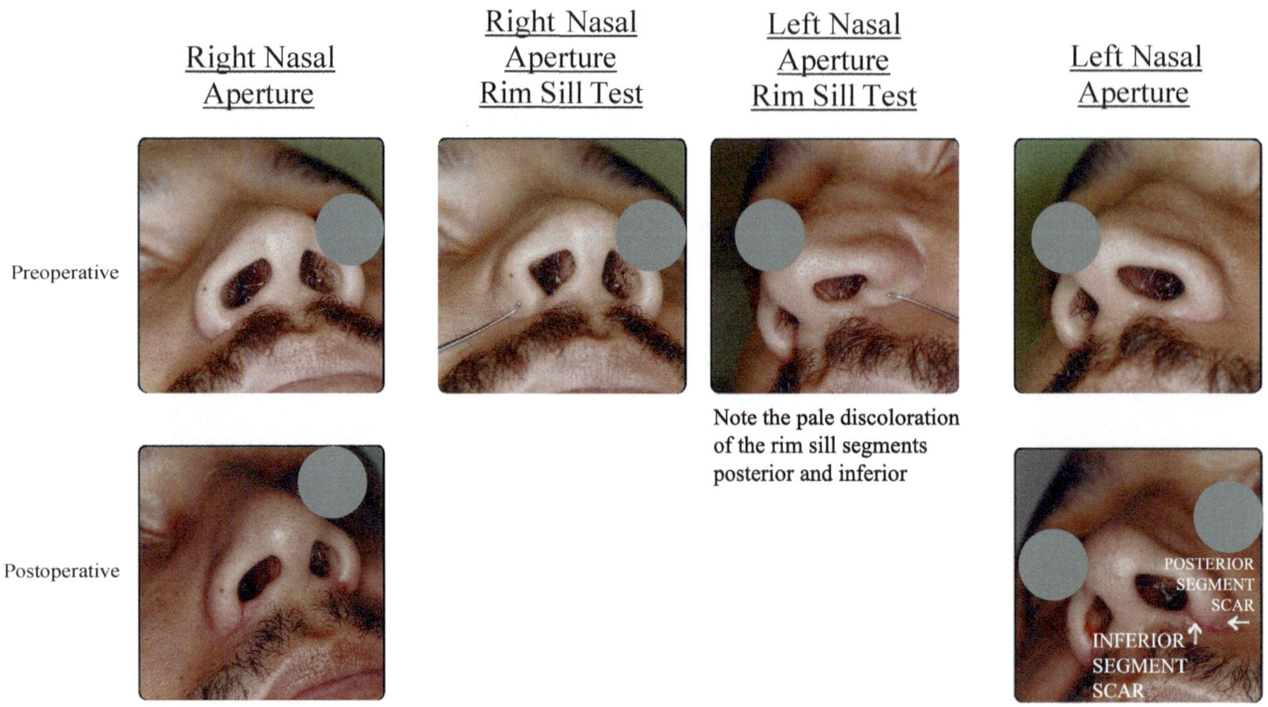
Right Nasal Aperture
Right Nasal Aperture Rim Sill Test
Left Nasal Aperture Rim Sill Test
Left Nasal Aperture
Preoperative
Postoperative
Note the pale discoloration of the rim sill segments posterior and inferior
POSTERIOR SEGMENT SCAR
INFERIOR SEGMENT SCAR

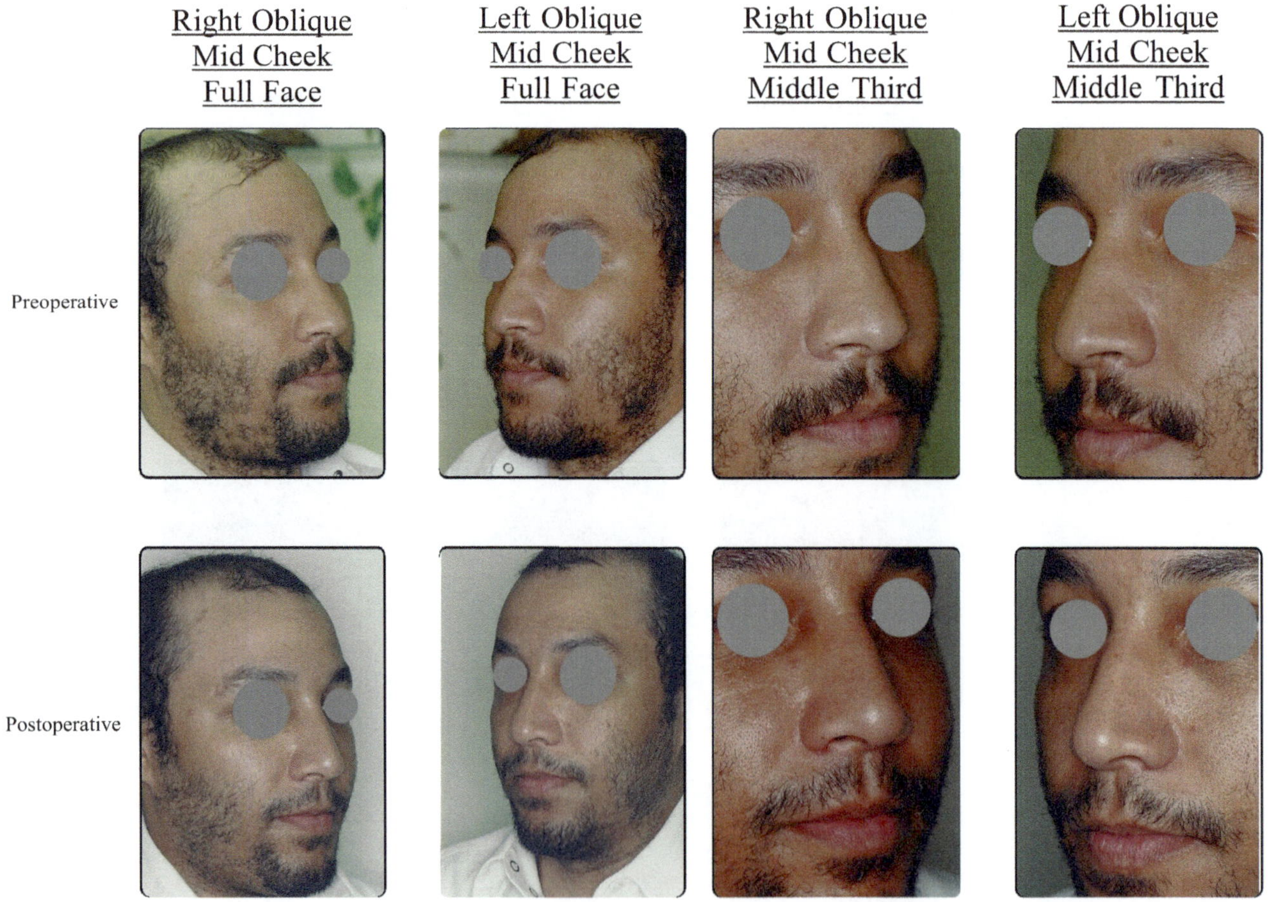
Right Oblique Mid Cheek Full Face
Left Oblique Mid Cheek Full Face
Right Oblique Mid Cheek Middle Third
Left Oblique Mid Cheek Middle Third
Preoperative
Postoperative

Right Oblique Cheek Margin Full Face | Left Oblique Cheek Margin Full Face | Right Oblique Cheek Margin Middle Third | Left Oblique Cheek Margin Middle Third

Preoperative

Postoperative

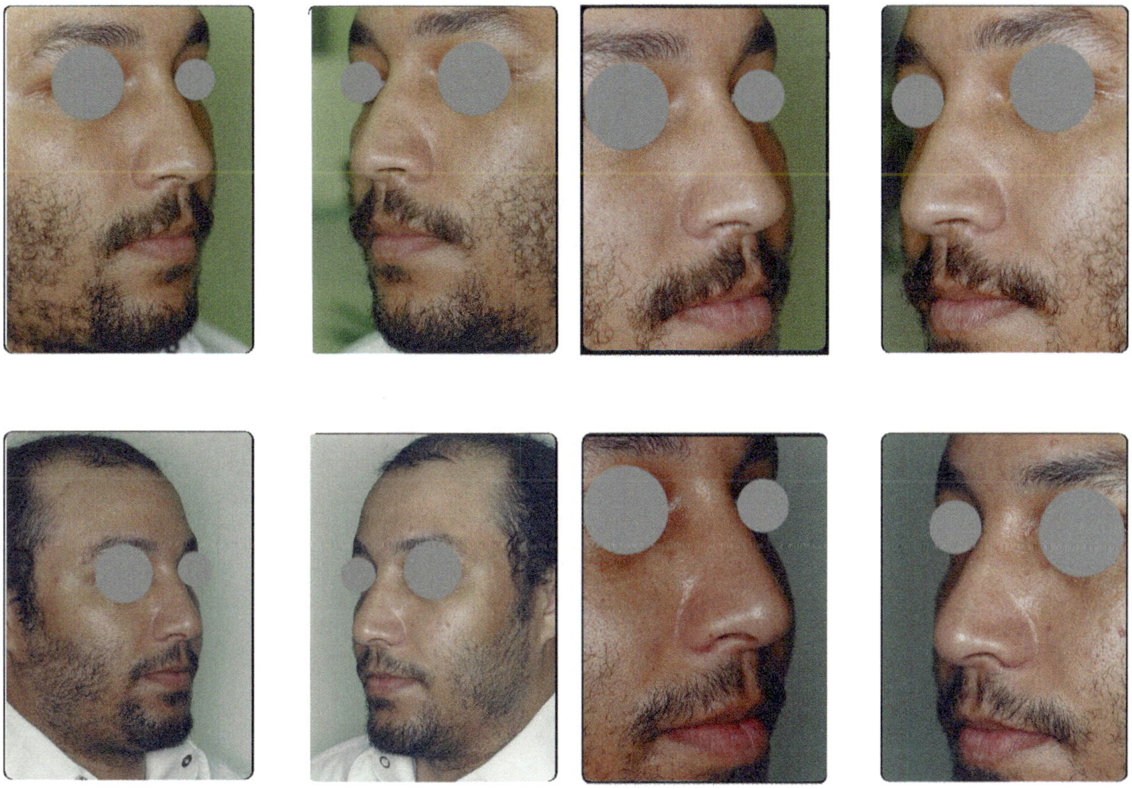

Right Lateral | Left Lateral | Right Lateral Smiling | Left Lateral Smiling

Preoperative

Postoperative

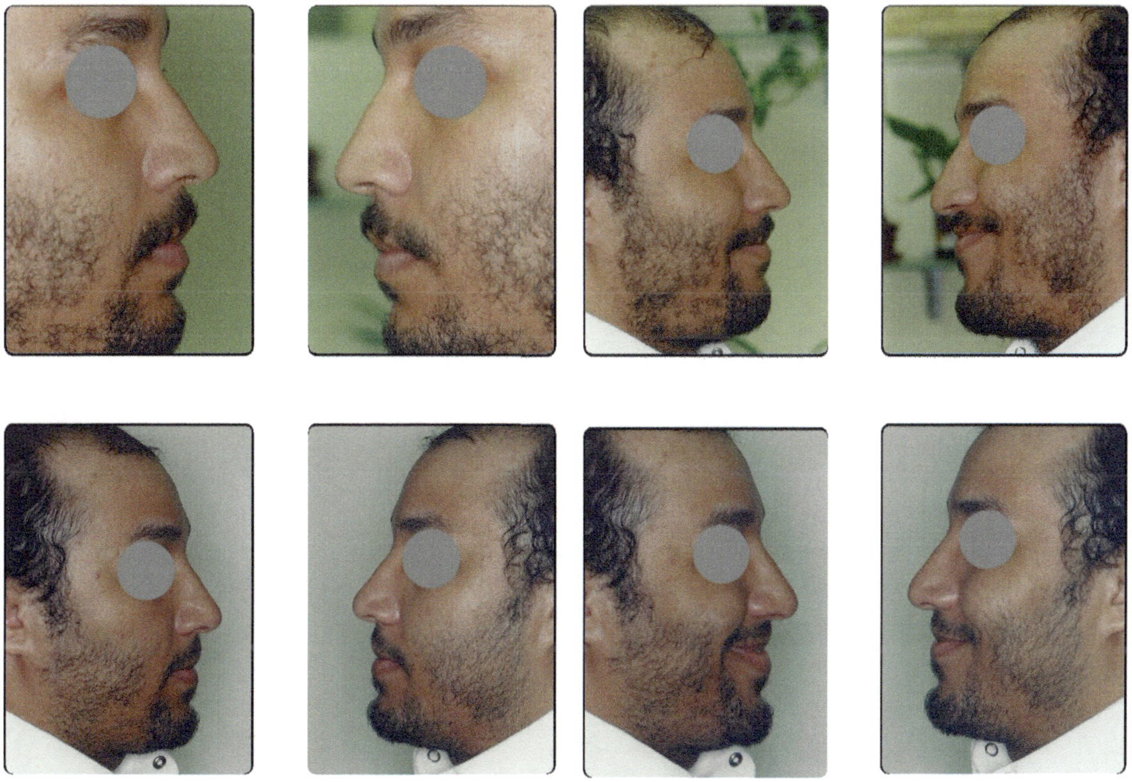

Right Lateral Middle Third | Left Lateral Middle Third

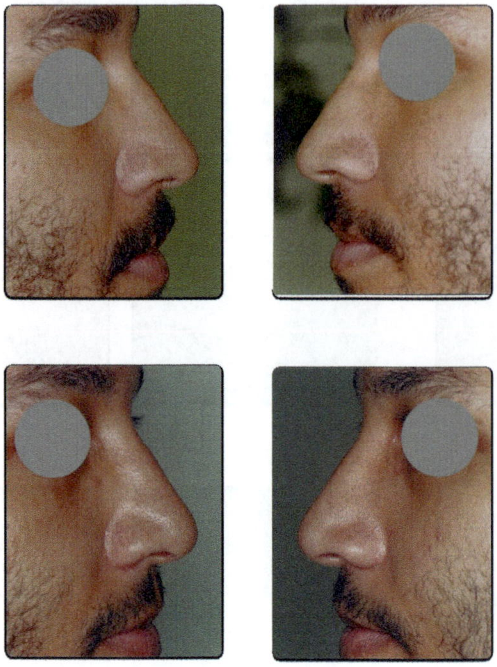

Preoperative

Postoperative

Part II: Clinical Case 9

11

Preoperative Assessment

1. **Frontolateral walls**
   a. Large and bulky tip with irregular surface (Frontal, Direct Dorsal and Overhead views).
   b. Bifid tip (Direct Dorsal and Backward Tilting Views). The tip light reflex shows two shining spots (Frontal and Backward Tilting Views).
2. **Medial Wall**
   Mobile nasal tip (Pre-operative Lateral Smiling Views).
3. **Boney pyramid**
   a. Wide base of the boney pyramid (Frontal, Direct Dorsal and Backward Tilting Views).
   b. Osteocartilaginous hump (Oblique and Lateral Views).
   c. Irregular dorsal light reflex (Preoperative Direct Dorsal Views).
4. **Alar base**
   Wide alar base. Note the pale rim-sill fold of skin in the rim-sill tests. Note the light reflexes in the nasal aperture views off the inferior alar margins, margins of the flat triangles and lateral crural margins.

Aims of Surgery

1. Reduce the size of the nose, tip, bony pyramid and alar base.
2. Abolish nasal tip bifidity.
3. Abolish nasal tip mobility.
4. Excise the osteocartilagenous hump.
5. Reduction of the alar base.

Surgical Plan

1. **Frontolateral Walls**
   a. DDD including the weak triangle to reduce the size and bulk of frontolateral walls And Supra tip area.
   b. Bilateral cephalic trim of lateral crurae to reduce the size of the nasal tip.
   c. Stitch the domes and medial crura to abolish the bifidity.
2. **Medial Wall**
   Division of the depressor septi muscles.
3. **Boney pyramid**
   a. Excision of the osteocartilaginous hump.
   b. Osteotomies and medialization of the lateral bony walls to reduce the width of the bony pyramid.
4. **Alar base**
   Excision of the inferior and posterior segments of the rim sill folds to reduce the size and the bulk of the alar base successively.

Surgical Procedure

a. As per Surgical Plan.
b. No stiching of the domes and medial crurae were necessary. No tip grafts.

Post-Operative Analysis

1. **Frontolateral Walls**
   a. Tip definition improved: the tip is slimmer and prominently well identified with thinner overlying skin. The alae nasi come into view to share in nasal

M. H. A. Shafy, *Atlas of Clinical Cases in Rhinoplasty*,
https://doi.org/10.1007/978-3-031-07504-9_11

aesthetics (Frontal, Direct Dorsal, Overhead, Backward Tilting and Basal Views).
   b. Bifidity disappeared after defatting and weakening of the domes without the need for stitching the two sides together.
   c. Tip projection: The nasal tip at the same level of the nasal dorsum with good aesthetic angle. This is coupled with good aesthetic nasolabial angle (lateral and oblique views).
   d. Tip light reflex is seen as one spot off the nasal tip. (Frontal and Backward Tilting Views).
2. **Medial Wall**
   Mobility of the tip was overcome.
3. **Bony Pyramid**
   a. Bony pyramid aesthetics: the nasal dorsum is straight and the sidewalls are smooth and narrow (all views except the Basal Views).
   b. Dorsal light reflex is seen as a regular one line off the nasal dorsum (Direct Dorsal Views).
4. **Alar Base**
   a. The superior alar grooves now clear off fat, become deeper, longer and more visible (Direct Dorsal, Oblique and Lateral Views).
   b. Posterior alar groove aesthetics improved by defatting as well as excising the posterior segments of the rim-sill folds. The impression of that flat tire appearance is no longer present. (Backward Tilting, Basal and Nasal Aperture Views).
   c. Nasal aperture aesthetics:
      i. The size of the nasal openings are reduced by defatting as well as excising the inferior segments of the rim-sill folds. (Backward Tilting, Basal and Nasal Aperture views).
      ii. The shape of nasal openings improved by defatting and excision of the rim-sill folds transforms the nasal apertures from thick walled wide and rounded openings with transverse long axes to thin walled small oval openings with anterior long axes. (Backward Tilting, Basal and Nasal Aperture views).
   d. Marginal light reflexes are clearly seen at:
      i. Inferior alar margins (Nasal Aperture Views).
      ii. Nasal sill bands (Oblique Views).
      iii. Lateral crural prominences (Lateral Views).

Commentary

The postoperative photos were taken only two months postoperatively, which explains the apparently protruding columella. This postoperative swelling of the columella is greatly reduced 4–6 months post operatively.

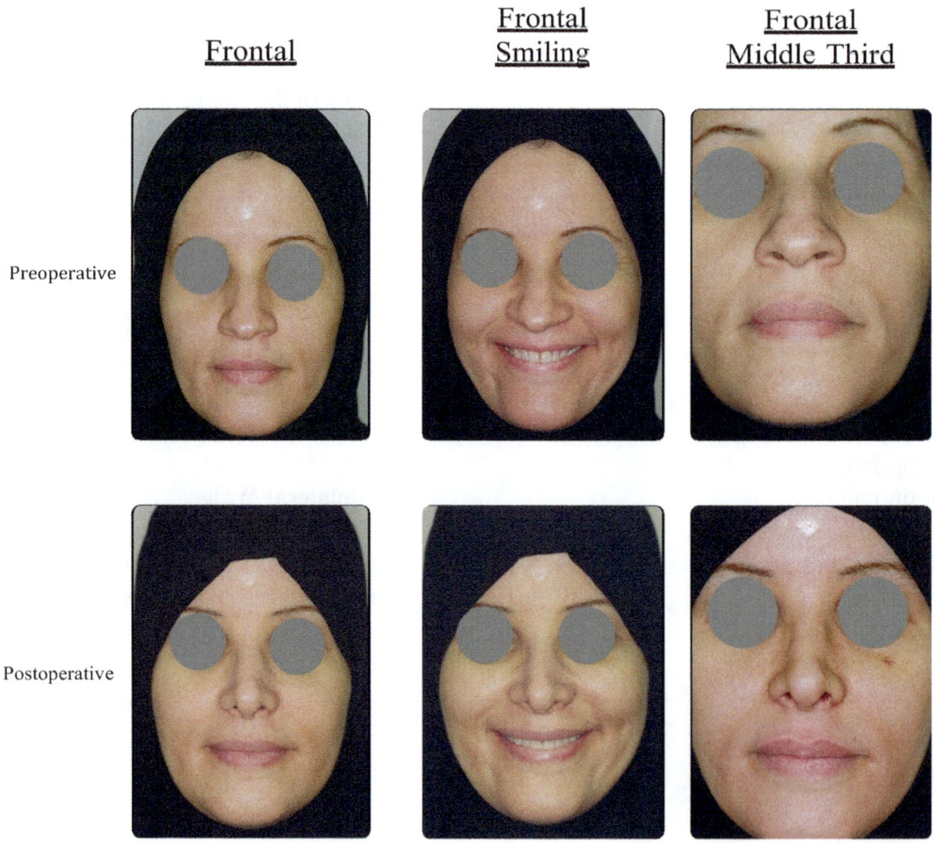

Direct Dorsal | Direct Dorsal Smiling | Overhead

Preoperative

Postoperative

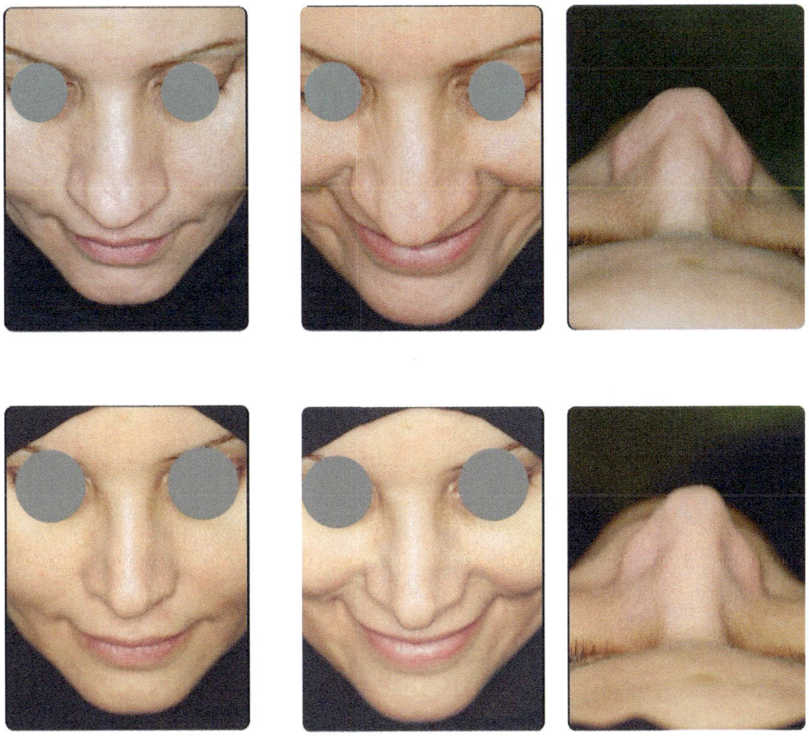

Backward Tilting | Steeper Backward Tilting | Basal

Preoperative

Postoperative

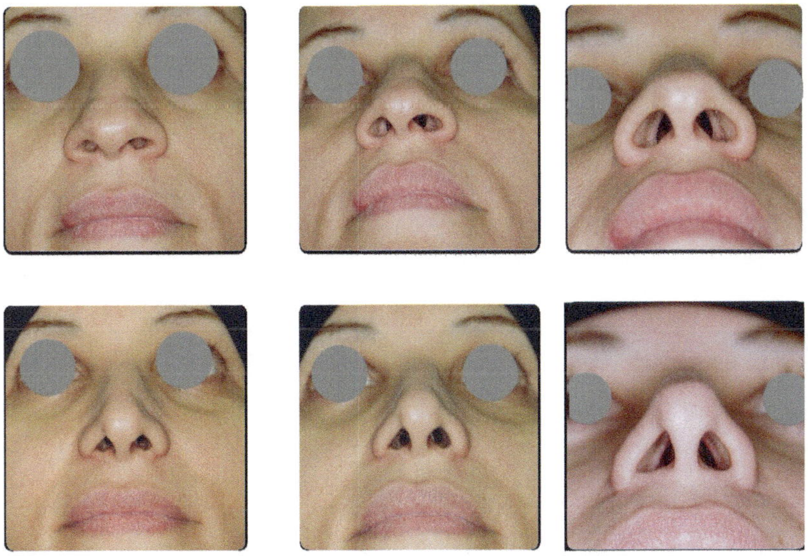

Right Nasal Aperture | Right Nasal Aperture Rim Sill Test | Left Nasal Aperture Rim Sill Test | Left Nasal Aperture

Preoperative

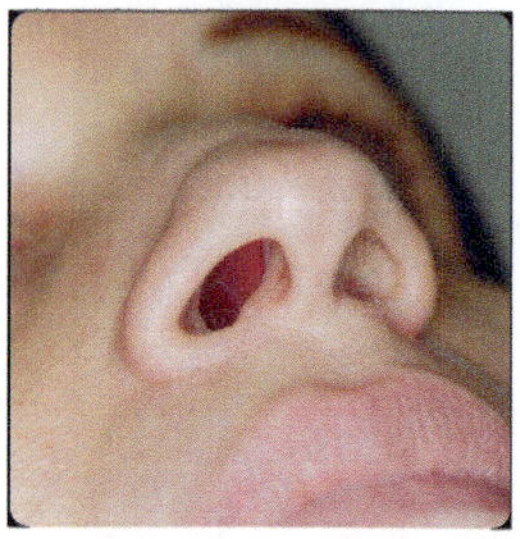

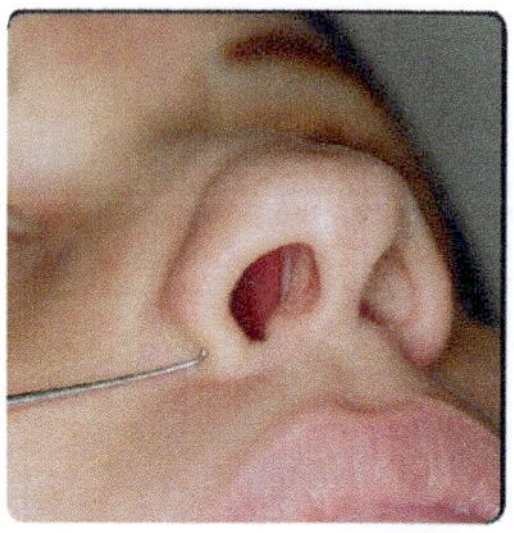

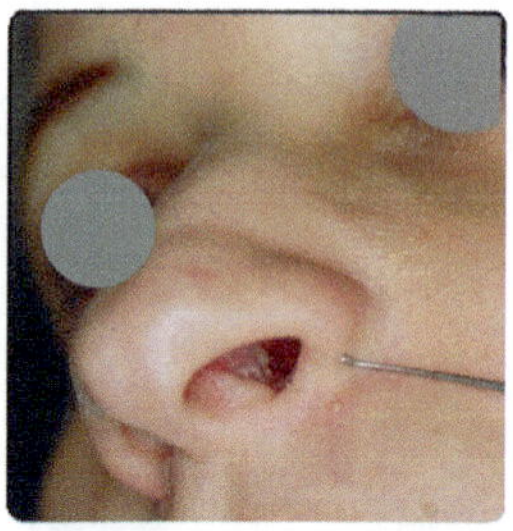

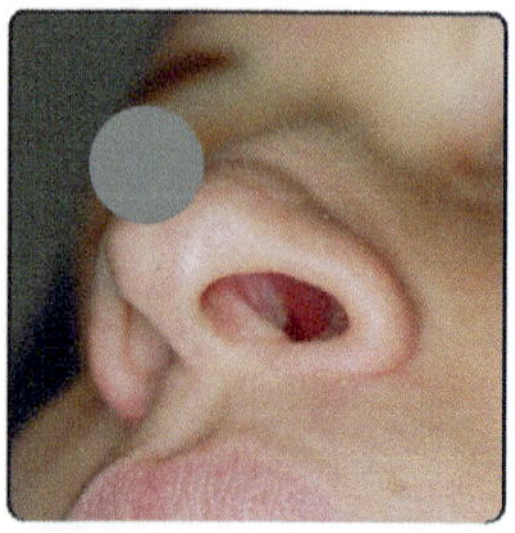

Note the pale discoloration of the rim sill folds, posterior and inferior

Postoperative

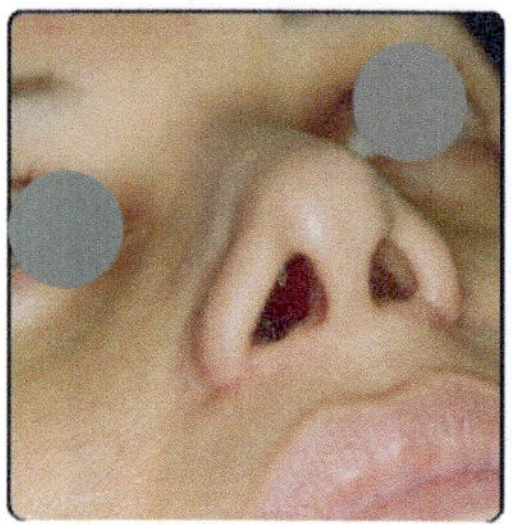

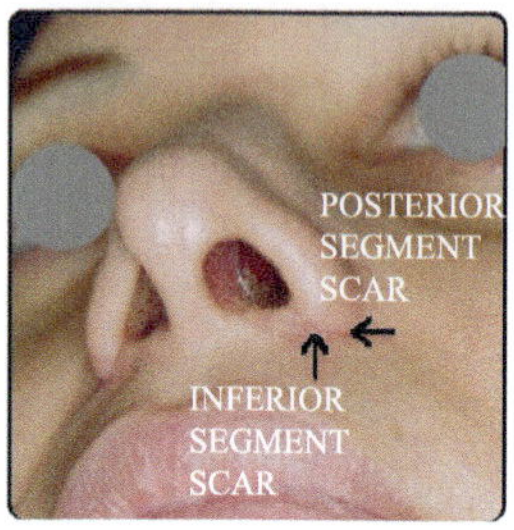

Right Oblique Mid Cheek Full Face | Left Oblique Mid Cheek Full Face | Right Oblique Mid Cheek Middle Third | Left Oblique Mid Cheek Middle Third

Preoperative

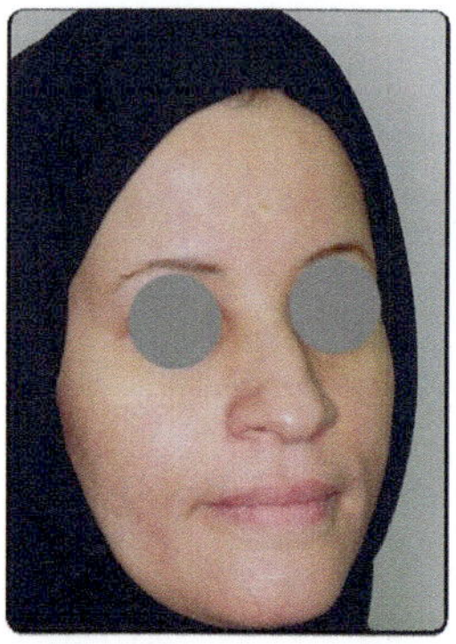

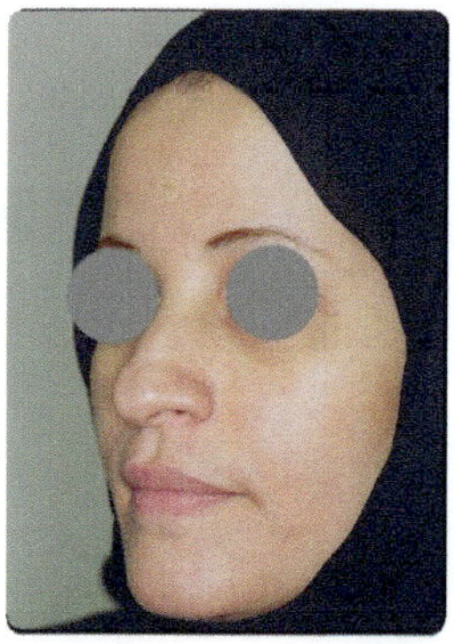

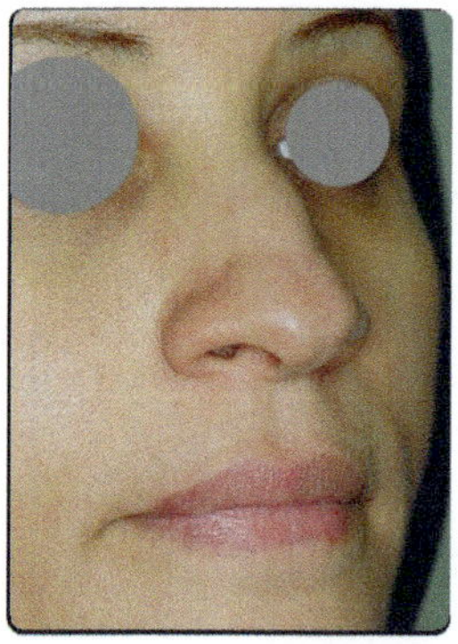

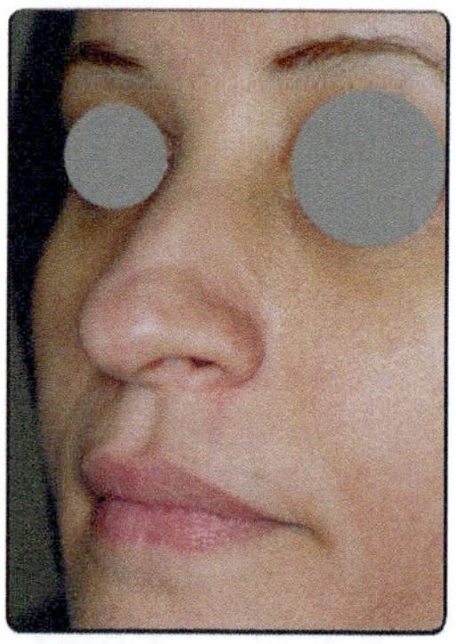

Postoperative

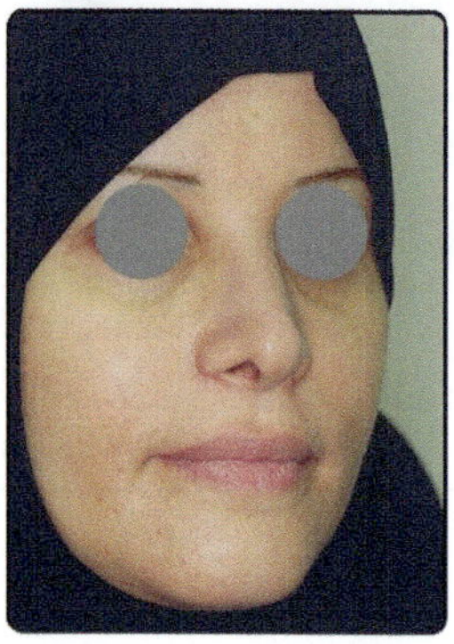

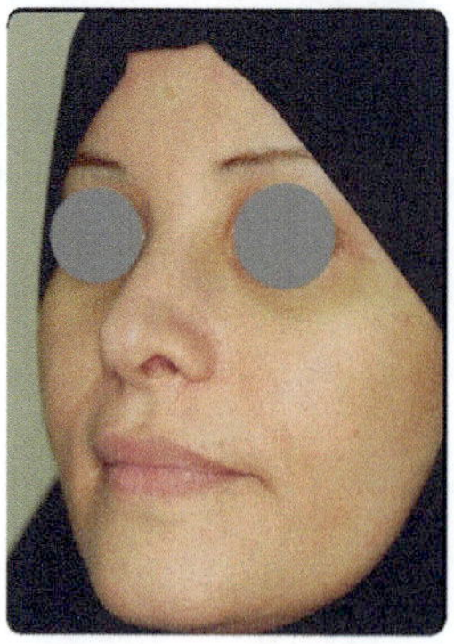

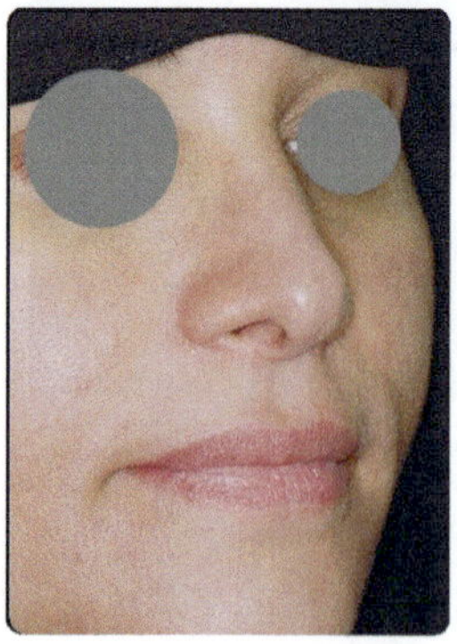

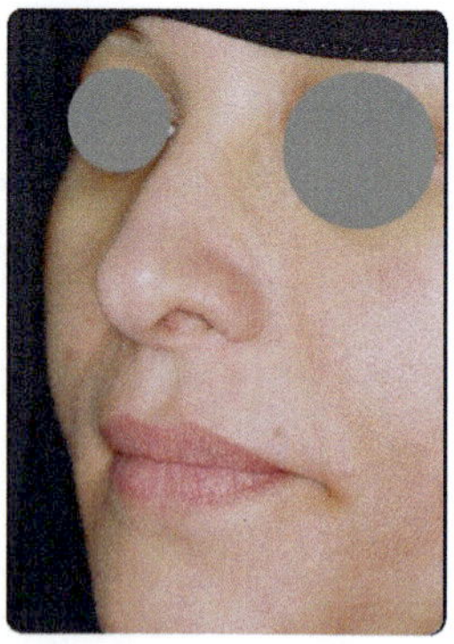

Right Oblique Cheek Margin Full Face | Left Oblique Cheek Margin Full Face | Right Oblique Cheek Margin Middle Third | Left Oblique Cheek Margin Middle Third

Preoperative

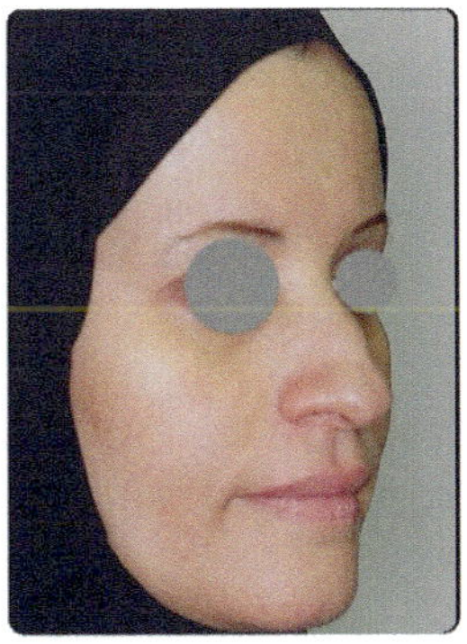
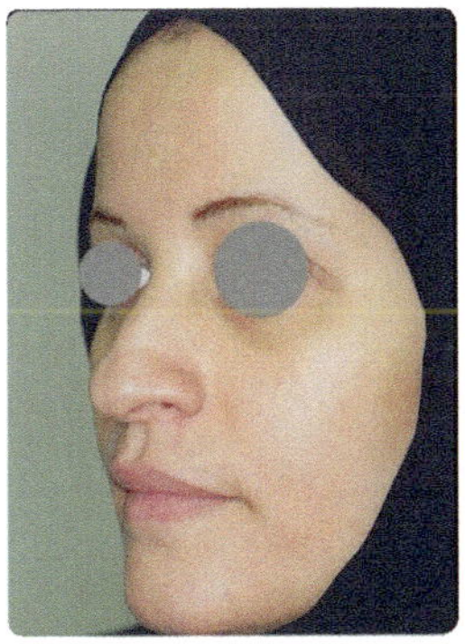
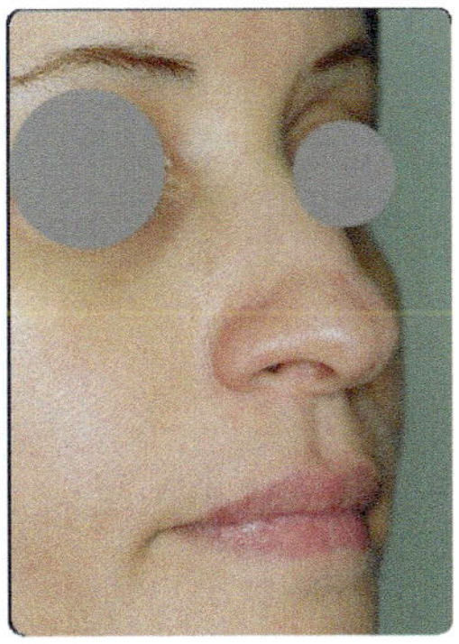
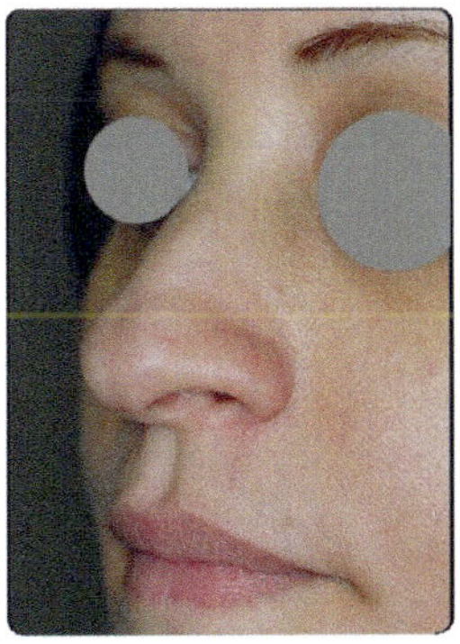

Postoperative

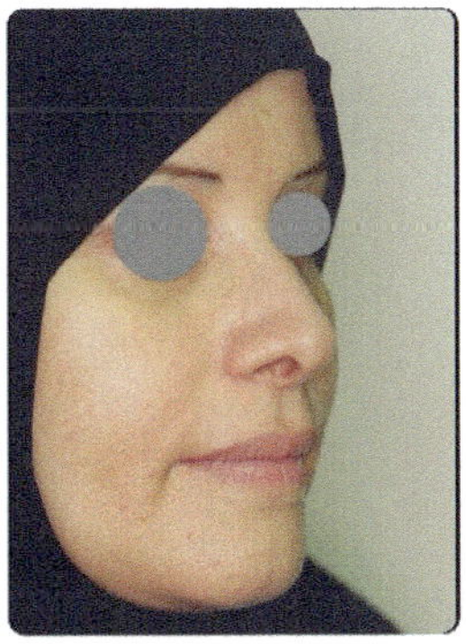
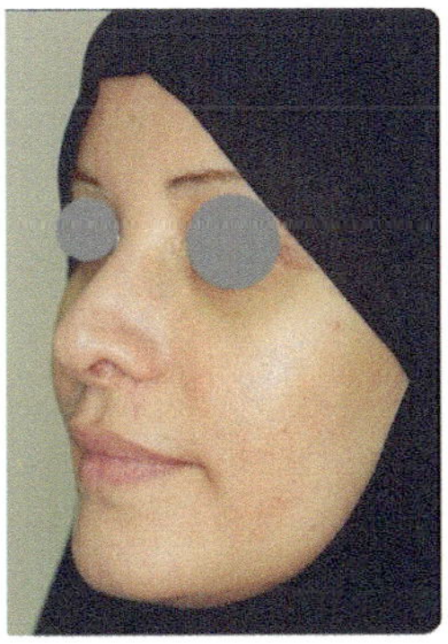
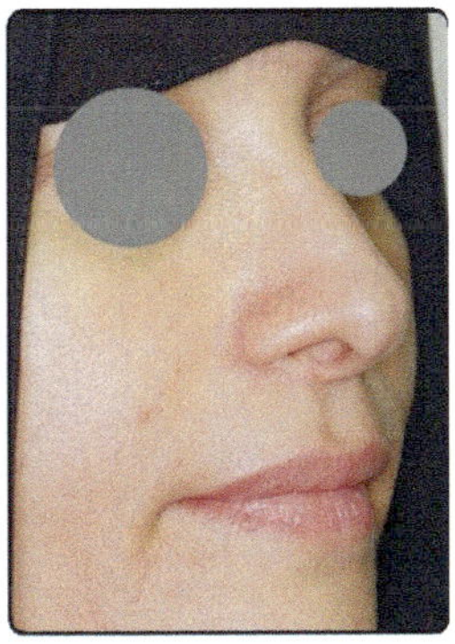
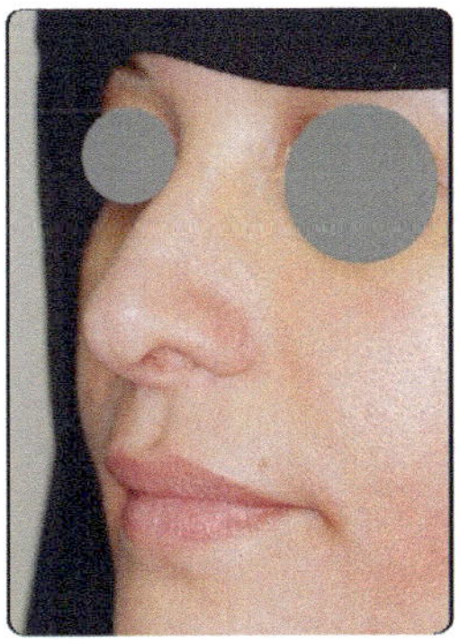

Right Lateral | Left Lateral | Right Lateral Smiling | Left Lateral Smiling

Preoperative

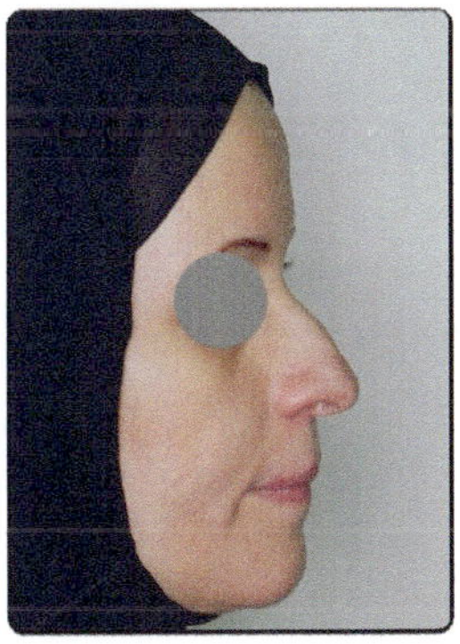
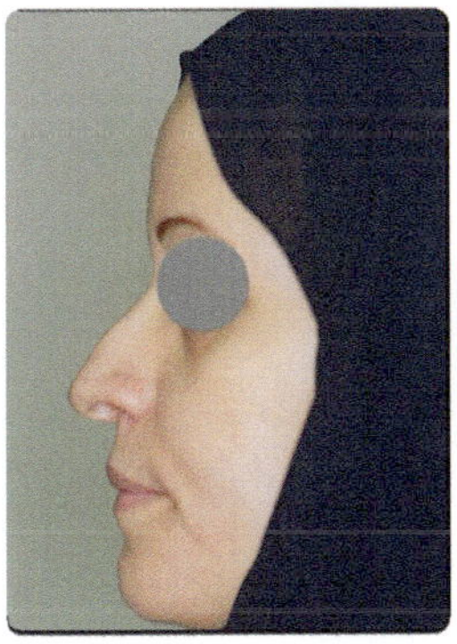
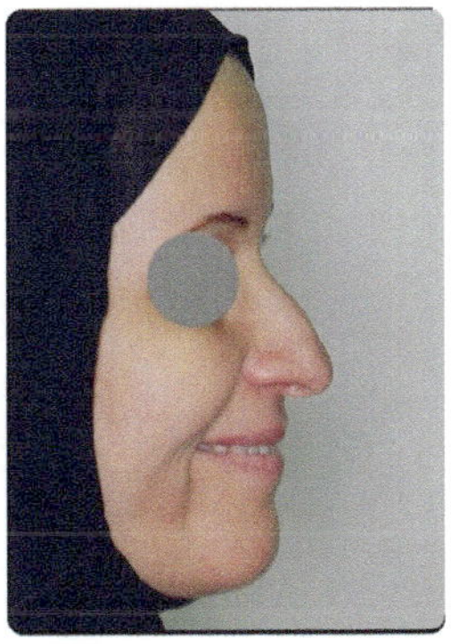
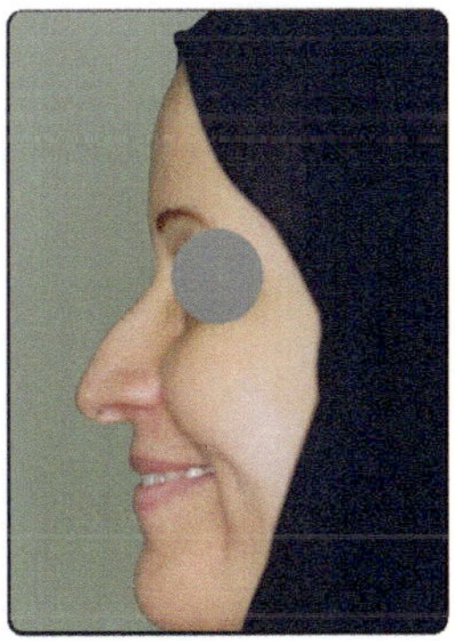

Postoperative

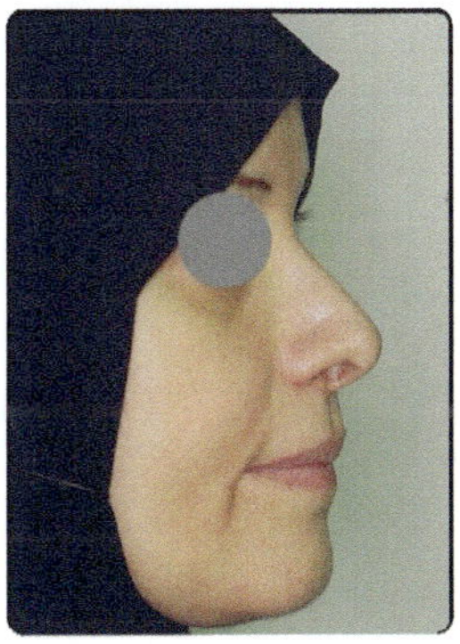
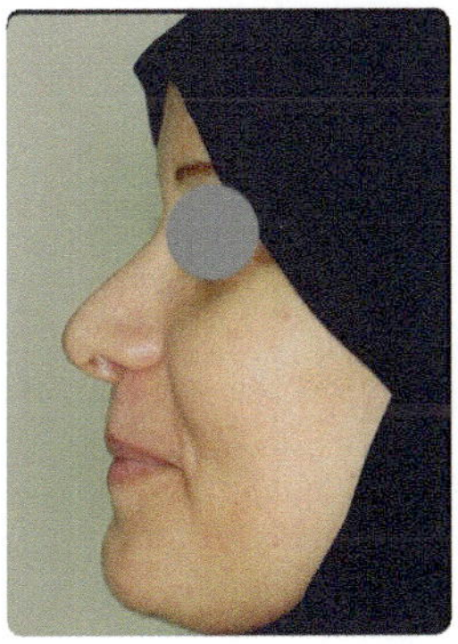
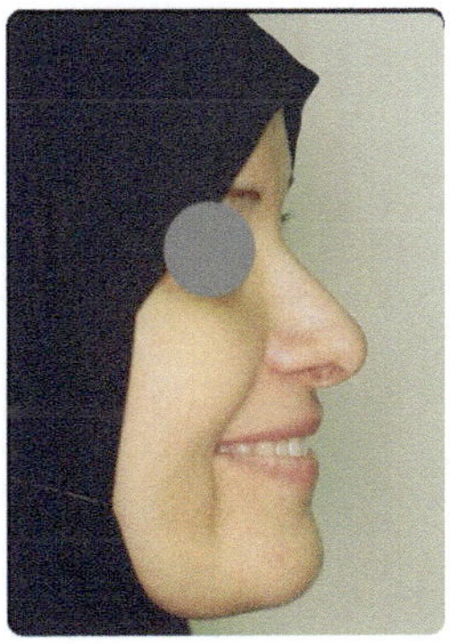
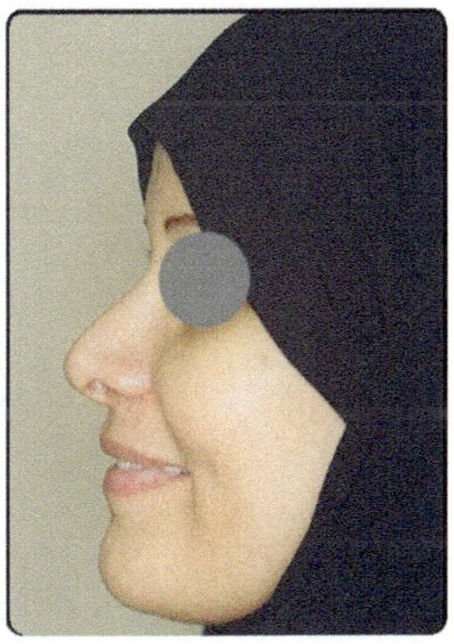

12 Part II: Clinical Case 10

Preoperative Assessment

1. **Frontolateral Walls**
   a. Large and long nose due to large lateral crurae which is, covered with thick irregular skin (Frontal and Lateral Views).
   b. The broad, large size and bulk of the nasal tip overshadowed the ale nasi (Direct Dorsal and Frontal Views).
2. **Media Wall**
   Nil of note.
3. **Boney pyramid**
   a. Osteocartilaginous hump oblique to the right due to bilateral maxillary asymmetry. The left cheek is wide and low while right cheek is narrow and high (backward tilting views).
   b. Wide base of the bony pyramid (Direct Dorsal and Backward Tilting Views).
   c. **Alar base**
   Wide alar base with laterally angulated alae nasi (Basal and Nasal Aperture Views).

Aims of Surgery

a. Overall reduction of the size of the nose.
b. Smoothen the irregularities of the external skin of the anterolateral walls.
c. Reduce the size of alar base. Nasal apertures were thick heavy and wide.

Surgical Plan

1. **Frontolateral Walls**
   a. DDD including the weak triangle to reduce the size and the bulk of the nasal tip and supra tip area.
   b. Bilateral cephalic trim of the lateral crurae to reduce the size of the nasal tip.
2. **Media Wall**
   Nil of note.
3. **Boney pyramid**
   a. Excision of the osteocartilaginous hump.
   b. Osteotomies and medialization of the lateral bony walls.
4. **Alar base**
   Excision of the inferior and posterior segments of the rim sill folds.

Surgical Procedure

As per Surgical Plan.

Post-Operative Analysis

1. **Frontolateral Walls**
   a. Tip definition improved: the tip is slimmer and prominently well identified with thinner overlying skin. The alae nasi come into view and share in nasal aesthetics (Frontal, Direct Dorsal, Overhead, Backward Tilting and Basal Views).
   b. Tip projection: the nasal tip at the same level of the nasal dorsum with good aesthetic angle. This is coupled with good aesthetic nasolabial angle (lateral and oblique views).
   c. Tip light reflex is seen as one spot off the nasal tip. (Frontal and Backward Tilting Views).
2. **Medial Wall**
   Nil of Note.
3. **Bony Pyramid**
   a. Bony pyramid aesthetics improved: the nasal dorsum is straight and the sidewalls are smooth and narrow (all views except the Basal Views).
   b. Dorsal light reflex is seen as an uninterrupted line off the nasal dorsum (Direct Dorsal Views).
4. **Alar Base**
   a. The superior alar grooves now clear off fat, become deeper, longer and visible (Direct Dorsal, Oblique and Lateral Views).

M. H. A. Shafy, *Atlas of Clinical Cases in Rhinoplasty*,
https://doi.org/10.1007/978-3-031-07504-9_12

b. Posterior alar groove aesthetics improved by defatting as well as excising the posterior segments of the rim-sill folds. The flat tire appearance is no longer present. (Backward Tilting, Basal and Nasal Aperture Views).
c. Alae nasi aesthetics improved. They are pulled medially become better seen, smaller and share in nasal aesthetics. (Nasal Aperture, Oblique and Lateral Views).
d. Nasal aperture aesthetics improved after defatting and excision of the rim-sill folds:
   i. The size of the nasal openings is smaller. (Backward Tilting, Basal and Nasal Aperture views).
   ii. The shapes of nasal opening become elegantly oval. Flat tire appearance is gone. (Backward Tilting, Basal and Nasal Aperture views).
e. Marginal light reflexes are clearly seen at:
   i. Inferior alar margins (Nasal Aperture Views).
   ii. Nasal sill bands (Oblique Views).
   iii. Lateral crural prominences (Lateral Views).

Commentary

a. Irregularities of the skin and cartridges of the frontal lateral walls become smooth as a result of the two step defatting of the middle and lateral crurae.
b. As well as the improvement in his nose, his teeth became white and shining after removing cigarette staining from them. (frontal smiling views).

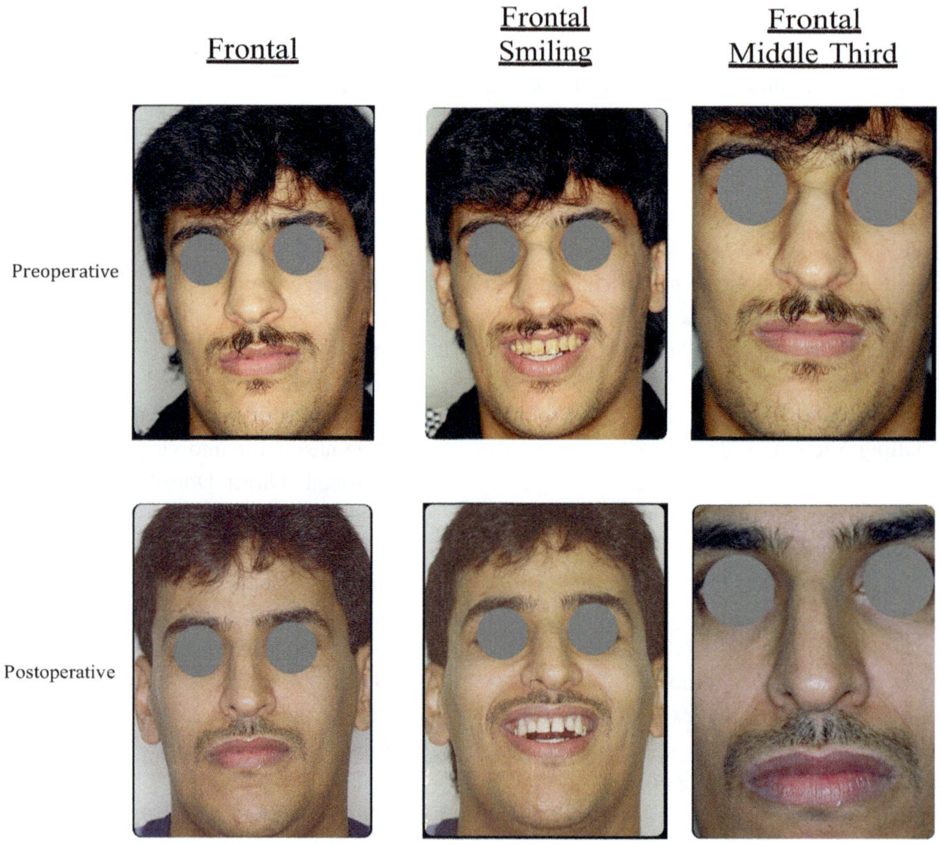

Direct Dorsal | Direct Dorsal Smiling

Preoperative

Postoperative

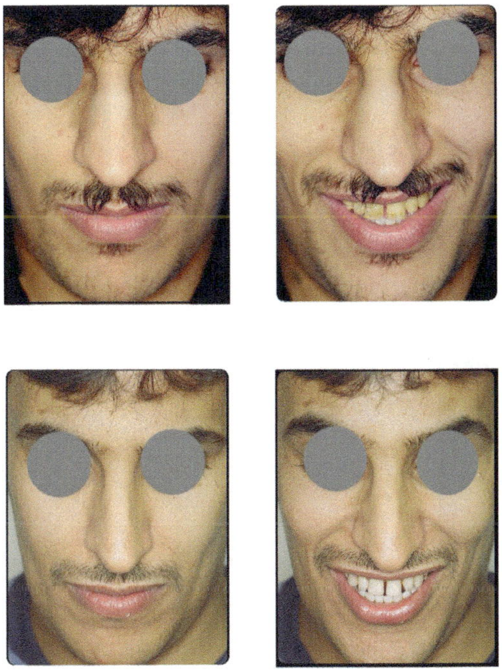

Backward Tilting | Steeper Backward Tilting | Basal | Basal Smiling

Preoperative

Postoperative

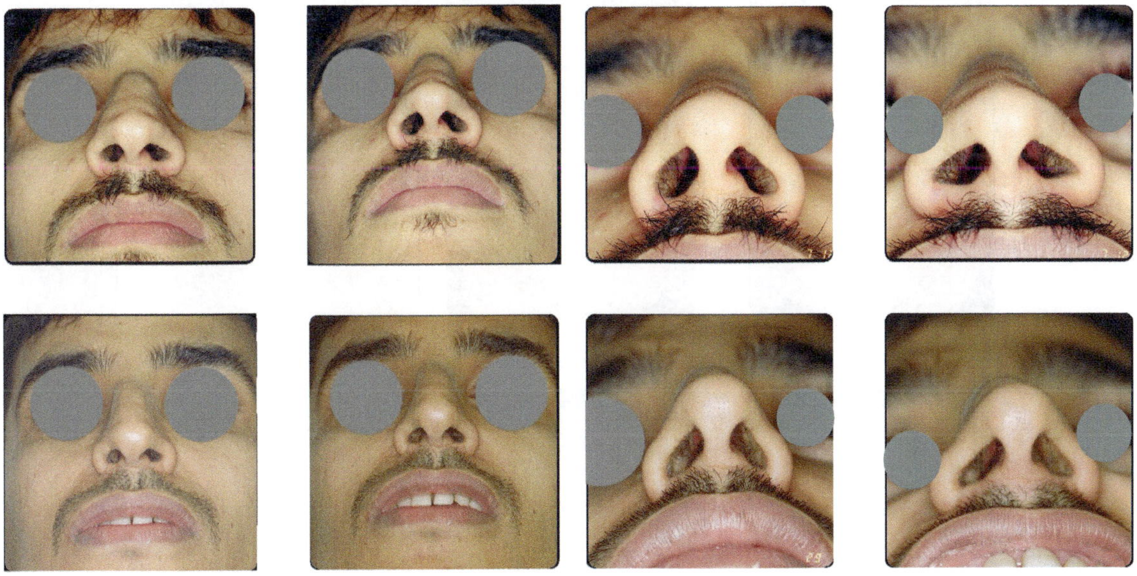

Right Nasal Aperture | Right Nasal Aperture Rim Sill Test | Left Nasal Aperture Rim Sill Test | Left Nasal Aperture

Preoperative

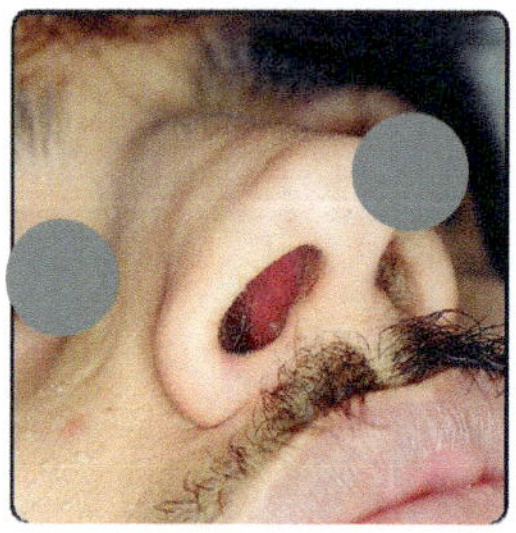
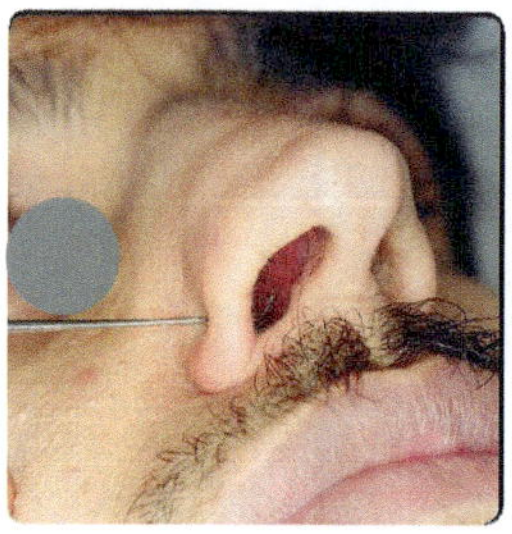
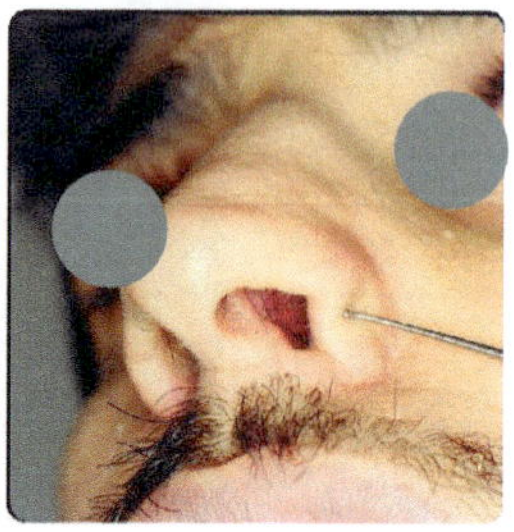
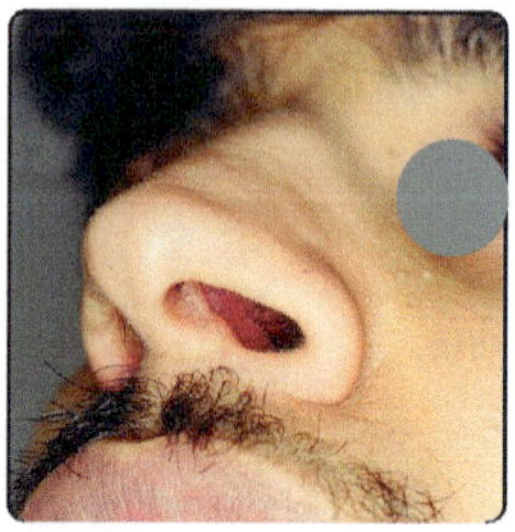

Postoperative

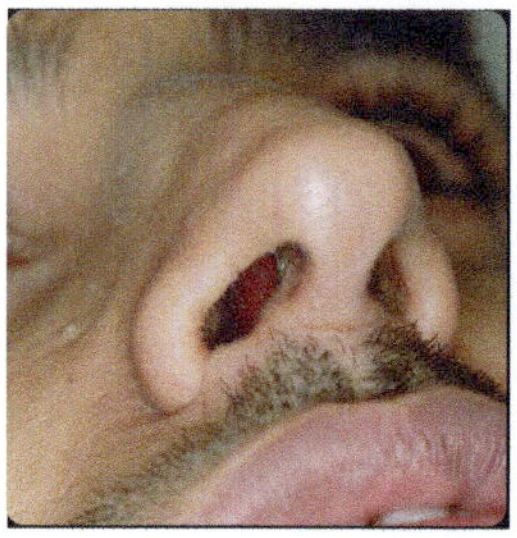
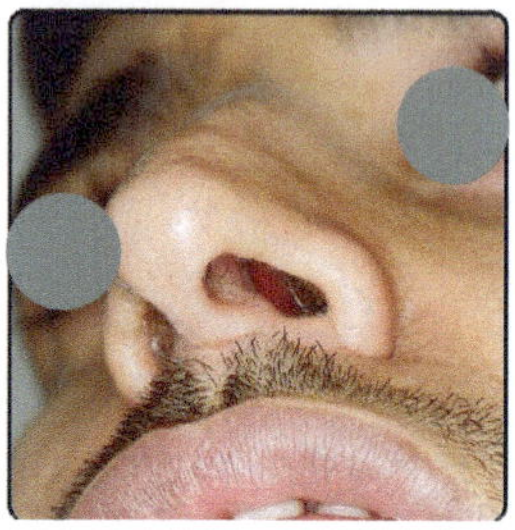

Right Oblique Mid Cheek Full Face | Left Oblique Mid Cheek Full Face | Right Oblique Mid Cheek Middle Third | Left Oblique Mid Cheek Middle Third

Preoperative

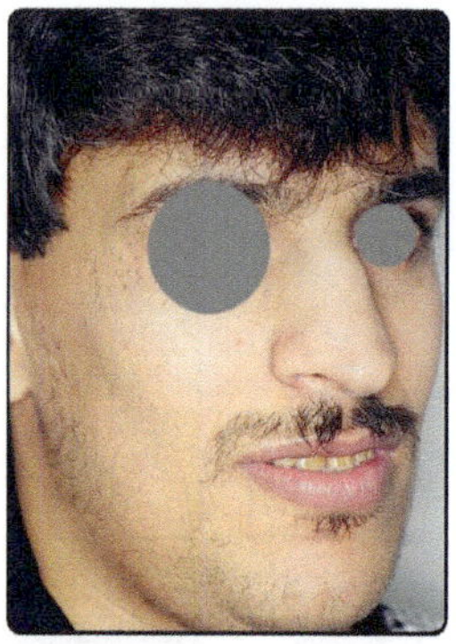
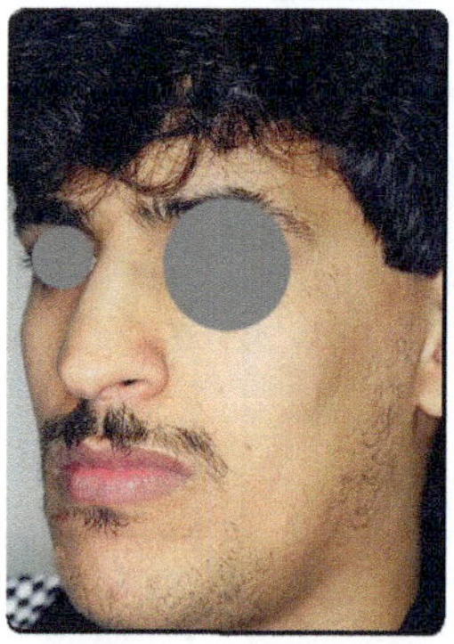
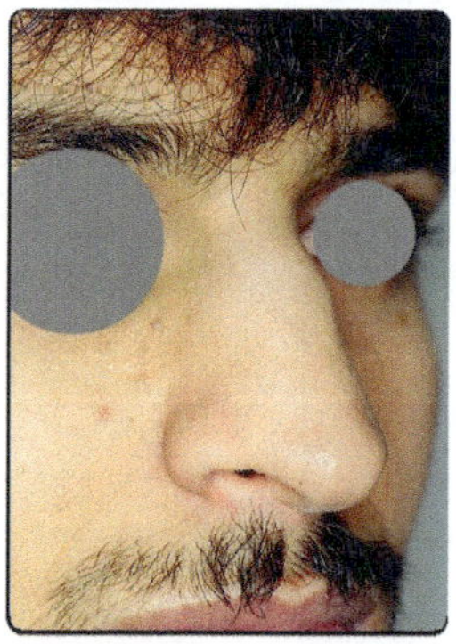
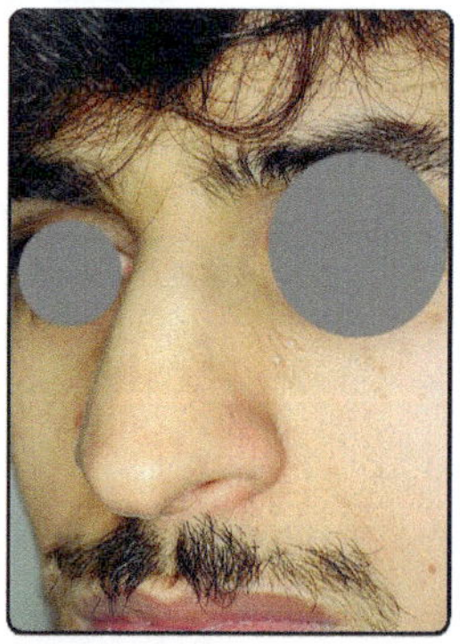

Postoperative

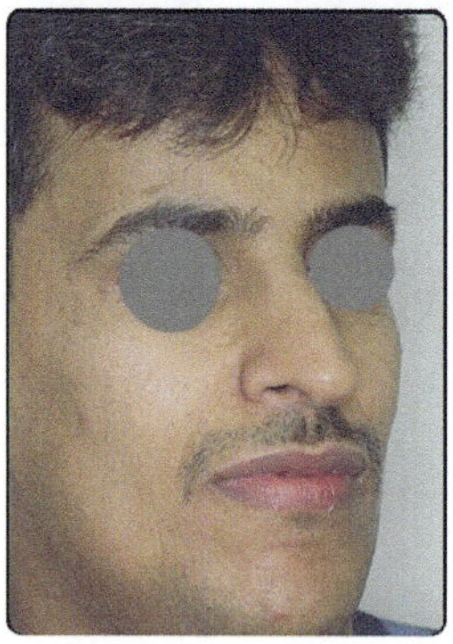
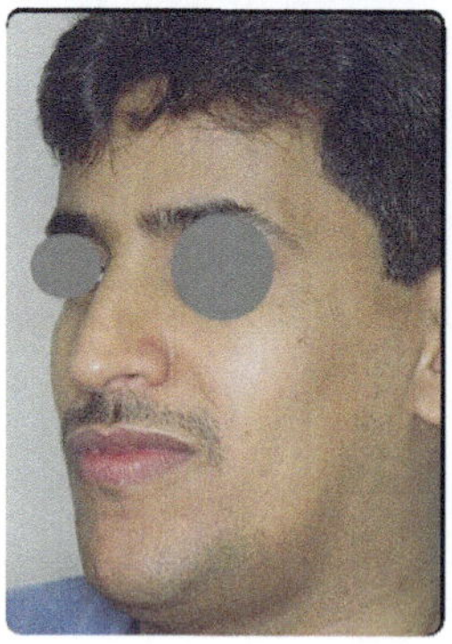
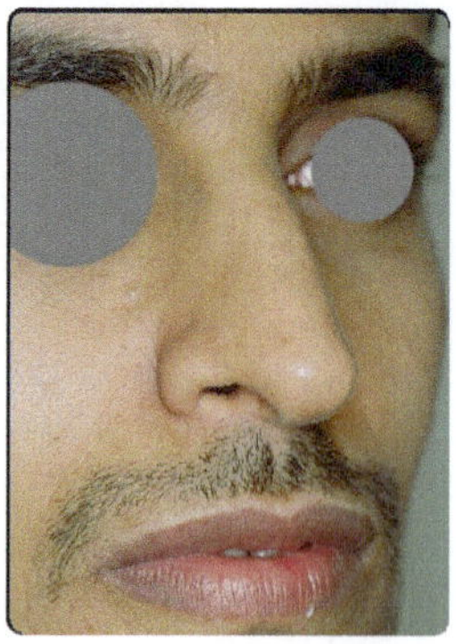
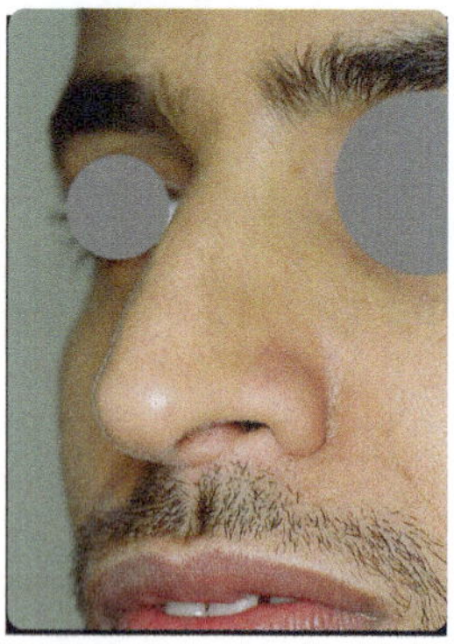

Right Oblique Cheek Margin Full Face | Left Oblique Cheek Margin Full Face | Right Oblique Cheek Margin Middle Third | Left Oblique Cheek Margin Middle Third

Preoperative

Postoperative

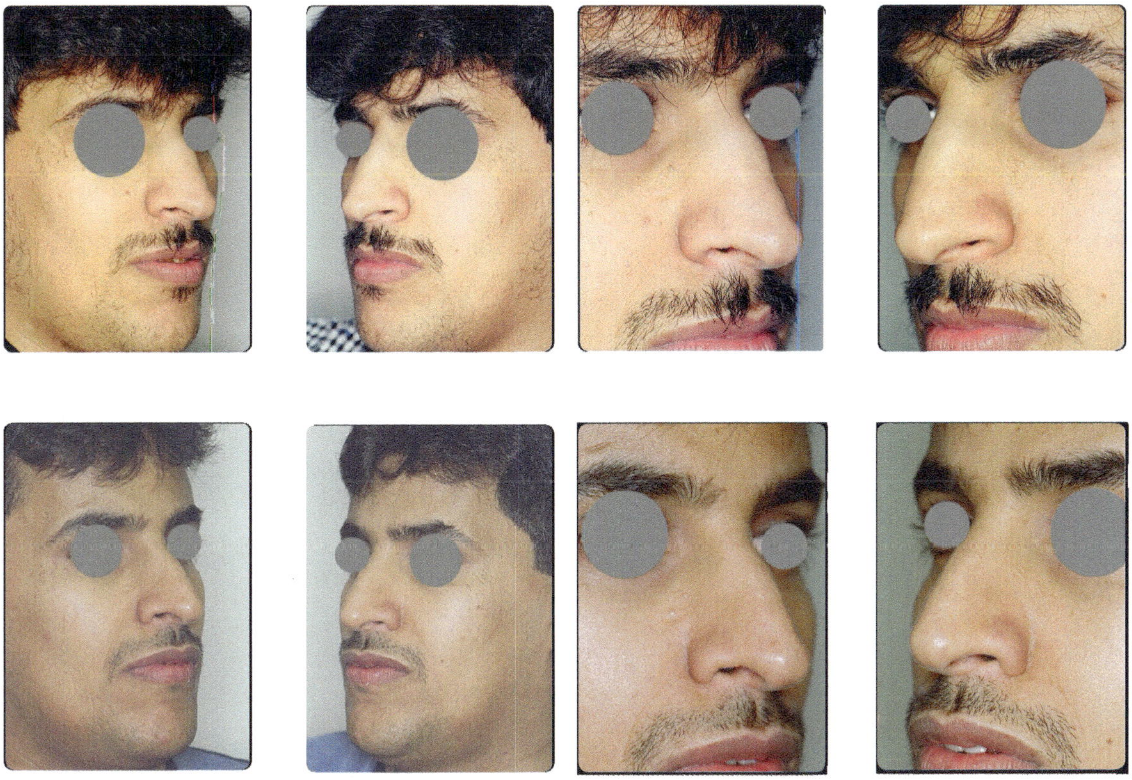

Right Lateral | Left Lateral | Right Lateral Middle Third | Left Lateral Middle Third

Preoperative

Postoperative

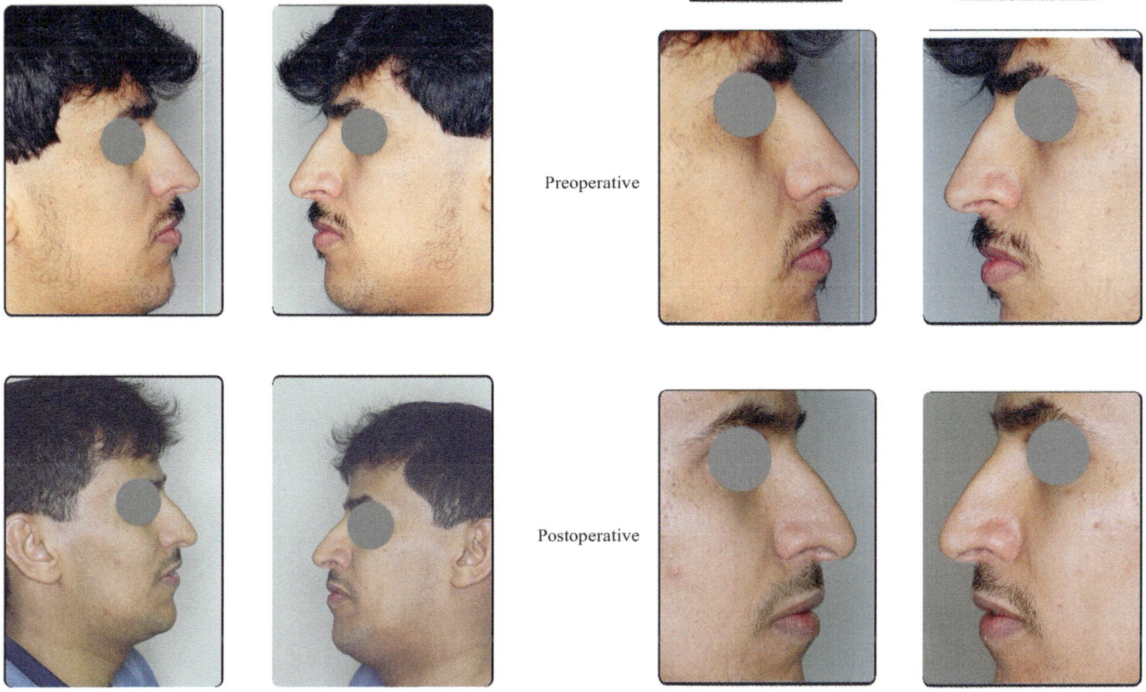

Part II: Clinical Case 11

13

Preoperative Assessment

1. **Frontolateral walls**
   Large thick frontolateral walls over shadowing the alae nasi (Frontal, Direct Dorsal and Overhead Views).
2. **Medial Wall**
   a. Right caudal septal deviation (Basal and Right Nasal Aperture Views).
   b. Mobile tip i.e. the nasal tip moves inferiorly on smiling (Lateral Smiling Views).
3. **Boney pyramid**
   a. Wide base of bony pyramid (Direct Dorsal and Backward Tilting Views).
   b. Osteocartilaginous hump which is oblique, but not deviated, to the right due to bilateral maxillary asymmetry. The right cheek is wide and low and the left cheek is narrow and high. (Backward Tilting Views).
   c. The light reflex of the nasal dorsum is absent (Direct Dorsal Views).
4. **Alar base**
   a. Wide nasal apertures due to long inferior segments of the rim-sill folds.
   b. Unequal alae nasi. The right ala is larger (Frontal, Direct Dorsal and Backward Tilting Views).
   c. A symmetrical smile: The left nasolabial fold is deeper than the right (Frontal Smiling View).

Aims of Surgery

1. Reduction of the overall size and bulk of the nose.
2. Abolish the mobile tip.
3. Reduction of the size of the bony pyramid and excision of the hump.
4. Reduction of the size of nasal apertures.

Surgical Plan

1. **Frontolateral walls**
   a. DDD Including the weak triangle to reduce the size and bulk of the nasal tip and supra tip area.
   b. Cephalic trim of lateral crurae to reduce the size.
2. **Nasal Septum**
   a. Septoplasty.
   b. Division of the depressor septi muscles.
3. **Boney pyramid**
   a. Excision of the osteocartilaginous hump.
   b. Osteotomies with Kassanjean maneuver to the left side i.e. cross fracture of the bony pyramid. (see Surgery of Bony Pyramid on the Text).
4. **Alar base**
   Excision of the inferior and posterior segments of the rim-sill folds.

Surgical Procedure

As per Surgical Plan.

Post-Operative Analysis

1. **Frontolateral Walls**
   a. Tip definition improved i.e. the tip is slimmer and prominently well identified. The alae nasi come into view to share in nasal aesthetics (Frontal, Direct Dorsal, Overhead, Backward Tilting and Basal Views).
   b. Tip projection: the nasal tip is at the same level of the nasal dorsum with good aesthetic angle. This is coupled with good aesthetic nasolabial angle (lateral and oblique views).

M. H. A. Shafy, *Atlas of Clinical Cases in Rhinoplasty*,
https://doi.org/10.1007/978-3-031-07504-9_13

c. Tip light reflex is seen as one spot off the nasal tip. (Frontal and Backward Tilting Views).

2. **Medial Walls**
   Mobility of the tip was overcome and abolished.
3. **Bony Pyramid**
   a. Bony pyramid aesthetics improved: the nasal dorsum is straight and the sidewalls are smooth and narrow (all views except the Basal Views).
   b. Dorsal light reflex is seen as a regular one line off the nasal dorsum (Direct Dorsal Views).
4. **Alar Base**
   a. Superior alar groove aesthetics improved by defatting. The grooves become longer and deeper (Oblique, Lateral and Direct Dorsal Views).
   b. Posterior alar groove aesthetics improved by defatting alone: the alae nasi are pulled medially and the angles of the posterior alar grooves with the upper lip become wider. Aesthetics of the alae nasi improve as they become clearly seen. (Backward Tilting and Nasal Aperture Views).
   c. Nasal aperture aesthetics:
      i. The size of the nasal openings are reduced by defatting as well as excising the inferior segments of the rim-sill folds. (Backward Tilting, Basal and Nasal Aperture views).
      ii. The shape of nasal openings improved. Defatting and excision of the rim-sill folds transformed the nasal apertures from thick walled wide and rounded openings with transverse long axes to thin walled small oval openings with anterior long axes. (Backward Tilting, Basal and Nasal Aperture views).
   d. The left ala nasi is developmentally smaller than the right one. Most cases of apparently different sizes of alae nasi, become closer in size and aesthetically acceptable after defatting. Unfortunely that was not the case in this lady's condition.
   e. Marginal light reflexes are clearly seen at:
      i. Inferior alar margins (Nasal Aperture Views).
      ii. Nasal sill bands (Oblique Views).
      iii. Lateral crural prominences (Lateral Views).

Commentary

a. This lady have had an overall successful surgery. The post-operative photographs are quiet good compared to the preoperative ones. All views are excellent except the frontal views. The frontal views are the most important of all views. They are quite unforgiving views. The unequal alae nasi almost always equalize after the defatting process. Unfortunately, it did not take place in this case and the difference was only noticeable postoperatively.
b. She was offered minimal surgery to augment the left ala nasi but she was quite satisfied and did not wish for any further aesthetic enhancement.
c. Patient's satisfaction is quite different from surgeon's satisfaction. Perfection is one of the greatest enemy of the surgeon.

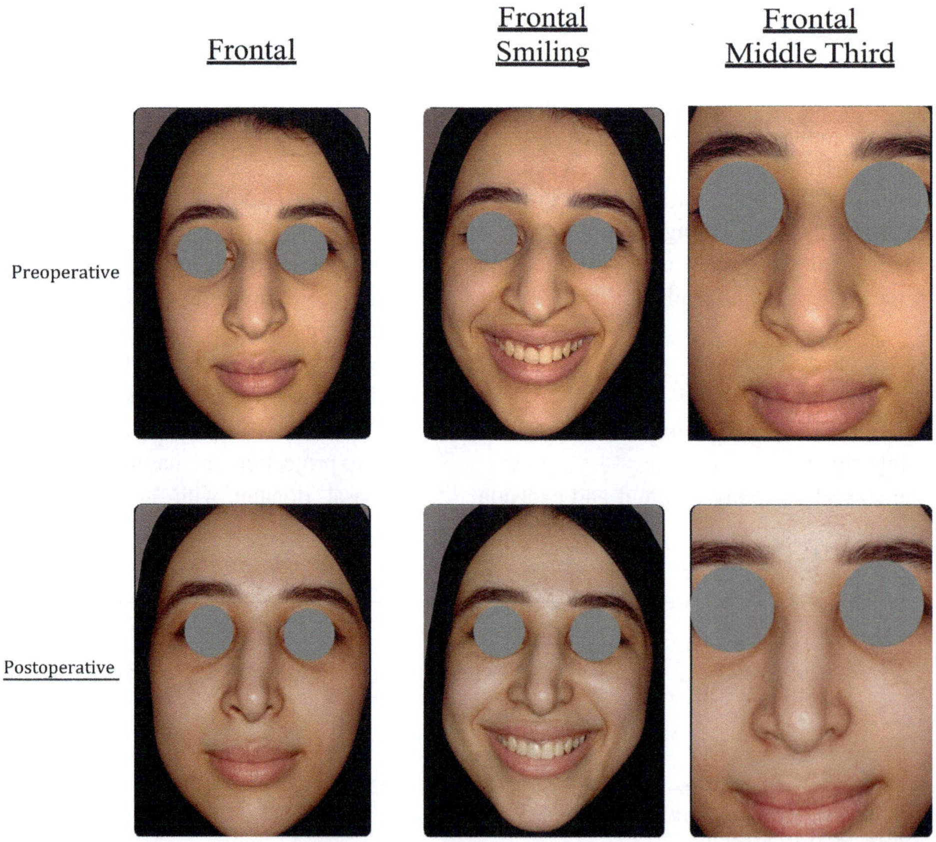

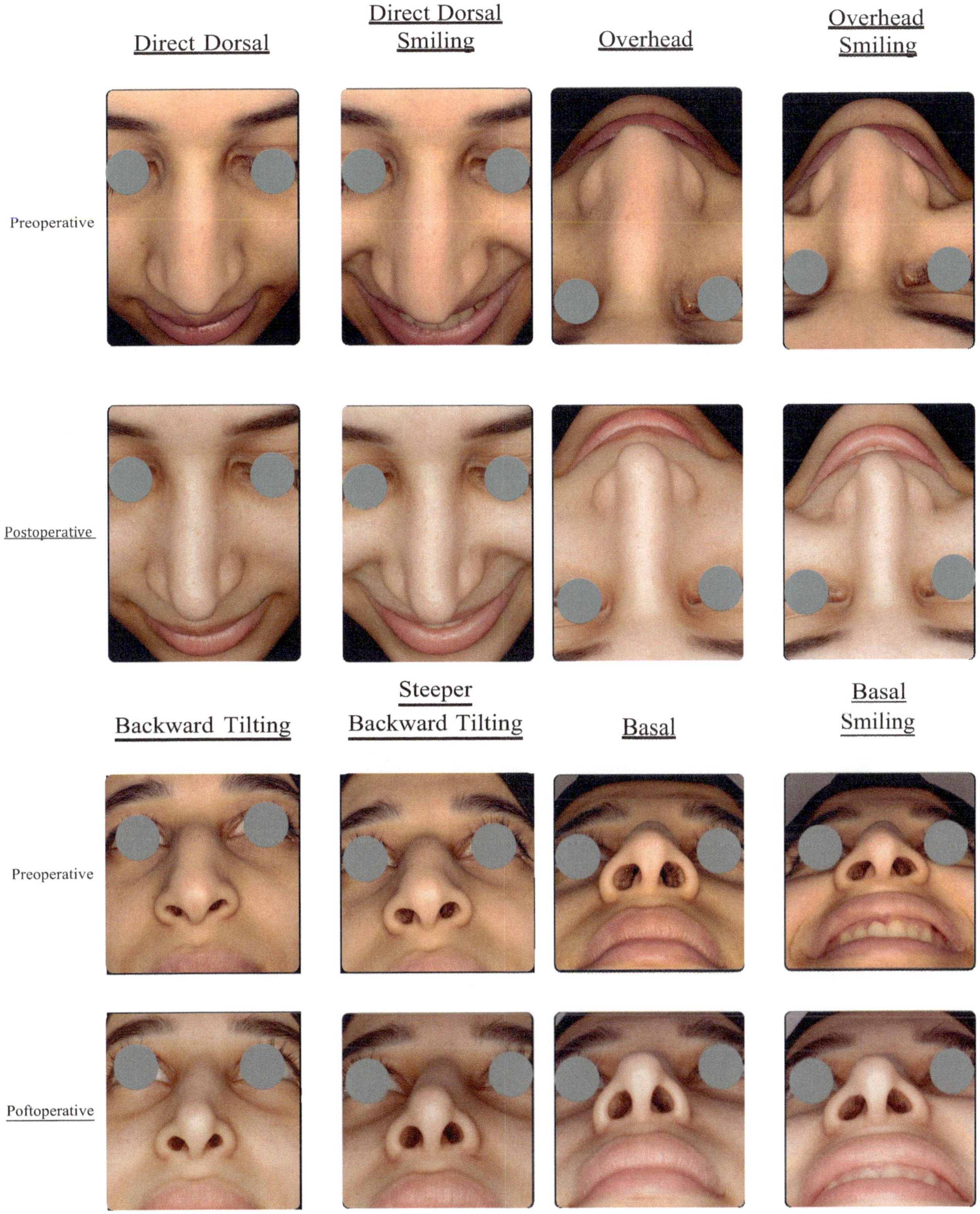
Direct Dorsal
Direct Dorsal Smiling
Overhead
Overhead Smiling
Preoperative
Postoperative
Backward Tilting
Steeper Backward Tilting
Basal
Basal Smiling
Preoperative
Poftoperative

	Right Nasal Aperture	Right Nasal Aperture Rim Sill Test	Left Nasal Aperture Rim Sill Test	Left Nasal Aperture
Preoperative				
Poftoperative				

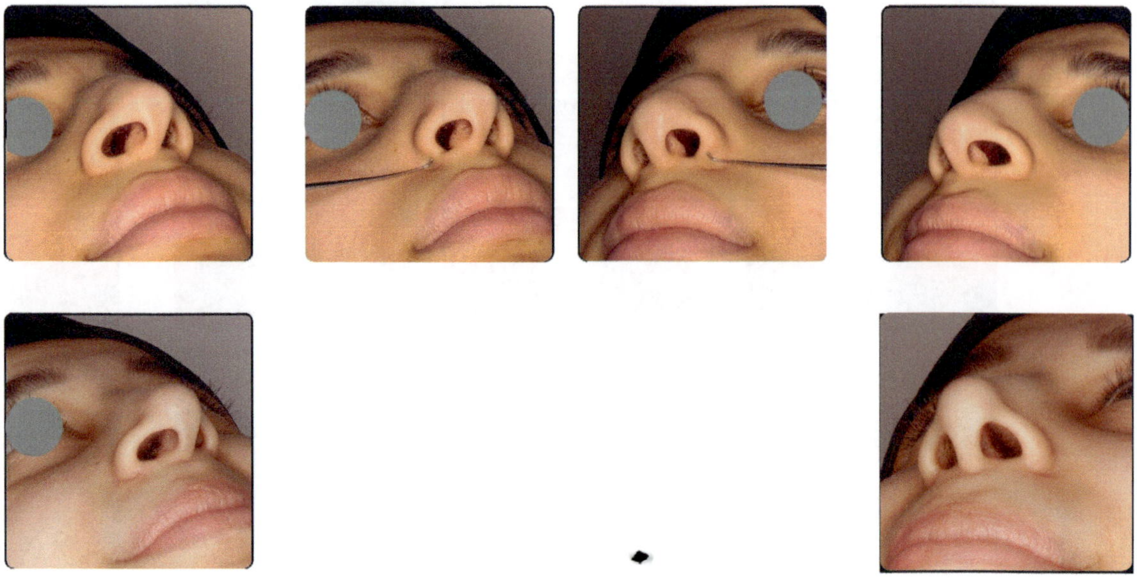

	Right Oblique Mid Cheek Full Face	Left Oblique Mid Cheek Full Face	Right Oblique Mid Cheek Middle Third	Left Oblique Mid Cheek Middle Third
Preoperative				
Poftoperative				

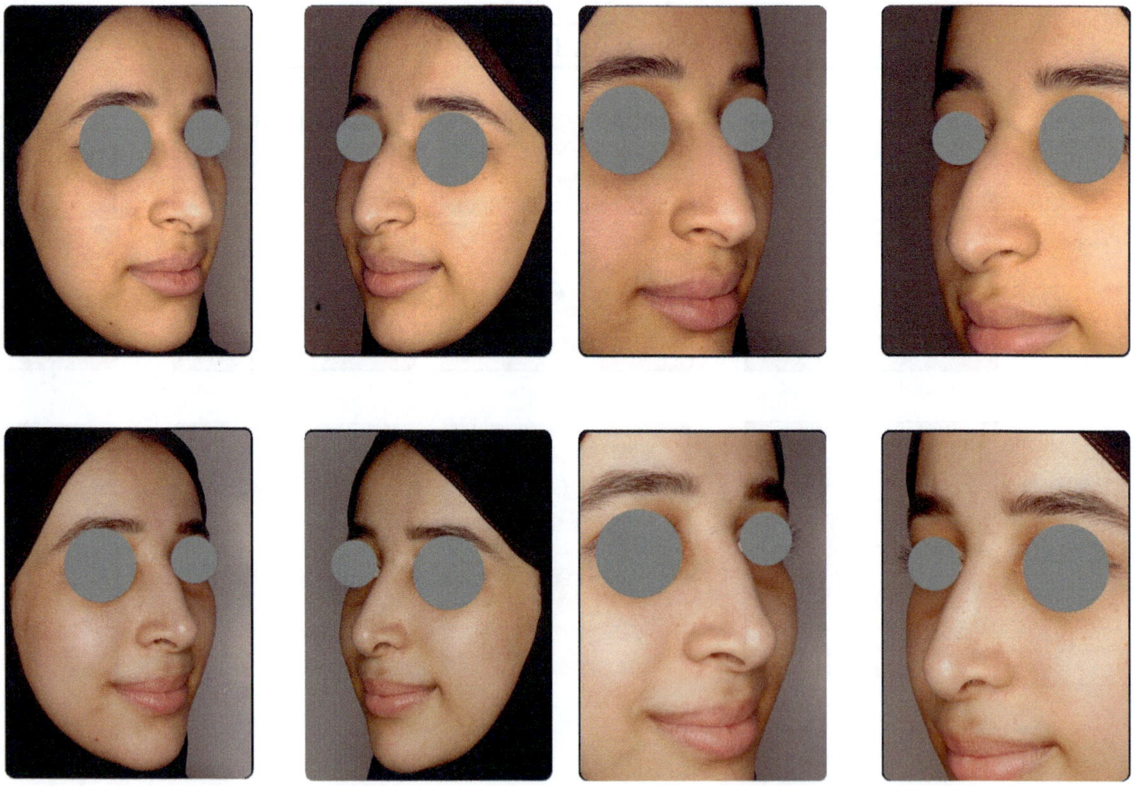

Right Oblique Cheek Margin Full Face | Left Oblique Cheek Margin Full Face | Right Oblique Cheek Margin Middle Third | Left Oblique Cheek Margin Middle Third

Preoperative

Poftoperative

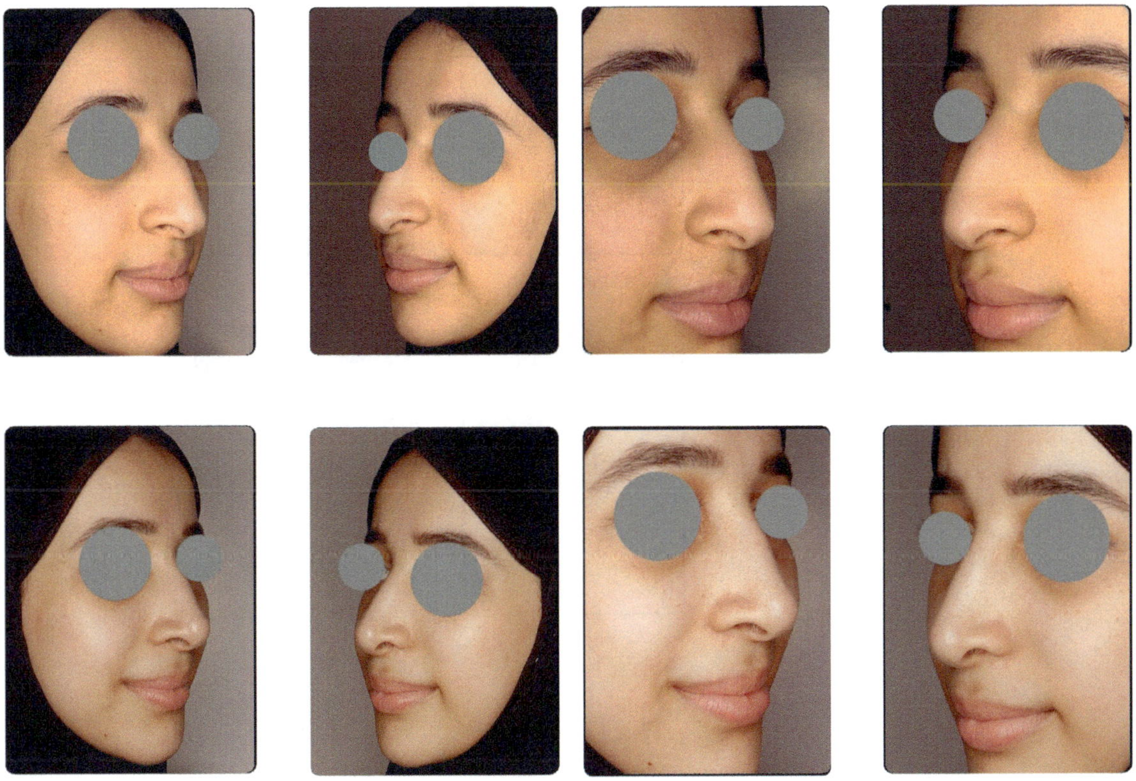

Right Lateral | Left Lateral | Right Lateral Smiling | Left Lateral Smiling

Preoperative

Poftoperative

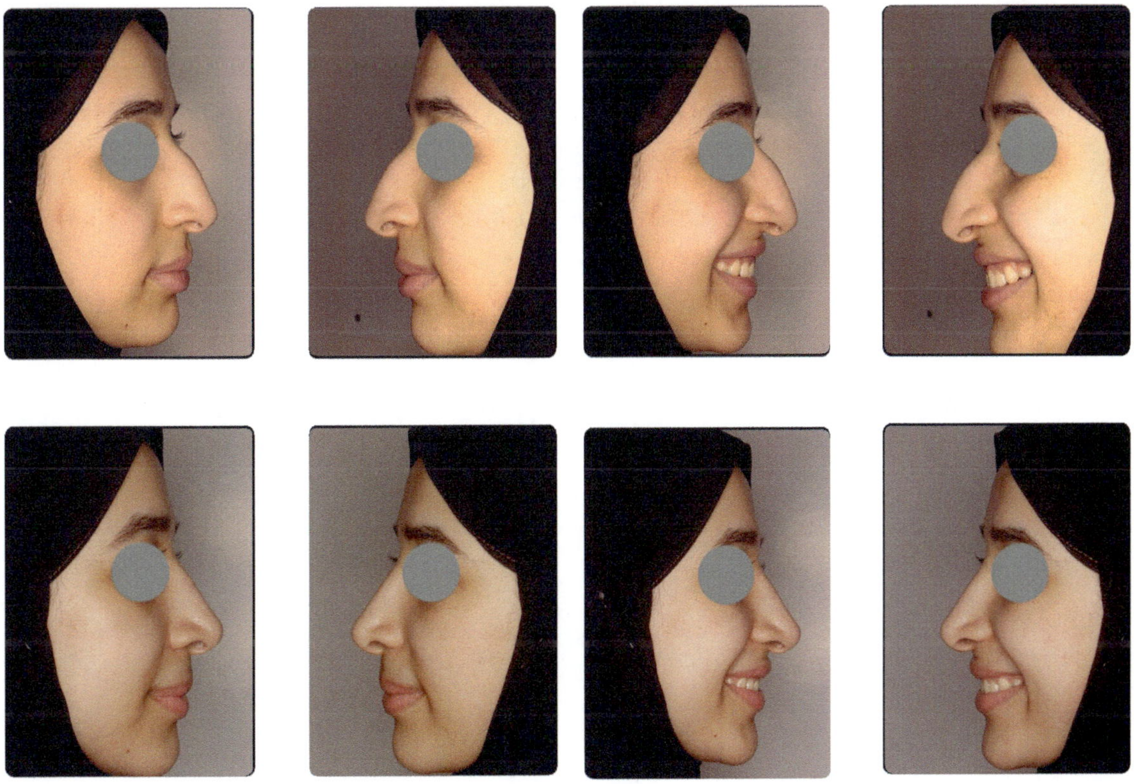

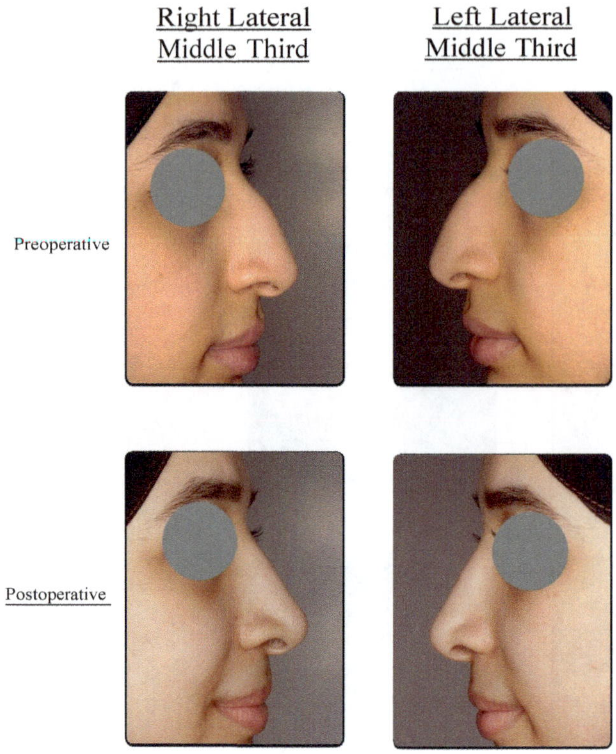
Right Lateral
Middle Third
Left Lateral
Middle Third
Preoperative
Postoperative

14 Part II: Clinical Case 12

Preoperative Assessment

1. **Frontolateral walls**
   a. Large and bulky nasal tip which was completely overshadowing the alae nasi (Frontal, Direct Dorsal and Backward Tilting Views).
   b. The nasal tip is deviated to the right side as a compensatory mechanism to the left deviation of the osteocartilaginous pyramid (Frontal Direct Dorsal and Backward Tilting Views).
2. **Medial Wall**
   Nil of note.
3. **Bony pyramid**
   a. Osteocartilaginous hump that is oblique and deviated to the left side due to bilateral maxillary symmetry. The left cheek is wide and low while the right cheek is narrow and high (Frontal, Direct Dorsal, and Backward Tilting Views). The nasal tip is counter deviated to the right.
   b. Wide base of bony pyramid (Frontal, Direct Dorsal and Backward Tilting Views).
4. **Alar base**
   Wide nasal openings due to long inferior segments of the rim sill folds.

Aims of Surgery

1. Reduce the size and the bulk of the frontolateral walls.
2. To centralize and reduce the size of the bony pyramid.
3. Excision of the nasal hump.
4. Reduction of the size of nasal openings.

Surgical Plan

1. **Frontolateral walls**
   a. DDD including the weak triangle to reduce the size and bulk of the nasal tip.
   b. Cephalic trim of the lateral crurae to reduce the size of the frontolateral walls.
2. **Medial Wall**
   Nil of note.
3. **Bony Pyramid**
   a. Excision of the osteocartilaginous hump down to the level of the anterior septal angle.
   b. Osteotomies and Kassanjean maneuver to the right i.e. cross fracture of the bony pyramid after osteotomies (see Surgery of the Bony Pyramid in Text).
   c. **Alar Base**
   Excision of the inferior segments of the rim sill folds.

Surgical Procedure

As per Surgical Plan.

Post-Operative Analysis

1. **Frontolateral Walls**
   a. Tip definition improved: the tip is slimmer and prominently well identified. The alae nasi come into view to share in nasal aesthetics (Frontal, Direct Dorsal, Overhead, Backward Tilting and Basal Views).
   b. Tip projection: the nasal tip is at the same level of the nasal dorsum with good aesthetic angle. This is coupled with good aesthetic nasolabial angle (lateral and oblique views).
   c. Tip light reflex is seen as one spot off the nasal tip (Frontal and Backward Tilting Views).
2. **Medial Walls**
   Nil of Note.
3. **Bony Pyramid**
   a. Bony pyramid aesthetics improved: the nasal dorsum is straight and the sidewalls are smooth and narrow (all views except the Basal Views).

M. H. A. Shafy, *Atlas of Clinical Cases in Rhinoplasty*,
https://doi.org/10.1007/978-3-031-07504-9_14

b. Dorsal light reflex is seen as a regular one line off the nasal dorsum (Direct Dorsal View).

4. **Alar Base**
   a. Superior and posterior alar groove aesthetics improved by defatting. The superior grooves become longer and deeper (Oblique, Lateral and Direct Dorsal grooves). Angles of the posterior alar grooves become wider.
   b. Nasal aperture aesthetics improved by defatting and excision of the inferior segments of the rim sill folds. The nasal openings became smaller oval in shape.
   c. Marginal light reflexes are clearly seen at:
      i. Inferior alar margins (Nasal Aperture Views).
      ii. Nasal sill bands (Oblique Views).
      iii. Lateral crural prominences (Lateral Views).

Commentary

a. This patient maintained her exact features post-operatively as she wished. The nose print is the same.
b. The smaller nose matches the sizes of the eyes, lips and chin.

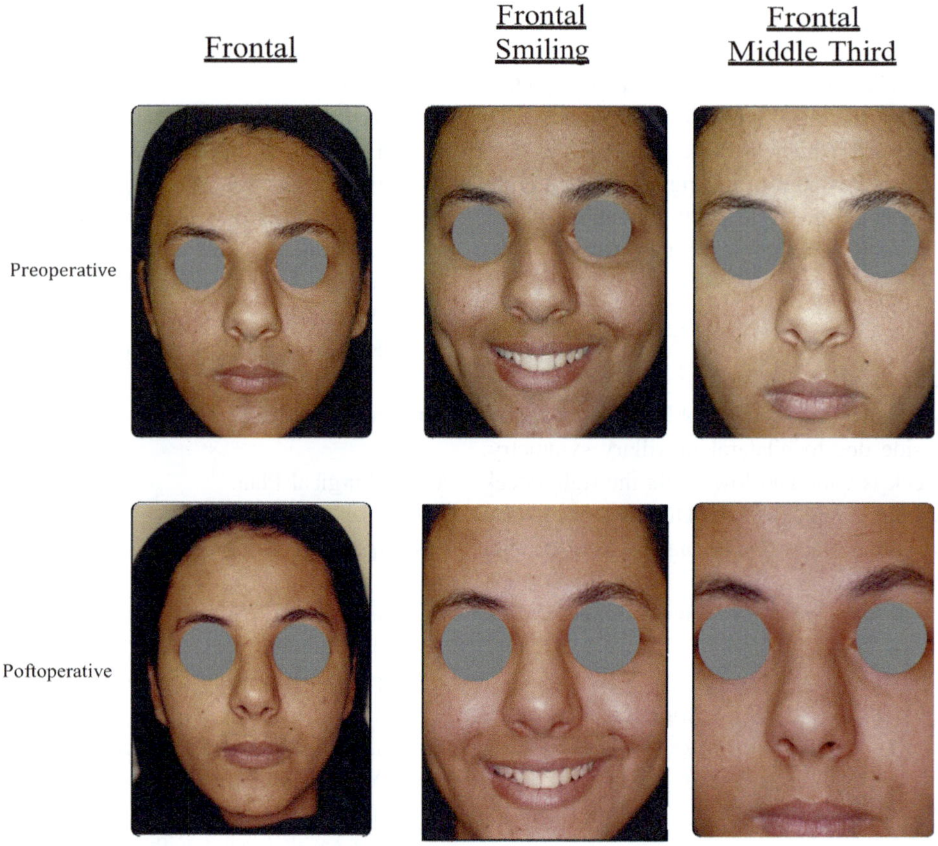

Direct Dorsal

Preoperative

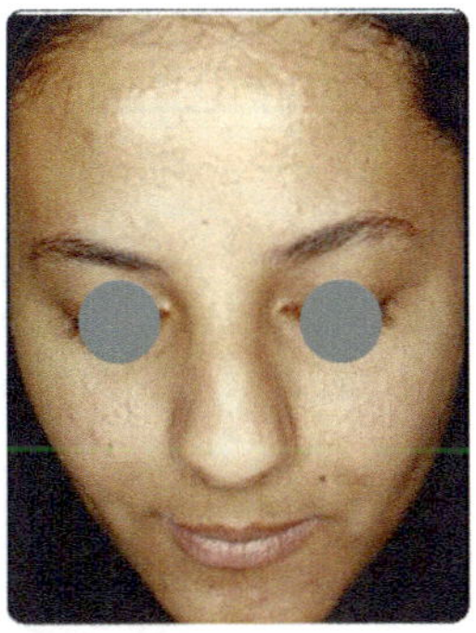

Poftoperative

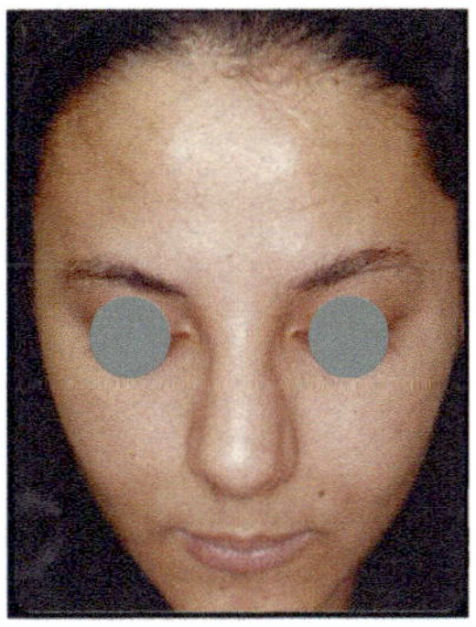

Backward Tilting / Steeper Backward Tilting

Preoperative

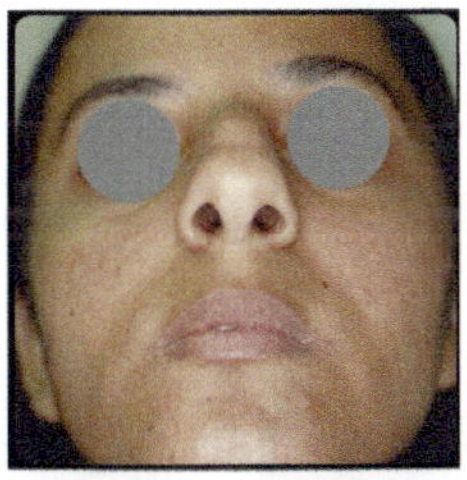

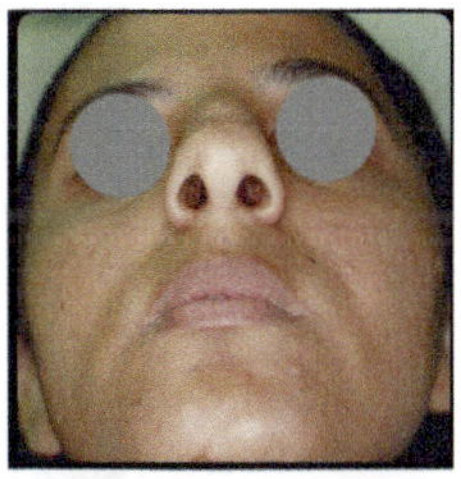

Poftoperative

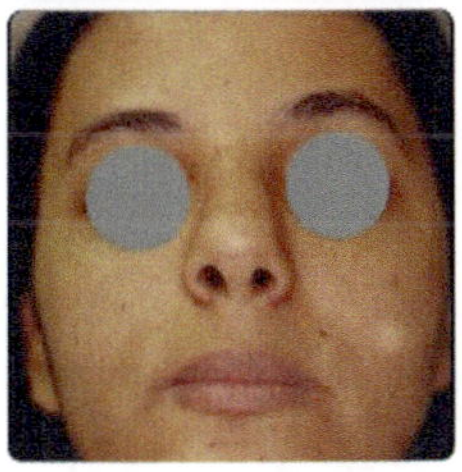

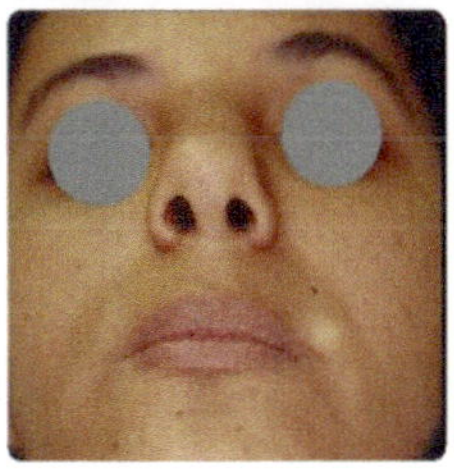

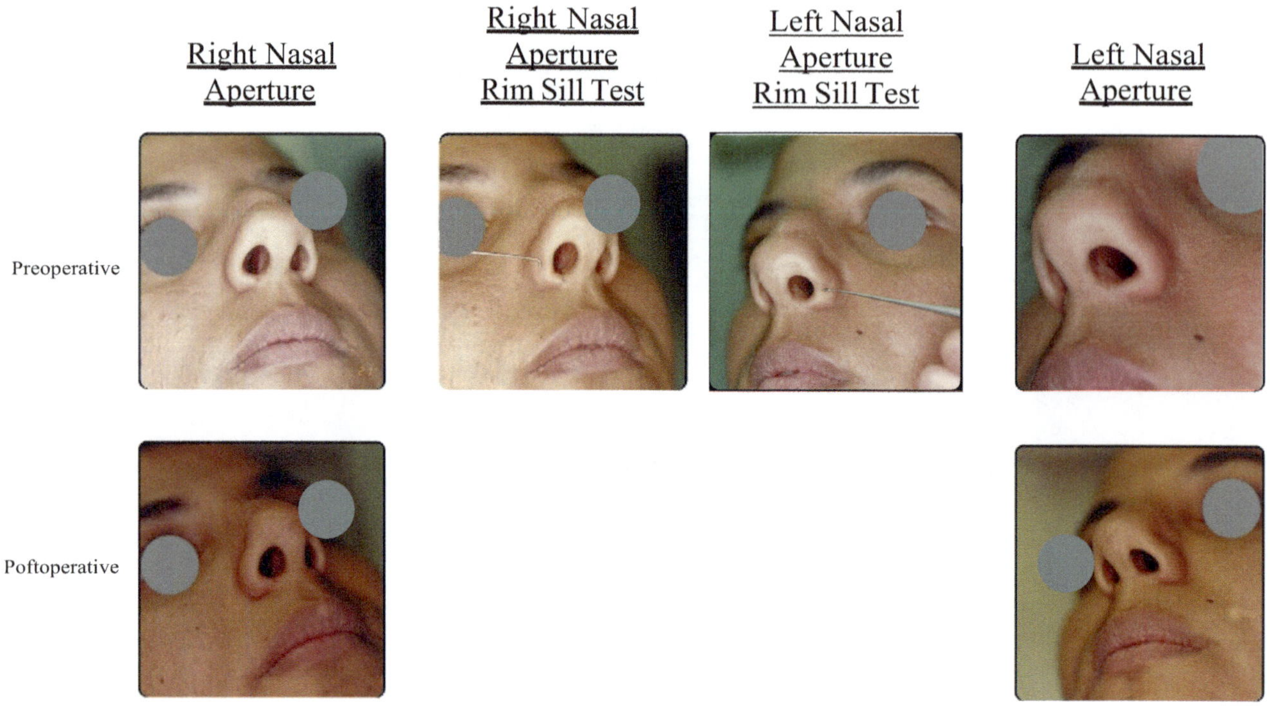
Right Nasal Aperture
Right Nasal Aperture Rim Sill Test
Left Nasal Aperture Rim Sill Test
Left Nasal Aperture
Preoperative
Poftoperative

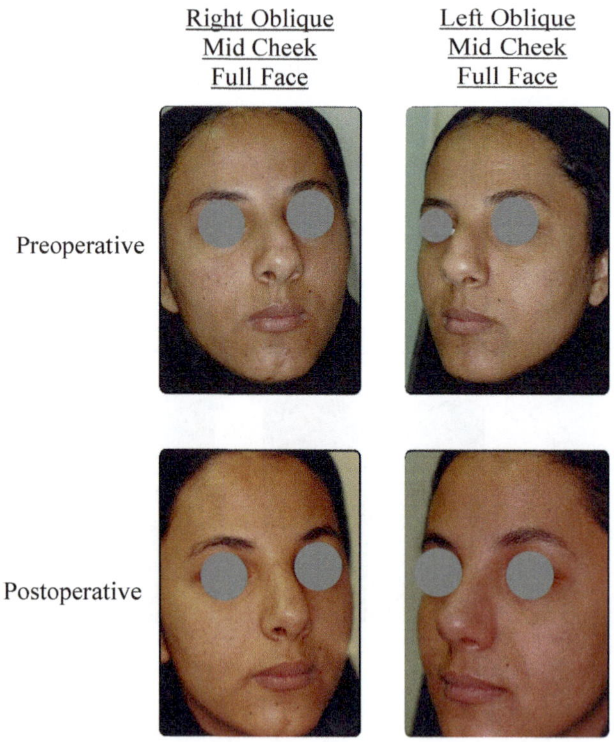
Right Oblique Mid Cheek Full Face
Left Oblique Mid Cheek Full Face
Preoperative
Postoperative

Right Oblique Cheek Margin Full Face | Left Oblique Cheek Margin Full Face | Right Oblique Cheek Margin Middle Third | Left Oblique Cheek Margin Middle Third

Preoperative

Postoperative

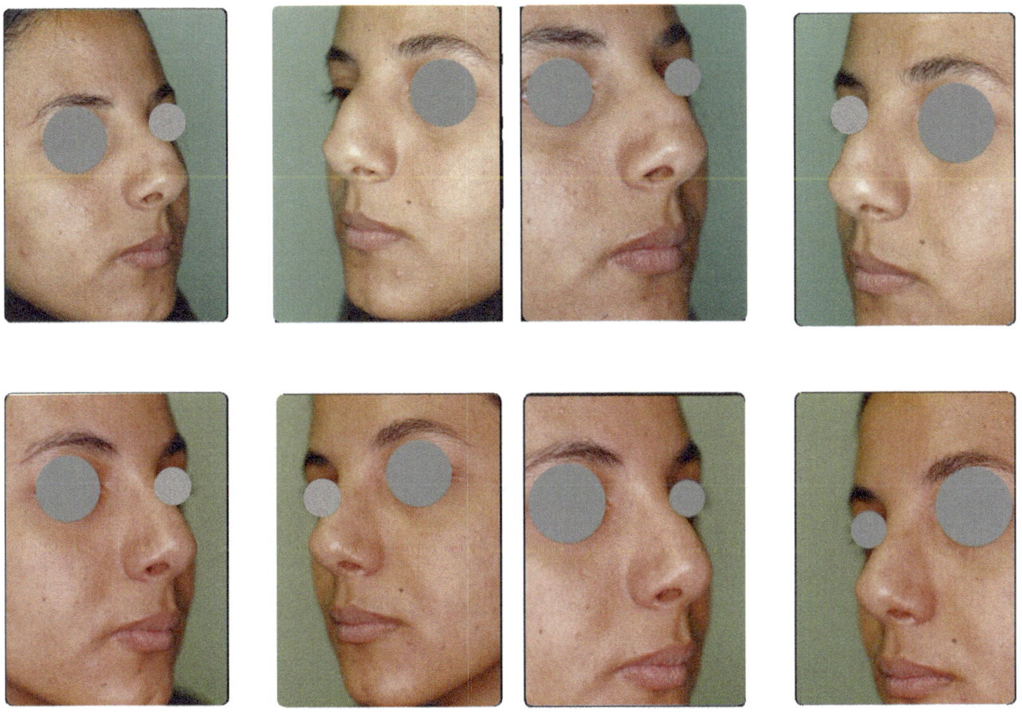

Right Lateral | Left Lateral | Right Lateral Smiling | Left Lateral Smiling

Preoperative

Postoperative

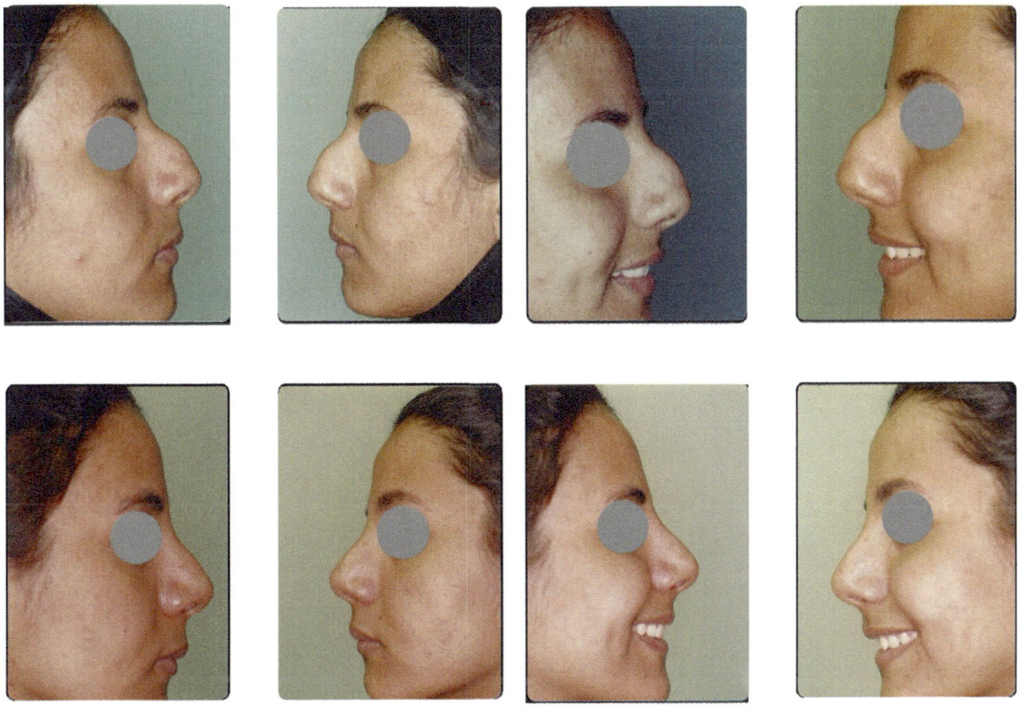

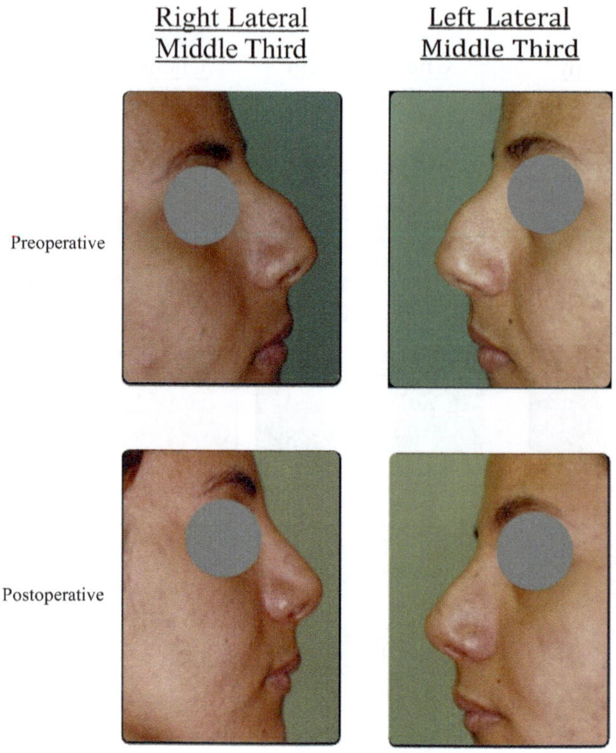
Right Lateral
Middle Third
Left Lateral
Middle Third
Preoperative
Postoperative

Part II: Clinical Case 13

15

Preoperative Assessment

1. **Frontolateral walls**
   a. The frontolateral walls: Large prominent bilobed lateral crurae with deep groove between them (Frontal, Direct Dorsal, Overhead and Backward Tilting Videos). The alae nasi disappeared behind the size and bulk of the alae nasi (Frontal, Direct Dorsal, and Overhead Views).
   b. Nasal tip deviated to the right side. The deviated caudal septum produced a prominent bulge of the right middle and lateral crurae (Backward Tilting Views).
2. **Medial Wall**
   a. Right caudal septal divination (Backward Tilting, Basal, and Right Nasal Apecture Views).
   b. Hanging columella (Right Lateral Views).
   c. Mobile tip (Lateral Smiling Views).
3. **Bony pyramid**
   a. High osteocartilaginous hump that is predominantly cartilaginous. It extended down to the anterior septal angle (Oblique and lateral Views).
   b. The hump is deviated to the right side due to bilateral maxillary asymmetry. The right cheek is wide and low while the left cheek is narrow and high (Backward Tilting Views).
   c. Wide base of the bony pyramid (Direct Dorsal and Backward Tilting Views).
   d. The dorsal light reflex was diffusely absent (preoperative Direct Dorsal Views).
4. **Alar base**
   a. Unequal alae nasi: the right ala nasi is apparently smaller than the left (Frontal and Direct Dorsal Views).
   b. Apparent unequal nasal openings due to right caudal septal deviation (Backward Tilting and Basal Views).

Aims of Surgery

1. Reduce the overall size and bulk of the nose and make its components proportionate to each other.
2. Produce a regular external surface with smooth skin.

Surgical Plan

1. **Frontolateral walls**
   a. DDD including the weak triangle to reduce the size and bulk of the frontolateral walls and supra tip area.
   b. Cephalic trim of the lateral crurae to reduce the size of the frontolateral walls.
2. **Medial Wall**
   a. Septoplasty to correct the caudal deviation.
   b. Correction of the hanging columella.
   c. Transnasal division of the depressor septi muscles.
3. **Bony pyramid**
   a. Excision of the osteocartilaginous hump down to the level of the anterior septal angle.
   b. Osteotomies with Kassanjean maneuver to the left to centralise the deviated bony pyramid i.e. cross fracture of the bony pyramid after osteotomies (see Surgery of the Bony Pyramid in Text).
4. **Alar base**
   Nil of Note.

Surgical Procedure

1. As per Surgical Plan.
2. Trimming of 2 mm of the caudal septum was sufficient to reduce the hanging columella. There was no need for direct surgical interference with the medial crurae.

Post-Operative Analysis

1. **Frontolateral Walls**
   a. Tip definition improved: the tip is slimmer and prominently well identified with smooth, thin overlying skin. The alae nasi come into view to share in nasal aesthetics (Frontal, Direct Dorsal, Overhead, Backward Tilting and Basal Views).
   b. Tip projection: The nasal tip is at the same level of the nasal dorsum with good aesthetic angle. This is

M. H. A. Shafy, *Atlas of Clinical Cases in Rhinoplasty*,
https://doi.org/10.1007/978-3-031-07504-9_15

coupled with good aesthetic nasolabial angle (Lateral and Oblique Views).
   c. Tip light reflex is seen as one spot off the nasal tip (Frontal and Backward Tilting Views).
2. **Medial Walls**
   a. Correction of right septal deviation have reduced the right lateral crural bulge and equalized the sizes of the nasal openings.
   b. Mobile tip is abolished.
   c. Hanging columella disappeared.
3. **Bony Pyramid**
   a. Bony pyramid aesthetics improved: the nasal dorsum is straight and the sidewalls are smooth and narrow (all views except the Basal Views).
   b. The light reflex is seen as a regular one line off the nasal dorsum (Direct Dorsal Views).
4. **Alar Base**
   a. Superior alar groove aesthetics improved by defatting. The grooves become longer and deeper (Oblique, Lateral and Direct Dorsal grooves).
   b. Nasal aperture aesthetics:
      i. The size of both apertures equalized after correction of the septal deviation (Backward Tilting and Basal Views).
      ii. The shapes of the apertures improved after defatting. They become elegantly oval (Backward Tilting, Basal and Nasal Aperture Views).
   c. Marginal light reflexes are clearly seen at:
      i. Inferior alar margins (Nasal Aperture Views).
      ii. Nasal sill bands (Nasal Aperture and Oblique Views).
      iii. Lateral crural prominences (Lateral Views).

Commentary

a. Having a regular external surface and smooth nasal skin was achieved by the combination of accurate resection of the osteocartilaginous hump, septoplasty, and reduction of the bulk of the nose by defatting as well as reducing the size of the front olateral walls by cephalic trimming of the lateral crurae.
b. The nasal tip became one smooth unit with both alae nasi on the sides contributing to nasal aesthetics. Although the alae nasi remain unequal (seen in frontal views only) yet they have no negative nasal aesthetics.

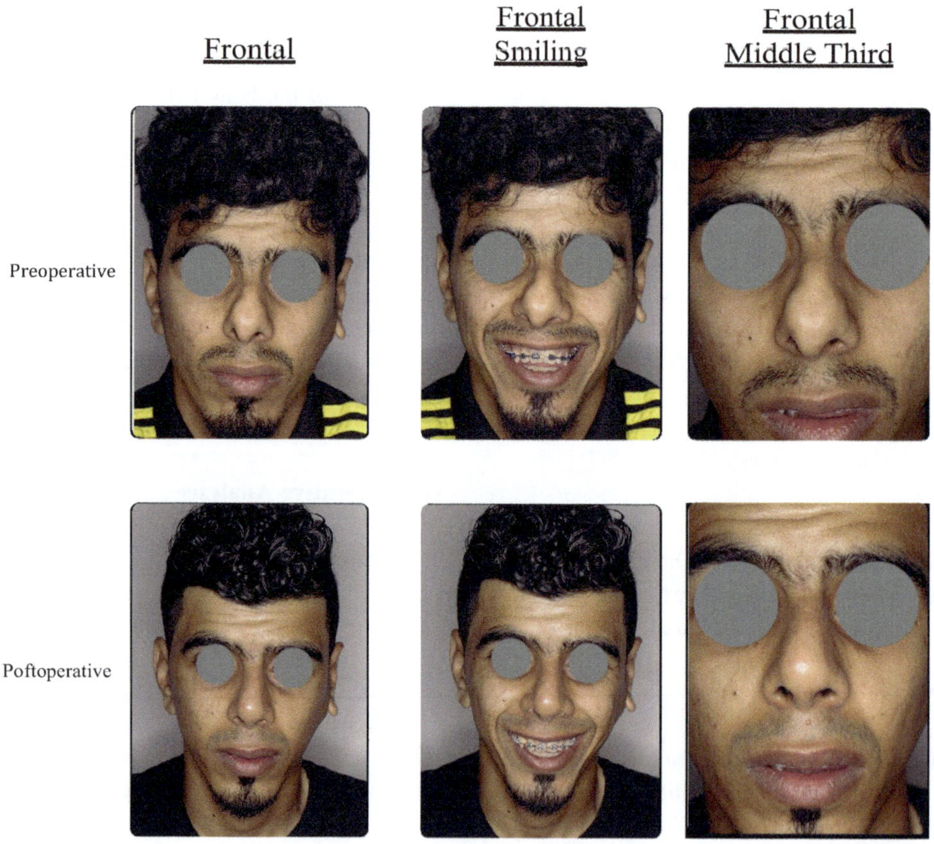

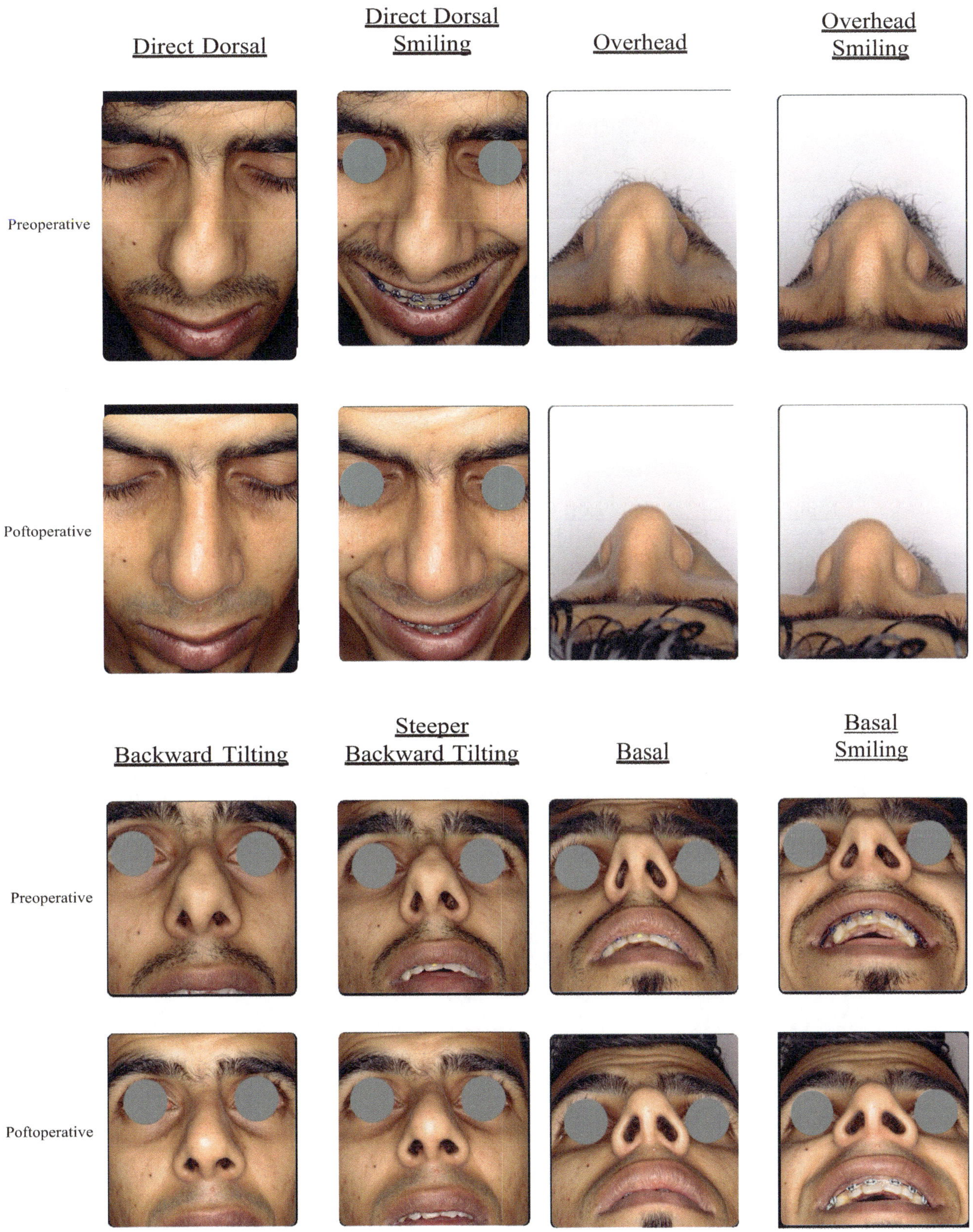
Direct Dorsal
Direct Dorsal Smiling
Overhead
Overhead Smiling
Preoperative
Poftoperative
Backward Tilting
Steeper Backward Tilting
Basal
Basal Smiling
Preoperative
Poftoperative

Right Nasal Aperture | Left Nasal Aperture

Preoperative

Poftoperative

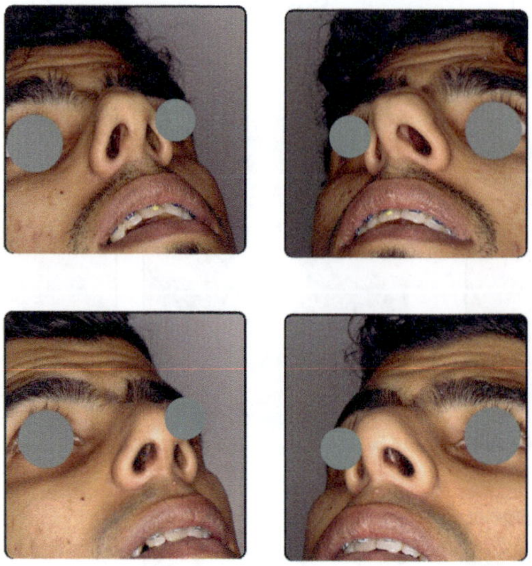

Right Oblique Mid Cheek Full Face | Left Oblique Mid Cheek Full Face | Right Oblique Mid Cheek Middle Third | Left Oblique Mid Cheek Middle Third

Preoperative

Poftoperative

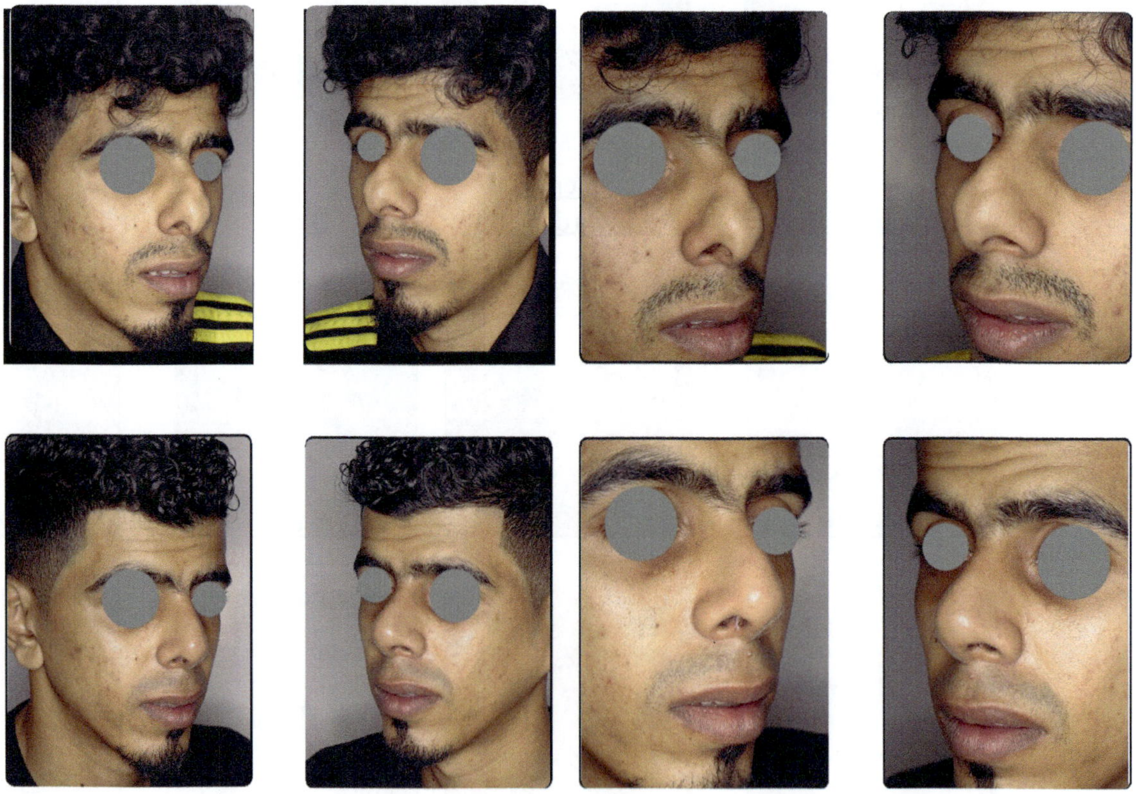

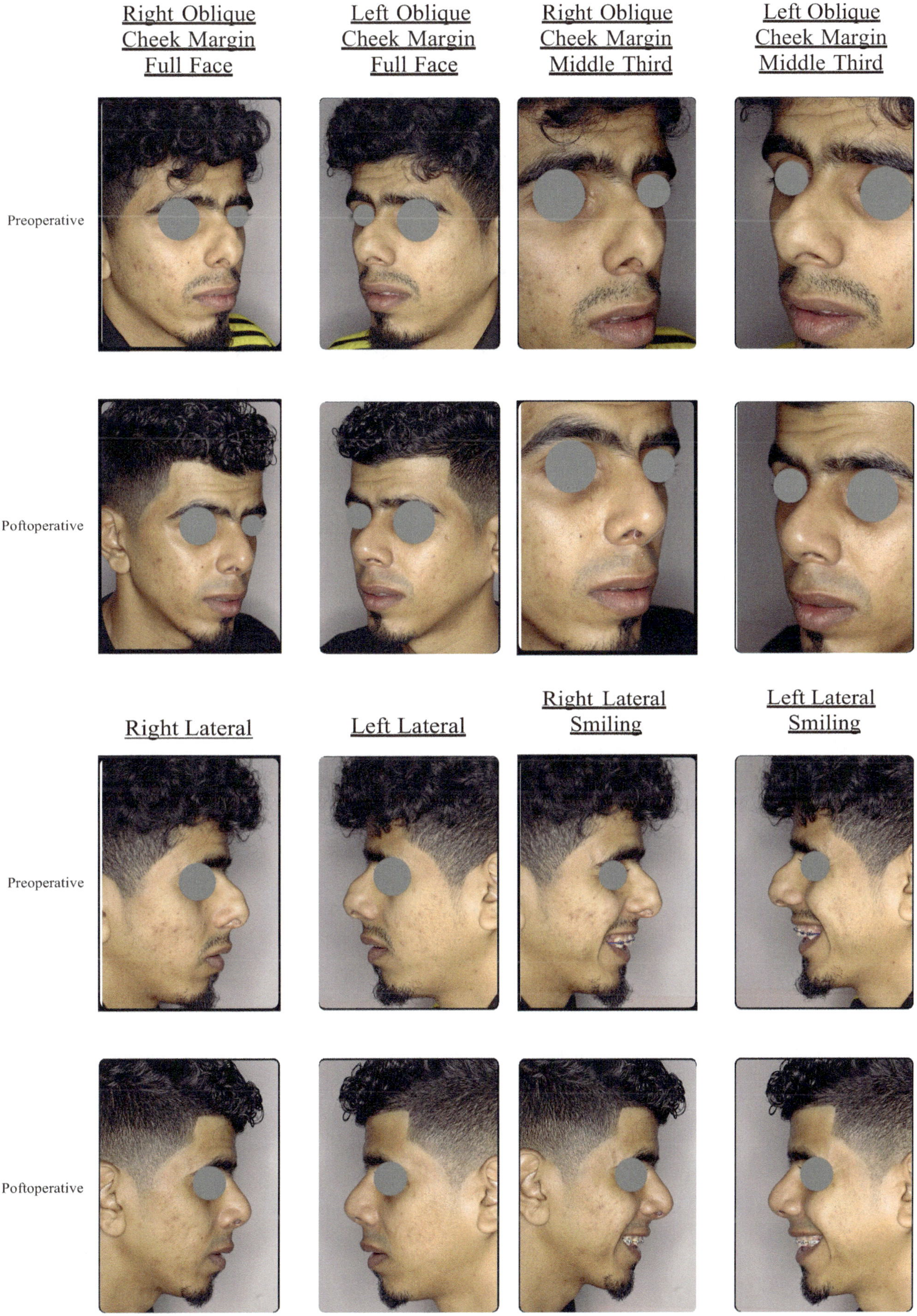
Right Oblique
Cheek Margin
Full Face
Left Oblique
Cheek Margin
Full Face
Right Oblique
Cheek Margin
Middle Third
Left Oblique
Cheek Margin
Middle Third
Preoperative
Poftoperative
Right Lateral
Left Lateral
Right Lateral
Smiling
Left Lateral
Smiling
Preoperative
Poftoperative

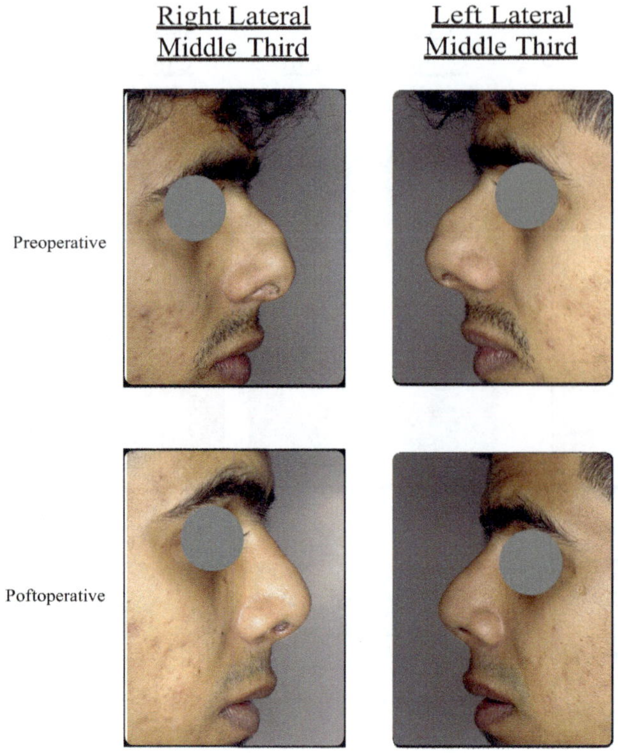
Right Lateral
Middle Third
Left Lateral
Middle Third
Preoperative
Poftoperative

Part III

Bulky Nose Rhinoplasty

16 Part III: Clinical Case 1

Preoperative Assessment

1. **Frontolateral walls**
   a. Bifid tip (Frontal, Direct Dorsal, Overhead, Backward Tilting and basal Views).
   b. Bulky frontolateral walls overshadowing the alae nasi (Frontal and Direct Dorsal Views).
   c. The bifid tip reflects two spots of light reflex (Frontal, Backward Tilting and Basal Views).
2. **Medial Wall**
   a. C-shaped deviation of the nasal septum to right side. The caudal margin is protruding to the left side. (Left Nasal Aperture view).
   b. The right side deviation of the cartilaginous septum caused a protrusion of the right side of the upper lateral cartilage, and a depression on the left side just above the left lateral crus (Left Nasal Aperture, Backward Tilting, Oblique and Overhead Views).
   c. Mobile tip (Lateral Smiling Views).
   d. Left caudal septal deviation (Left Nasal Aperture View).
3. **Bony pyramid**
   a. Wide base of the boney pyramid (Direct Dorsal and Backward Tilting Views).
   b. Osteocartilaginous hump (Backward Tilting, Oblique and Lateral Views).
4. **Alar base**
   Thick walled rounded nasal openings.

Aims of Surgery

a. Reduction of the bulk and bifidity of nasal tip.
b. Abolish mobility of tip.
c. Excision of bony hump and reduction of the size of bony pyramid.

Surgical Plan

1. **Frontolateral walls**
   a. DDD including the weak triangle to reduce the bulk and size of the nasal tip and supra tip area.
   b. Cephalic trim of lateral crurae to reduce the size of the fronto-lateral walls.
   c. Abolish the bifidity.
2. **Medial Wall**
   a. Septoplasty.
   b. Division of the Depressor septi muscles.
3. **Bony pyramid**
   a. Excision of the osteocartilaginous hump.
   b. Osteotomies and medialization of the lateral bony walls to reduce the size of the bony pyramid.
4. **Alar base**
   Nil of note.

Surgical Procedure

a. As per Surgical Plan.
b. The two inferior margins of the medial crurae were stitched together to abolish their bifidity effects.

Post-Operative Analysis

1. **Frontolateral Wall**
   a. Tip definition improved: the tip is slimmer and prominently well identified with thinner and smoother overlying skin. The alae nasi come into view to share in nasal aesthetics (Frontal, Direct Dorsal, Overhead, Backward Tilting and Basal Views).
   b. Tip projection improved (lateral and smiling lateral views) the nasal tip is at the same level as the nasal dorsum.

M. H. A. Shafy, *Atlas of Clinical Cases in Rhinoplasty*,
https://doi.org/10.1007/978-3-031-07504-9_16

c. Tip light reflex: the double light reflex transformed into single spot of light reflex (Frontal, Backward Tilting and Basal Views).

2. **Medial Wall**
   a. Tip mobility abolished (Lateral Views).
   b. The left caudal deviation was corrected.
   c. Correction of the septal deviation immediately balanced the height of the two sides of the upper lateral cartilage, so that the bulge on the right side and the depression on the left side became on the same level.
3. **Bony Pyramid**
   a. Bony pyramid aesthetics: the nasal dorsum is straight and the sidewalls are smooth and narrow (all views except the Basal Views).
   b. Dorsal light reflex is seen as an uninterrupted line off the nasal dorsum (Direct Dorsal Views).
4. **Alar Base**
   a. Superior alar groove aesthetics improved by defatting. The grooves become longer and deeper (Oblique, Lateral and Direct Dorsal grooves).
   b. Posterior alar groove aesthetics improved by defatting. The alae nasi are pulled medially and the angles of the posterior alar groove became wider.
   c. Aesthetics of alae nasi improved by defatting. They are better seen and share elegantly in nasal aesthetics.
   d. Nasal aperture aesthetics improved by defatting alone:
      i. The size of nasal aperture did not change.
      ii. The shapes became more elegantly oval (Backward Tilting, Basal, and Nasal Aperture Views).
   e. Marginal light reflexes are clearly seen at:
      i. Inferior alar margins (Nasal Aperture Views).
      ii. Nasal sill bands (Oblique Views).
      iii. Lateral crural prominences (Lateral Views).

Commentary

There was overall reduction in the size and bulk of the nose while keeping its exact image and nasal print.

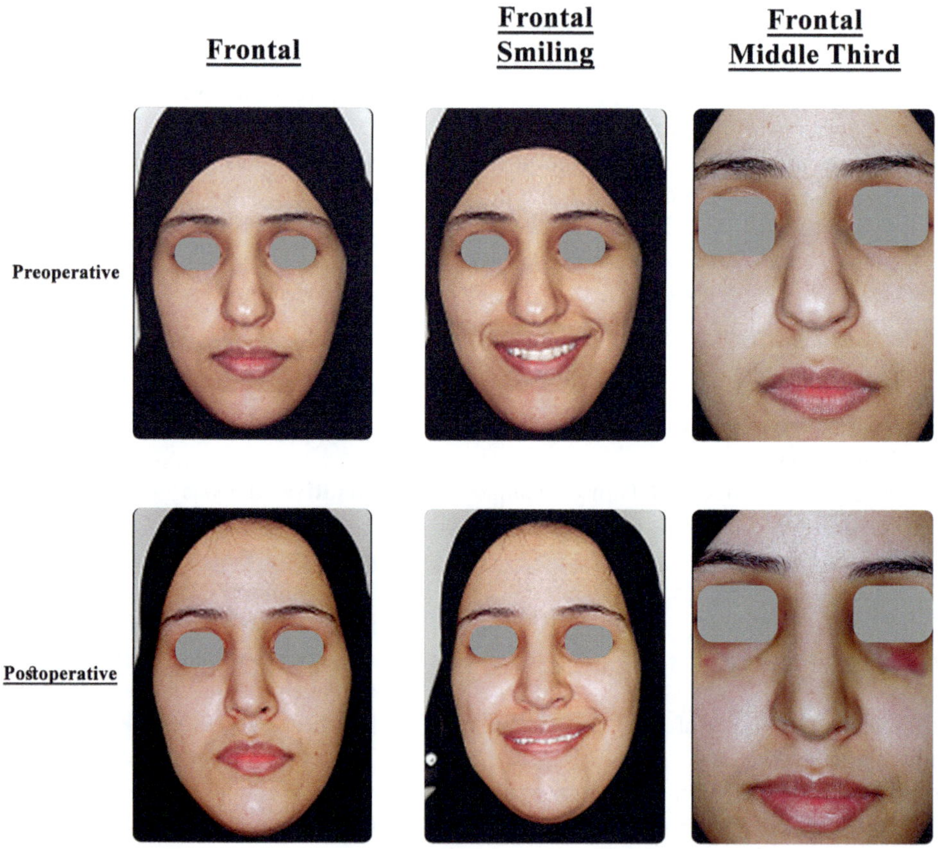

Direct Dorsal **Overhead**

Preoperative

Postoperative

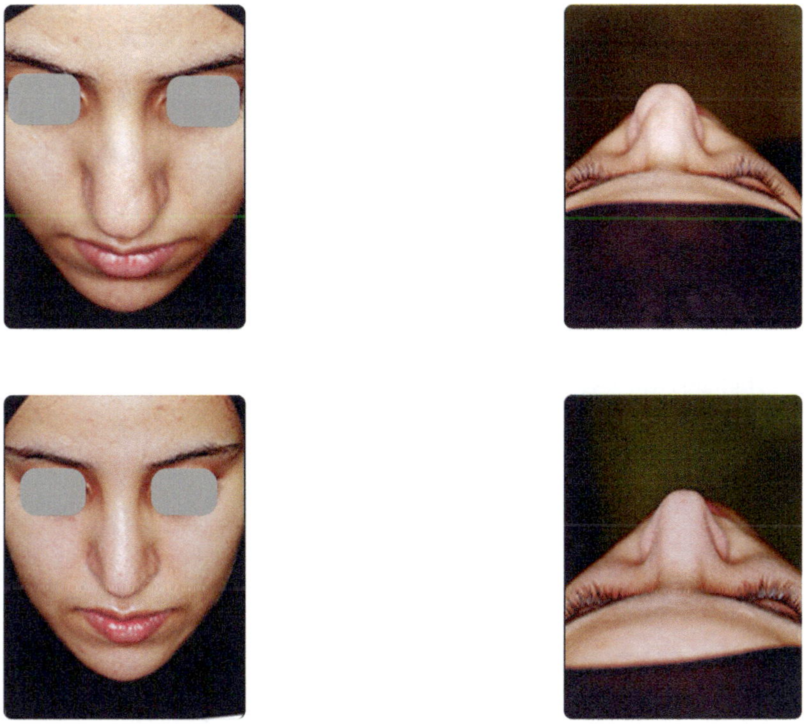

Steeper
Backward Tilting **Backward Tilting** **Basal**

Preoperative

Postoperative

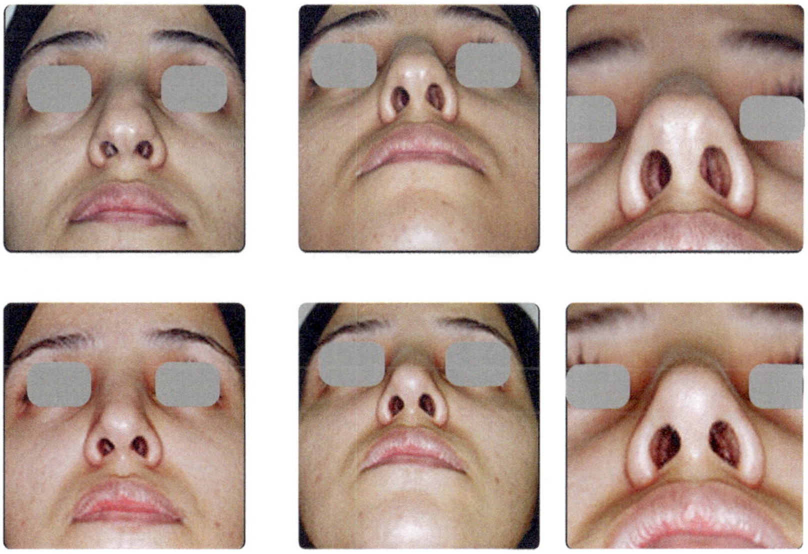

Right Nasal Aperture | **Right Nasal Aperture Rim Sill Test** | **Left Nasal Aperture Rim Sill Test** | **Left Nasal Aperture**

Preoperative

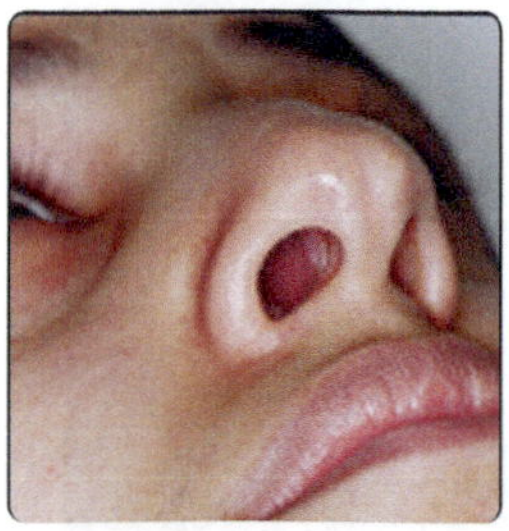
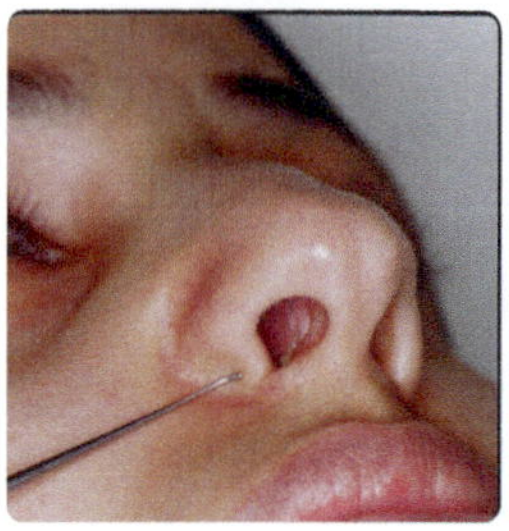
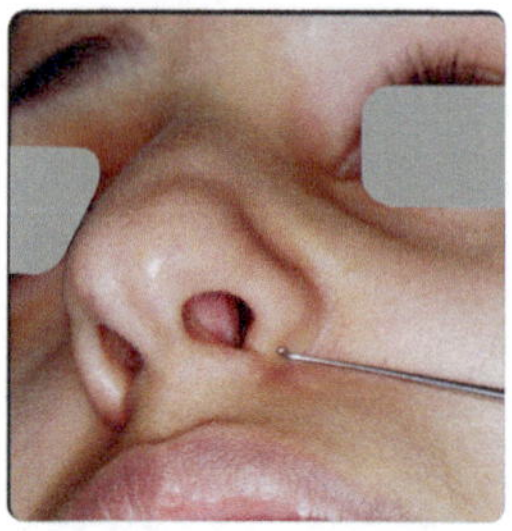
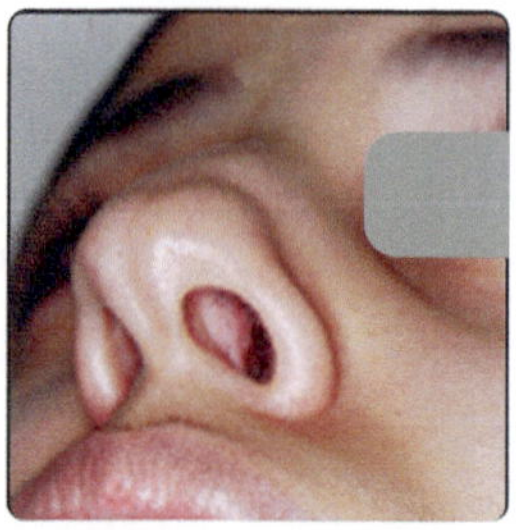

Postoperative

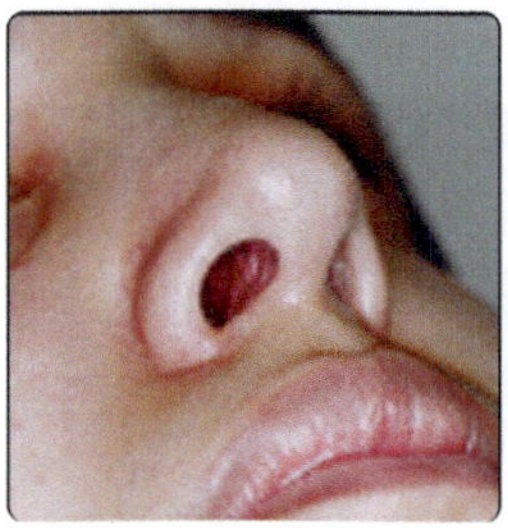
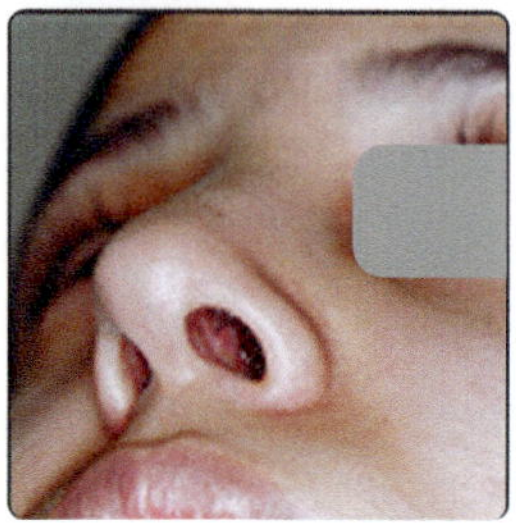

Right Oblique Mid Cheek Full Face | **Left Oblique Mid Cheek Full Face**

Preoperative

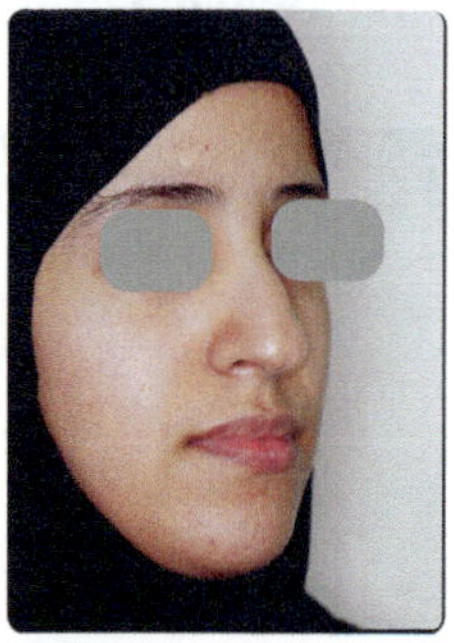
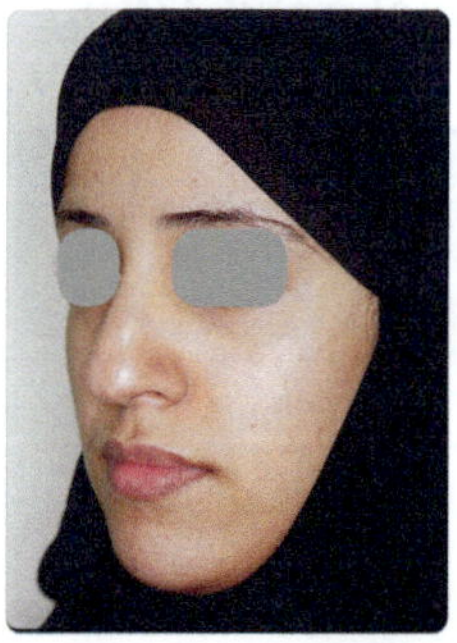

Postoperative

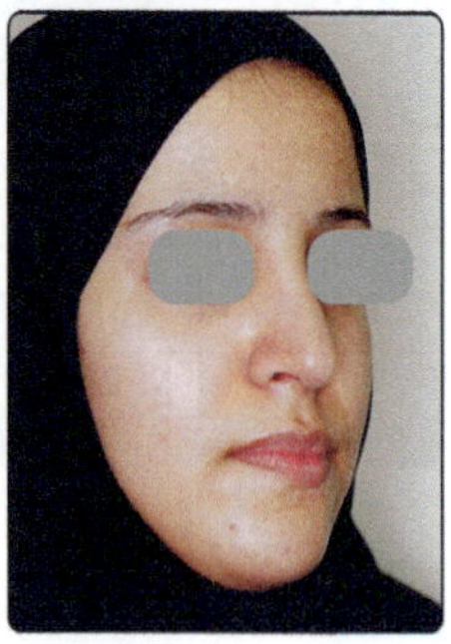
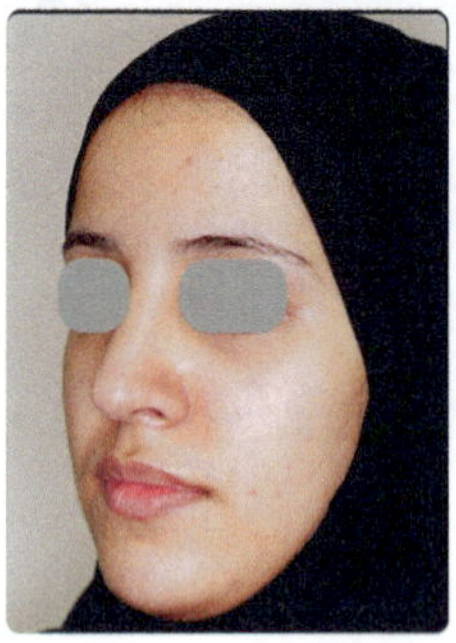

Right Oblique Cheek Margin Full Face | **Left Oblique Cheek Margin Full Face** | **Right Oblique Cheek Margin Middle Third** | **Left Oblique Cheek Margin Middle Third**

Preoperative

Postoperative

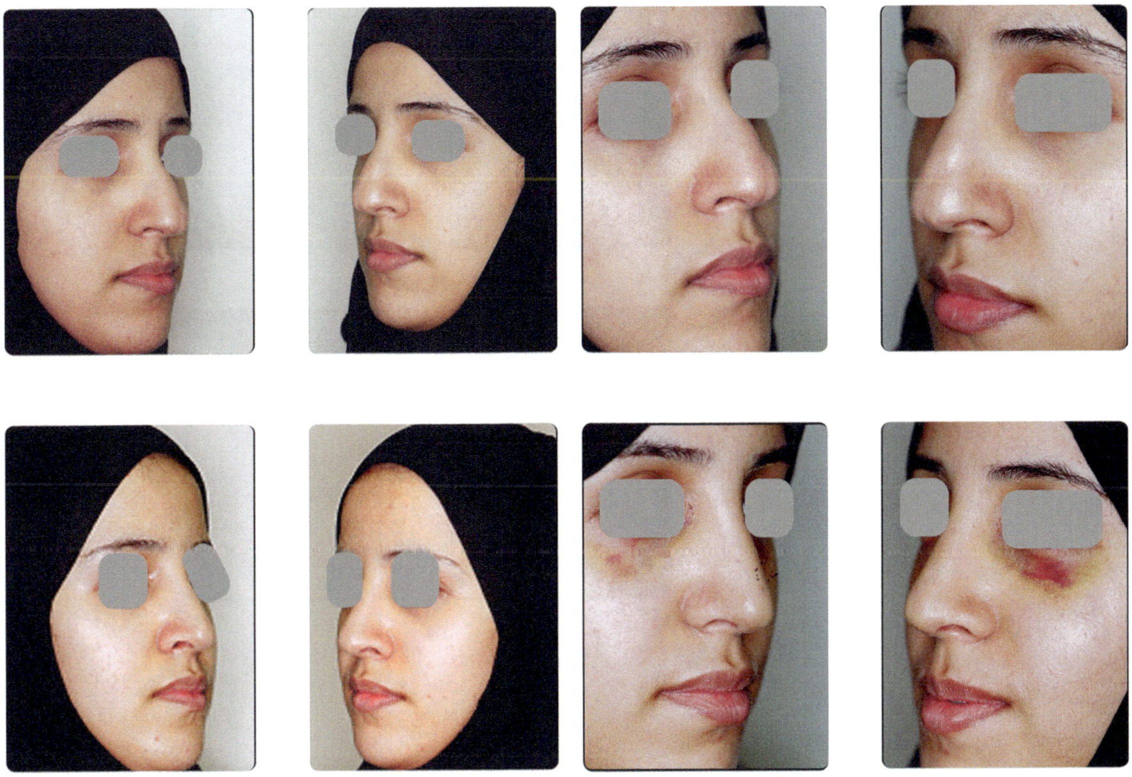

Right Lateral | **Left Lateral** | **Right Lateral Smiling** | **Left Lateral Smiling**

Preoperative

Postoperative

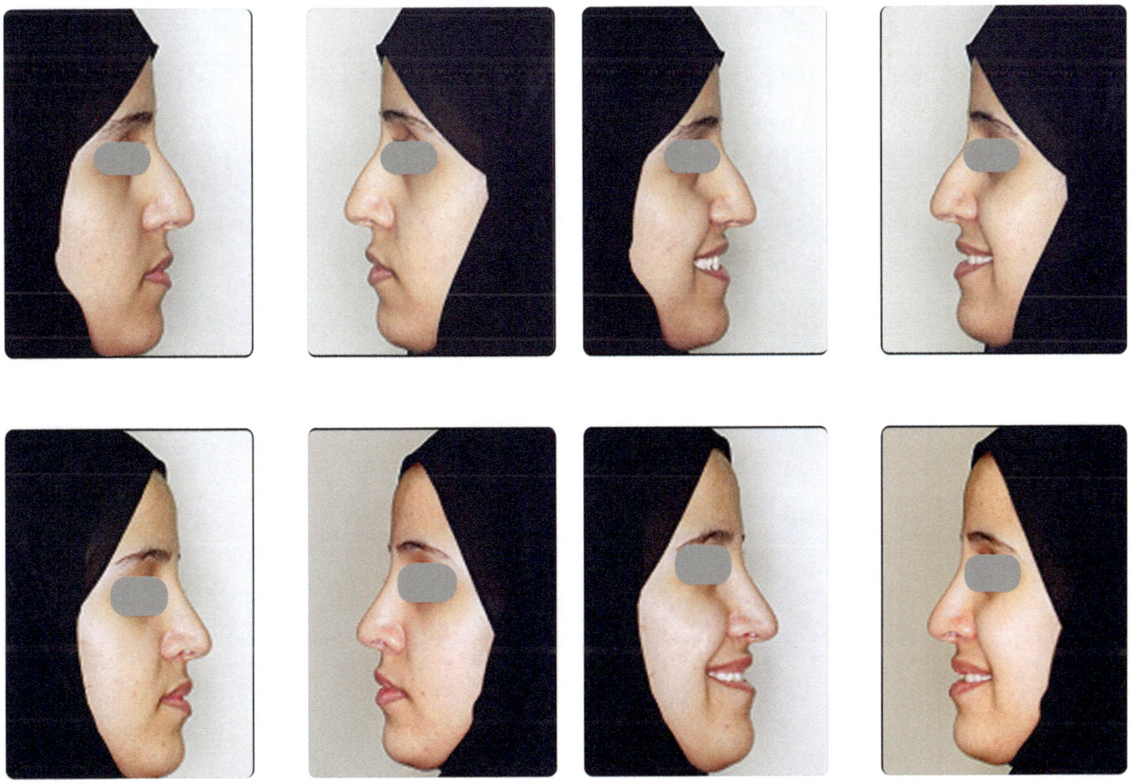

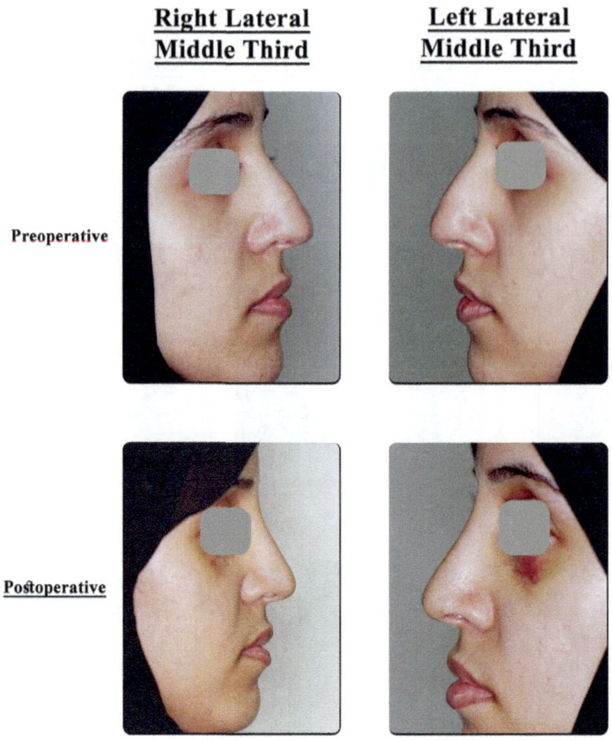
Right Lateral Middle Third
Left Lateral Middle Third
Preoperative
Postoperative

Part III: Clinical Case 2

17

Preoperative Assessment

1. **Frontolateral walls**
   a. Bulky fronto-lateral walls overshadowing the alae nasi (Frontal and Direct Dorsal Views).
   b. The tip light reflex is defuse (Frontal and Backward Tilting Views).
2. **Medial Wall**
   Nil of note.
3. **Boney pyramid**
   a. Wide base of the boney pyramid (Direct Dorsal and Backward Tilting Views).
   b. There is a small osteocartilaginous hump (Backward Tilting and Oblique views). This is due to the natural concavoconvex anatomy of the nasal bones from above downwards (See Anatomy Section).
   c. The middle third of the nose is bulky due to excess fat in the weak triangle and over the lower part of the upper lateral cartilage.
4. **Alar base**
   a. Wide alar base caused by the inferior segments of the rim-sill folds (Backward Tilting, Basal, and Nasal Aperture Views).
   b. Bulky alar base caused by the bulky posterior segments of the rim-sill folds. The acute angle of the alae nasi with the upper lip give the impression of a flat tire appearance (Backward Tilting, Basal, and Nasal, Aperture of Views).
   c. Note the pale areas of skin in the left rim-sill test.

Aims of Surgery

1. Overall reduction of the size and bulk of the lower two thirds of the nose to give more features to the different areas of the nose.
2. Reduction in the width and bulk of the alar base.

Surgical Plan

1. **Frontolateral walls**
   a. DDD including the weak triangle and the fat over the lower part of the upper lateral cartilage to reduce the bulk of the nasal tip and midvault.
   b. Cephalic trim of the lateral crurae to reduce the size of the frontolateral walls.
2. **Medial Wall**
   Nil of note.
3. **Boney pyramid**
   a. Excision of the osteocartilaginous hump i.e. reducing the natural convexities of the nasal bones.
   b. Osteotomies and medialization of the lateral bony walls.
4. **Alar base**
   Excision of the inferior and posterior segments of the rim sill folds.

Surgical Procedure
As per Surgical Plan.

Post-Operative Analysis

1. **Frontolateral Wall**
   a. Tip definition: the nasal tip is slimmer, prominent and well identified from the alae nasi. The nasal tip is covered with thinner skin. The alae nasi become more visible to share in nasal aesthetics (Frontal, Direct Dorsal, Backward Tilting and Basal Views).
   b. Tip projection: The nasal tip is at the same level of the nasal dorsum (Lateral and Oblique views).
   c. Tip light reflex is seen as one spot off the nasal tip (Frontal and Backward Tilting Views).
2. **Medial Wall**
   Nil of Note.

M. H. A. Shafy, *Atlas of Clinical Cases in Rhinoplasty*,
https://doi.org/10.1007/978-3-031-07504-9_17

3. **Bony Pyramid**
    a. Bony pyramid aesthetics improved: the dorsum is straight and the side walls are smooth and narrow (all views except Basal Views).
    b. Dorsal light reflex is seen as an uninterrupted line off the nasal dorsum (Direct Dorsal Views).
4. **Alar Base**
    a. The superior alar grooves aesthetics improved: after defatting they become deeper, longer and more visible (Direct Dorsal, Oblique and Lateral Views).
    b. Posterior alar groove aesthetics improved by defatting as well as excising the posterior segments of the rim-sill folds. The flat tire appearance is no longer present (Backward Tilting, Basal and Nasal Aperture Views).
    c. Alae nasi aesthetics improved. They are pulled medially become better seen, smaller and share in nasal aesthetics (NasalAperture, Oblique and Lateral Views).
    d. Nasal aperture aesthetics improved by defatting and excision of rim-sill folds:
        i. The size of the nasal openings are smaller (Backward Tilting, Basal and Nasal Aperture views).
        ii. The shape of nasal openings changed from thick heavy wide and round openings with transverse long axes to thin delicate small oval openings with anterior long axes (Backward Tilting, Basal and NasalAperture views).
    e. Marginal light reflexes are clearly seen at:
        i. Inferior alar margins (Nasal Aperture Views).
        ii. Nasal sill bands (Oblique Views).
        iii. Lateral crural prominences (Lateral Views).

Commentary

a. Keeping her original features and the exact nasal print, the post-operative photographs shows closer aesthetic matching with her mouth, cheeks and chin. This can be seen especially in the frontal and direct dorsal views.
b. The amorphously bulky large nose is transformed to a nose that has the features of its different components i.e. nasal tip, nasal dorsum and slim bony side walls. The alae nasi have better aesthetics with clearer superior and posterior alar grooves.

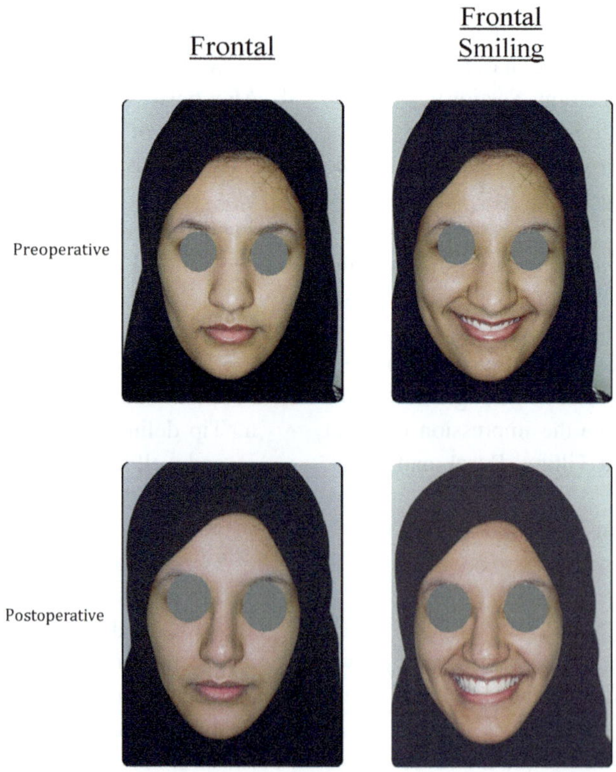

Direct Dorsal | Direct Dorsal Smiling

Preoperative

Postoperative

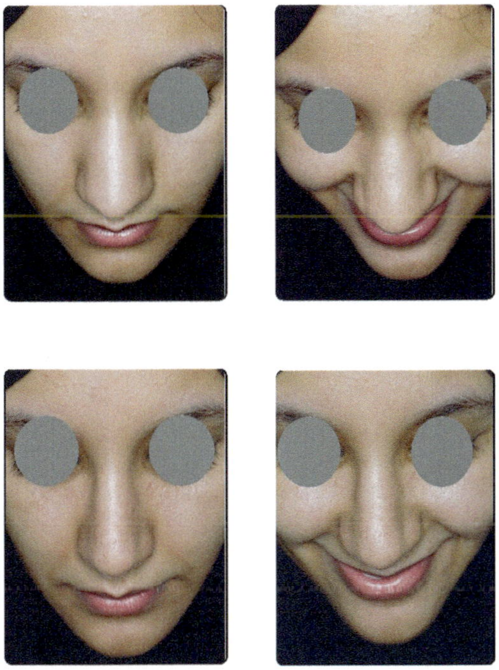

Backward Tilting | Steeper Backward Tilting | Basal | Basal Smiling

Preoperative

Postoperative

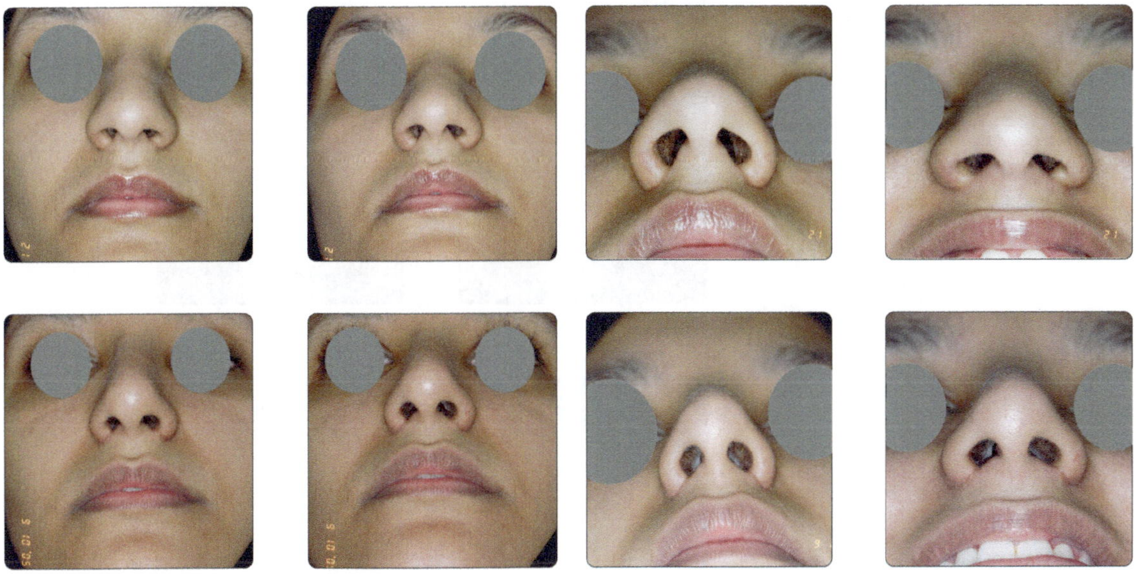

Right Nasal Aperture | Right Nasal Aperture Rim Sill Test | Left Nasal Aperture Rim Sill Test | Left Nasal Aperture

Preoperative

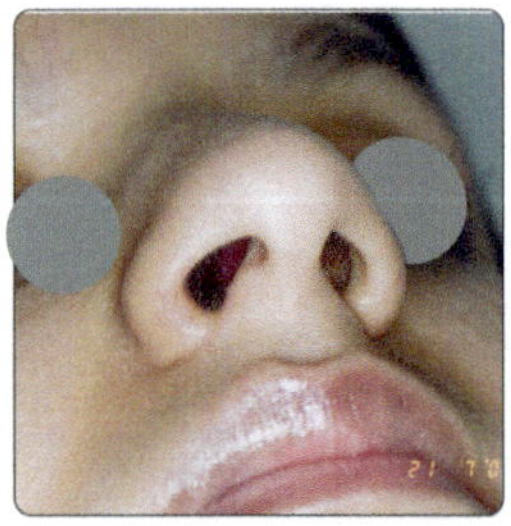
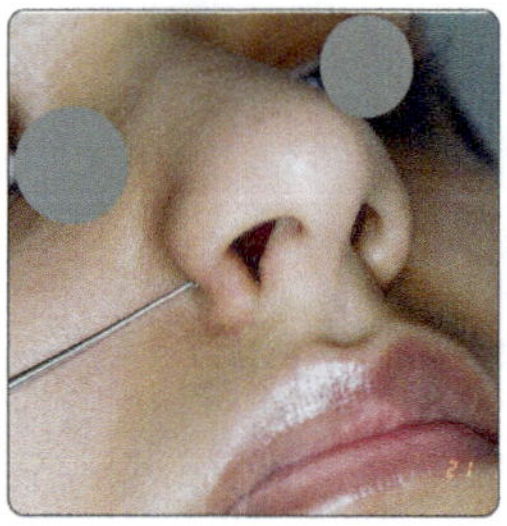
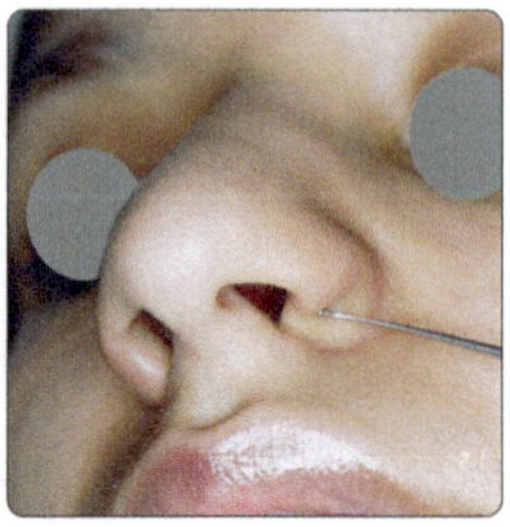
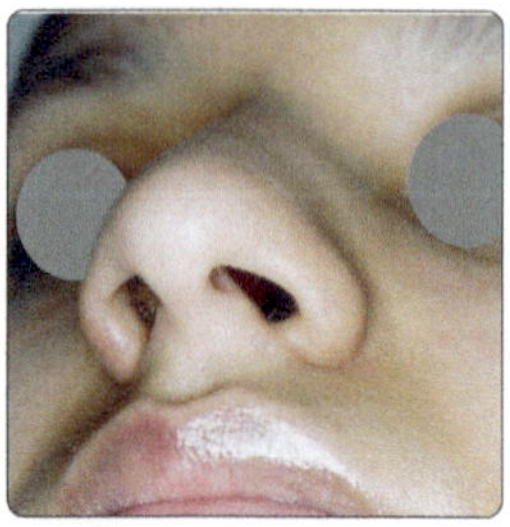

Postoperative

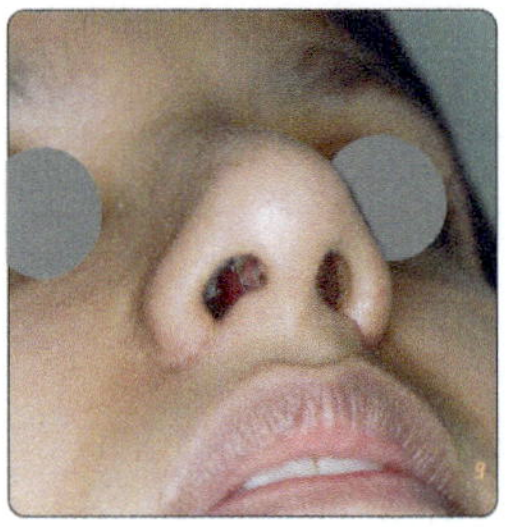
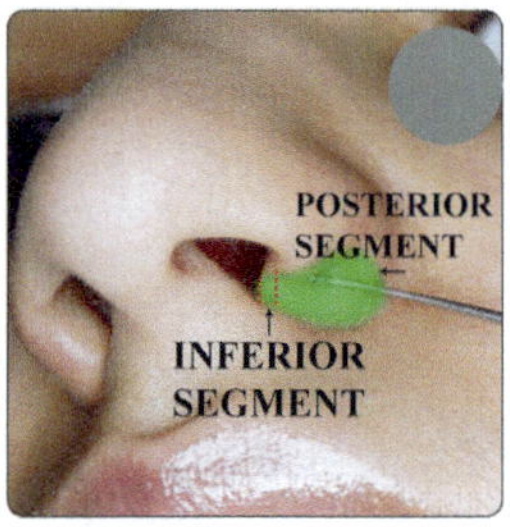

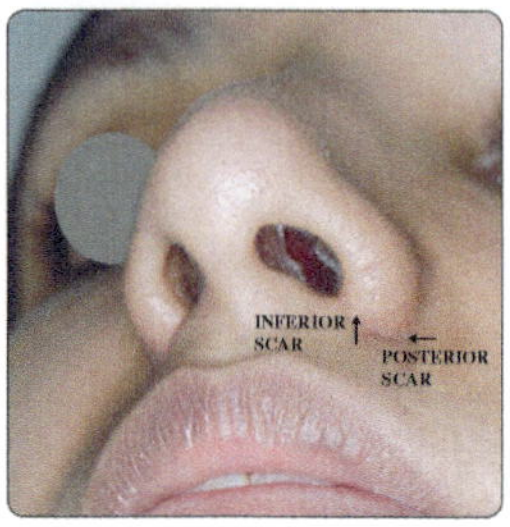

Right Oblique Mid Cheek Full Face | Left Oblique Mid Cheek Full Face

Preoperative

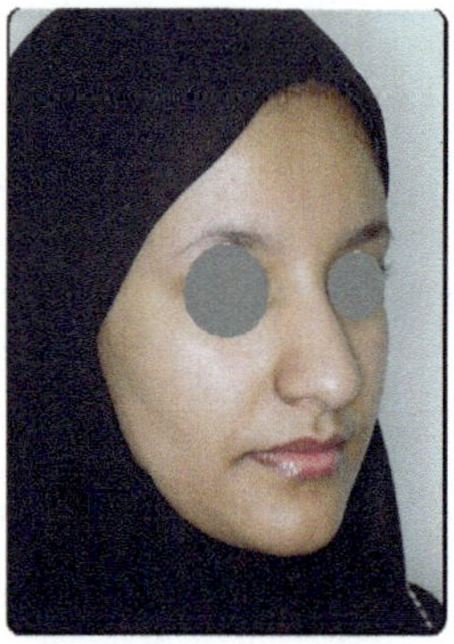
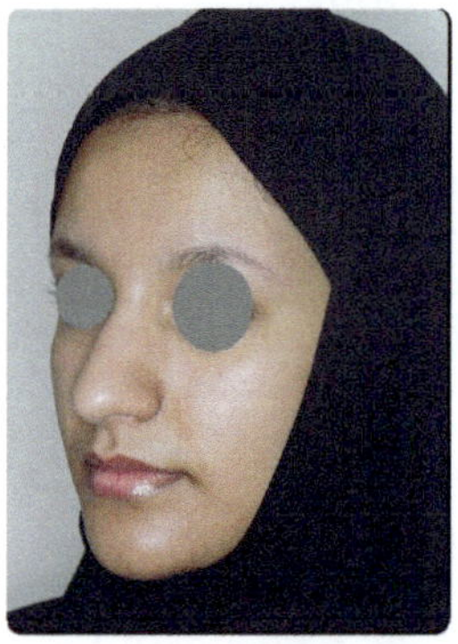

Postoperative

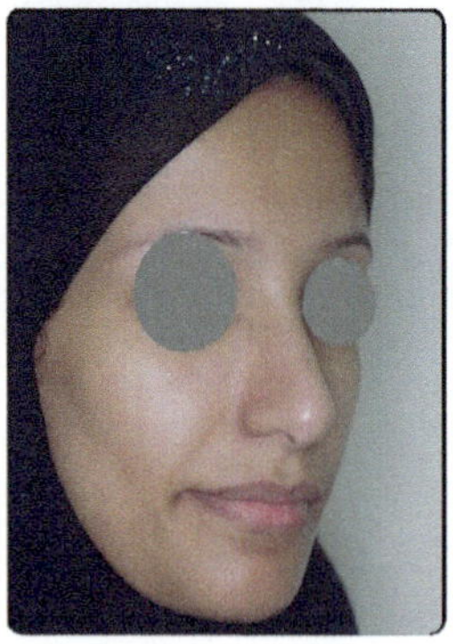
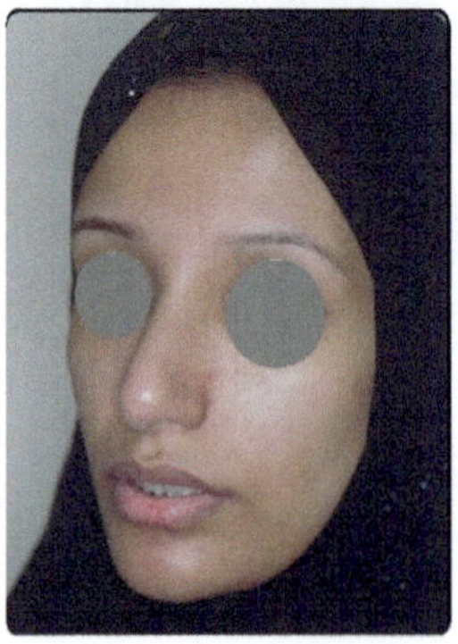

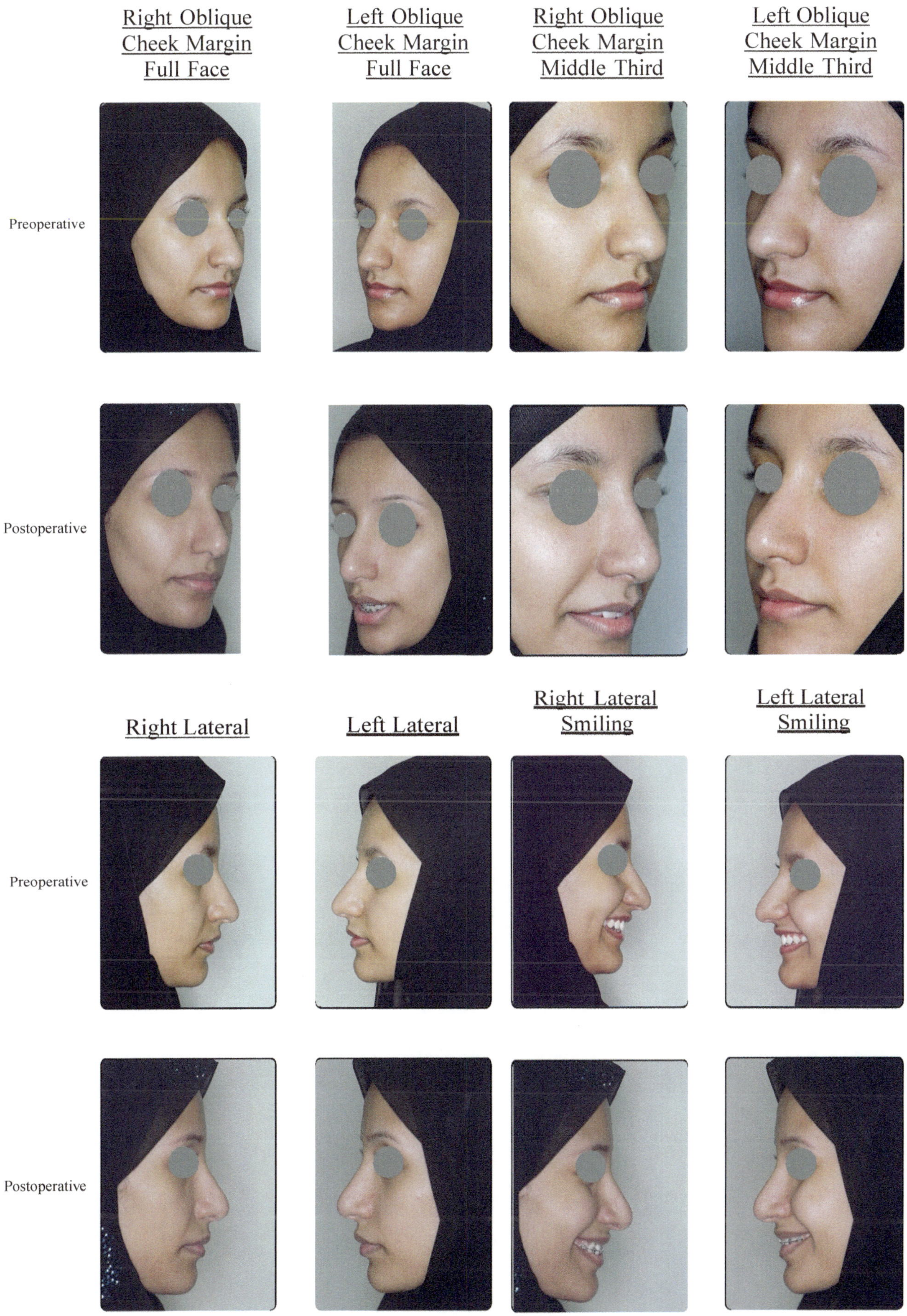
Right Oblique Cheek Margin Full Face
Left Oblique Cheek Margin Full Face
Right Oblique Cheek Margin Middle Third
Left Oblique Cheek Margin Middle Third
Preoperative
Postoperative
Right Lateral
Left Lateral
Right Lateral Smiling
Left Lateral Smiling
Preoperative
Postoperative

Part III: Clinical Case 3

18

Preoperative Assessment

1. **Frontolateral walls**
   a. Bulky frontolateral walls overshadowing the alae nasi (Frontal, Direct Dorsal and Overhead Views).
   b. Minimal bifid tip (Frontal, Direct Dorsal, Backward Tilting and Nasal Aperture Views).
2. **Medial Wall**
   a. Mobile tip i.e. the nasal tip moves downwards on smiling (Smiling Lateral Views).
   b. Sliding tip i.e. the nasal tip moves backwards (posteriorly) on smiling (Smiling Lateral Views).
3. **Bony pyramid**
   a. Wide base of the boney pyramid (Frontal, Direct Dorsal and Overhead Views).
   b. Osteocartilaginous hump deviated to the right due to bilateral maxillary asymmetry. The right cheek is wide and low and the left cheek is narrow and high (Backward Tilting, Oblique and Lateral Views).
   c. The middle third of the nose is bulky due to excess fat in the weak triangle and over the lower part of the upper lateral cartilage.
4. **Alar base**
   Although nasal apertures were small yet they had unaesthetic thick walls and rounded in shape (Backward Tilting and Basal Views).

Aims of Surgery

1. Reduce the bulk of the frontolateral walls.
2. Abolish the mobile and the sliding tip.
3. Excision of the osteocartilaginous hump.

Surgical Plan

1. **Frontolateral walls**
   a. D.D.D. including weak triangle to reduce the bulk and size of the nasal tip and supra tip area.
   b. Bilateral cephalic trim of the lateral crurae to reduce the size.
2. **Medial Wall**
   a. Division of the Depressor Septi muscles.
   b. Trim of the membranous septum and fixing the caudal cartilagenous septum to the medial crurae.
3. **Bony pyramid**
   a. Excision of the osteocartilaginous hump down to the anterior septal angle.
   b. Osteotomies and medialization of the lateral bony walls.
   c. Kasanjian maneuver to the left.
4. **Alar base**
   Nil of note.

Surgical Procedure

a. As per Surgical Plan.
b. No surgery was necessary to the membranous septum to correct the sliding tip. Division of the Depressor Septi muscles was sufficient to overcome both mobile and sliding tip.
c. There was mild maxillary asymmetry. After osteotomies the boney pyramid was deviated to the right side. The Kasanjian maneuver was necessary to the left to bring the boney pyramid to the mid line.

Post-Operative Analysis

1. **Frontolateral Wall**
   a. Tip definition improved i.e. slimmer and prominently well identified. The overlying skin is thinner. The alae nasi come into view to share in nasal aesthetics (Frontal, Direct Dorsal, Overhead, Backward Tilting and Basal Views).
   b. The nice narrow projecting tip was the result of defatting procedure. No grafts were used and no direct stitching were made to the lower lateral cartilages.

M. H. A. Shafy, *Atlas of Clinical Cases in Rhinoplasty*,
https://doi.org/10.1007/978-3-031-07504-9_18

c. Bifidity of the nasal tip was abolished after defatting procedure.
d. Tip projection: nasal tip is high at the end of the nasal dorsum with nice aesthetic angle (Lateral and Oblique views). This is coupled with aesthetic nasolabial angle.
e. Tip light reflex is seen as one spot off the nasal tip (Frontal and Backward Tilting Views).

2. **Medial Wall**
   a. Mobile tip abolished.
   b. Sliding tip disappeared.
3. **Bony Pyramid**
   a. Bony pyramid aesthetics improved: the nasal dorsum is straight and the sidewalls are smooth and narrow (all views except the Basal Views).
   b. Dorsal light reflex is seen as an uninterrupted line off the nasal dorsum (Direct Dorsal Views).
4. **Alar Base**
   a. The superior alar grooves now clear off fat, become deeper, longer and visible (Direct Dorsal, Oblique and Lateral Views).
   b. Posterior alar groove aesthetics improved by defatting. Their angle with the upper lip became wider.
   c. Alae nasi aesthetics improved. They are pulled medially become better seen, smaller and share in nasal aesthetics (Nasal Aperture, Oblique and Lateral Views).
   d. Nasal Aperture aesthetics improved: the shapes of the nasal aperture improved by defatting. They became thin walled, elegantly oval without the change in their size (Backward Tilting, Nasal Aperture and Basal Views).
   e. Marginal light reflexes are clearly seen at:
      i. Inferior alar margins (Nasal Aperture Views).
      ii. Nasal sill bands (Oblique Views).
      iii. Lateral crural prominences (Lateral Views).

Commentary

a. Postoperative photographs are taken two month after surgery. Better long term results are expected.
b. The subdermal fat of the weak triangle, middle and lateral crurae was both thick and irregular. Together with irregularities of the broad bony sidewalls in a small nose, all together, have resulted in the thick irregular bulky nose.

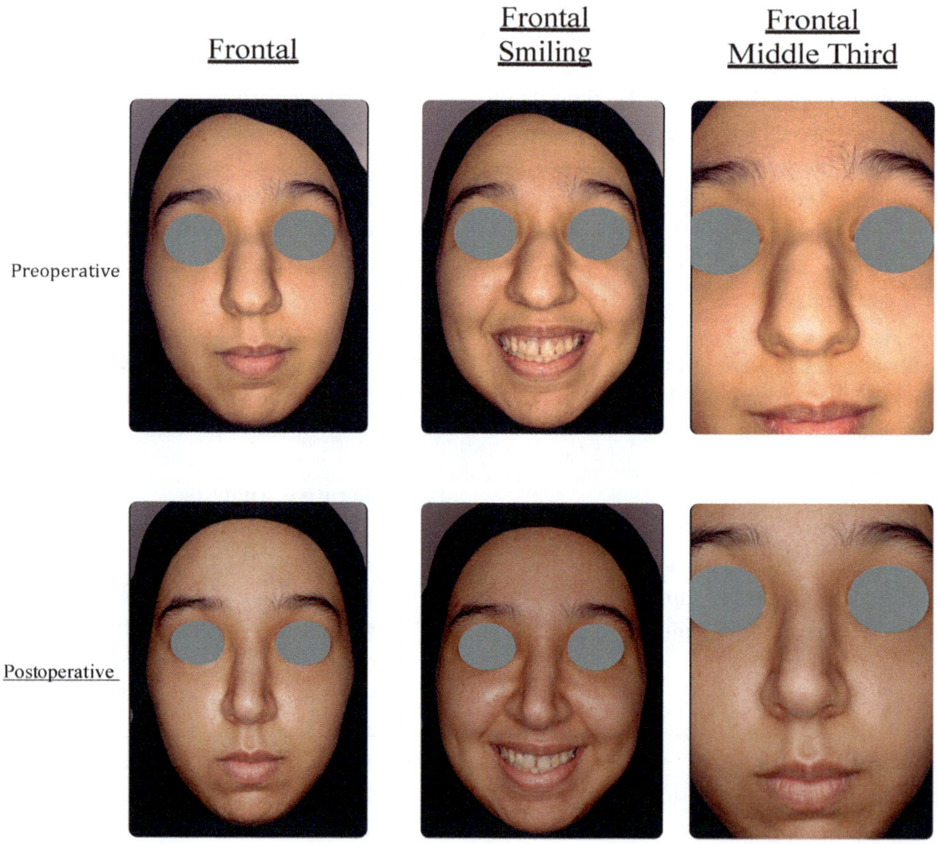

Direct Dorsal | Direct Dorsal Smiling | Overhead | Overhead Smiling

Preoperative

Postoperative

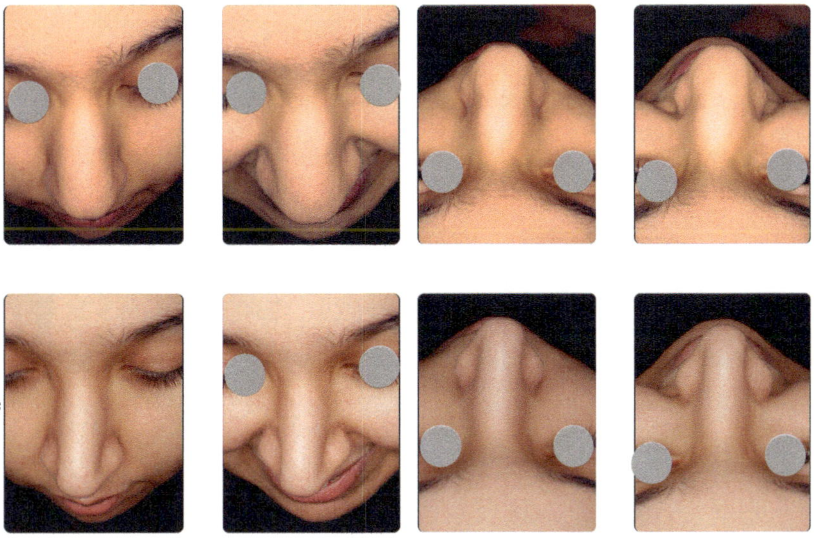

Backward Tilting | Steeper Backward Tilting | Basal | Basal Smiling

Preoperative

Postoperative

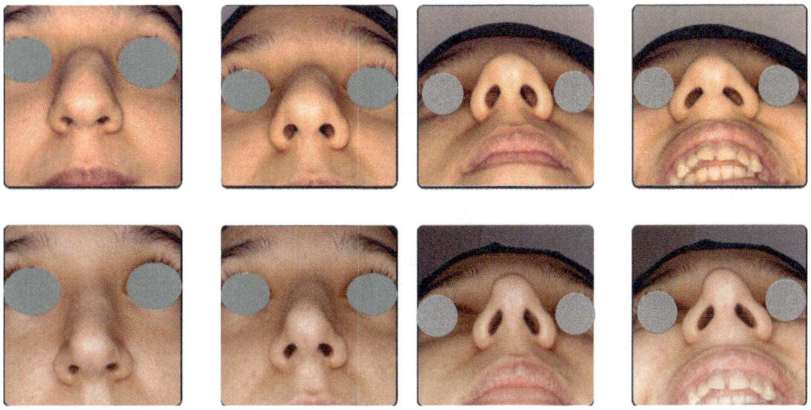

Note: The change in the shapes of the nasal tip and nasal openings after defatting process.

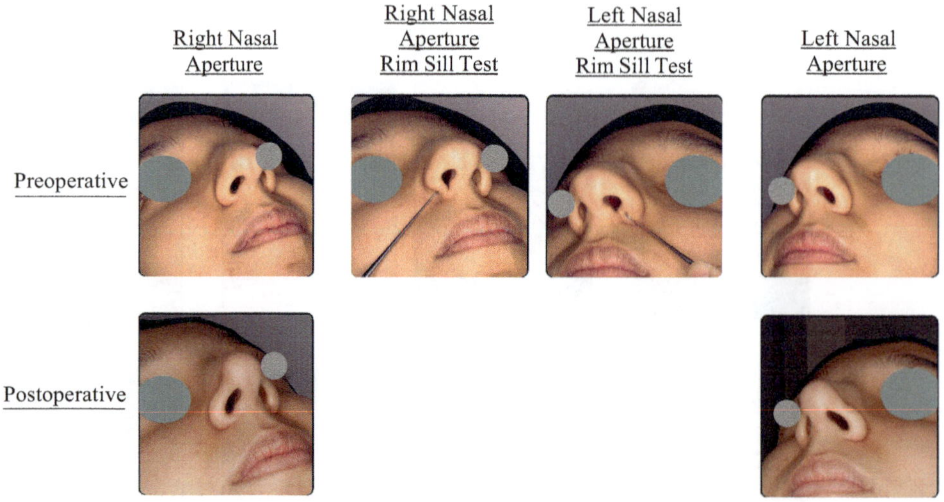
Right Nasal Aperture
Right Nasal Aperture Rim Sill Test
Left Nasal Aperture Rim Sill Test
Left Nasal Aperture
Preoperative
Postoperative

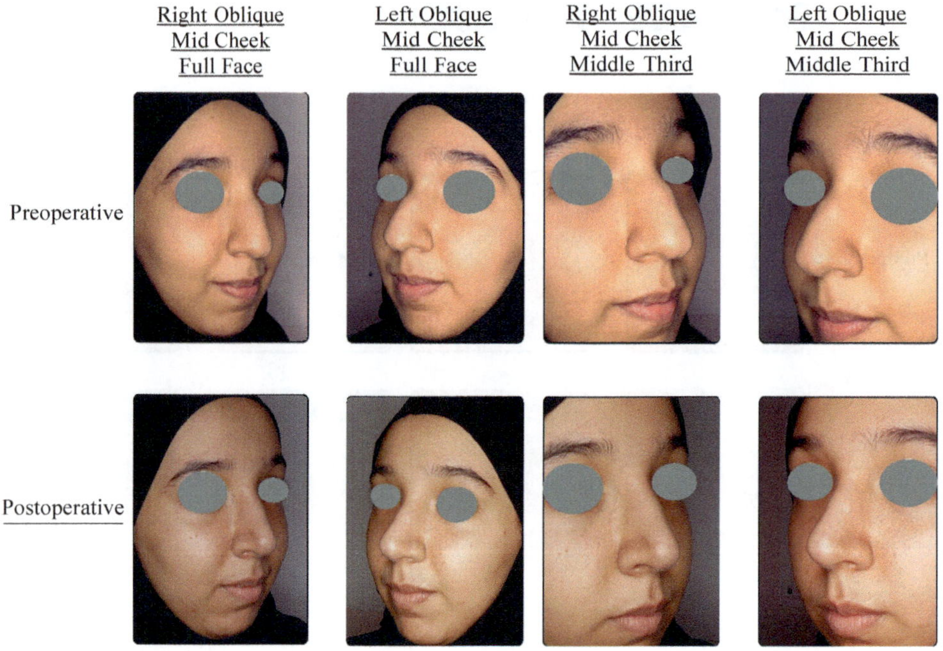
Right Oblique Mid Cheek Full Face
Left Oblique Mid Cheek Full Face
Right Oblique Mid Cheek Middle Third
Left Oblique Mid Cheek Middle Third
Preoperative
Postoperative

Right Oblique Cheek Margin Full Face | Left Oblique Cheek Margin Full Face | Right Oblique Cheek Margin Middle Third | Left Oblique Cheek Margin Middle Third

Preoperative

Postoperative

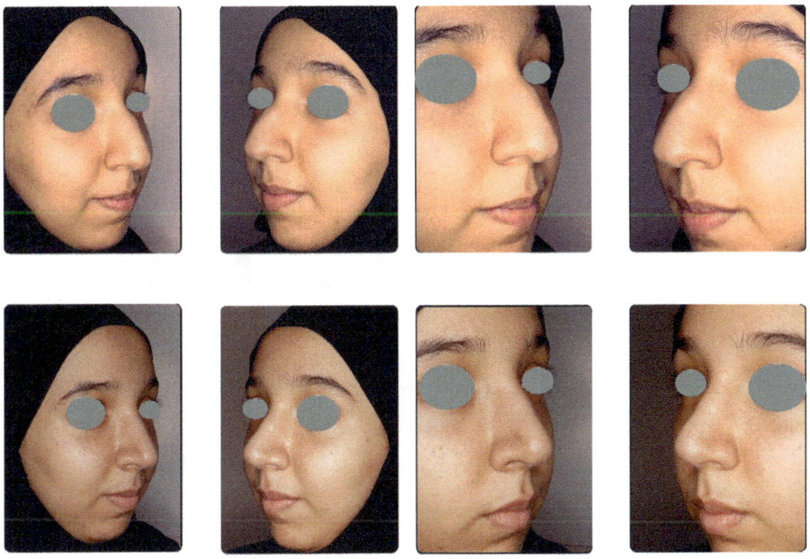

Right Lateral | Left Lateral | Right Lateral Smiling | Left Lateral Smiling

Preoperative

Postoperative

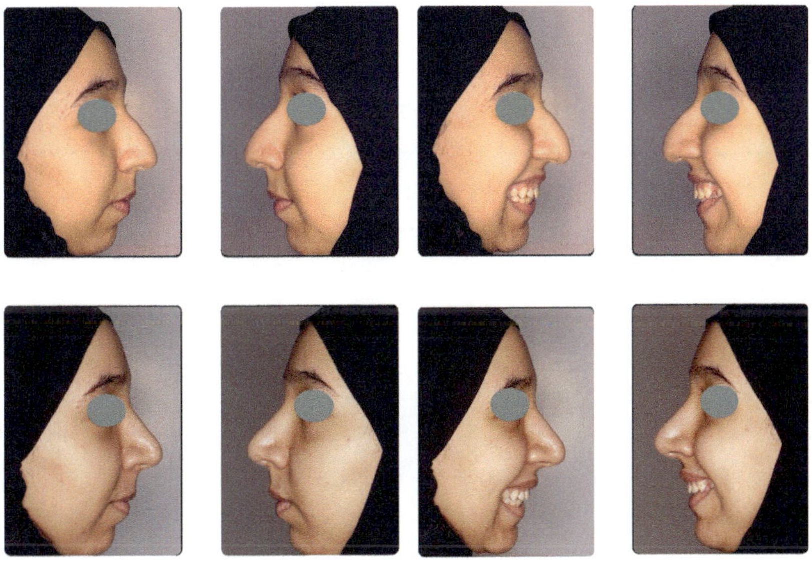

Right Lateral Middle Third

Left Lateral Middle Third

Preoperative

Postoperative

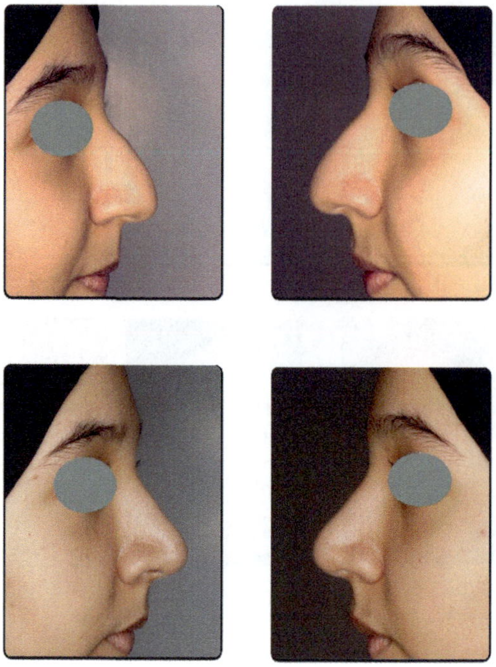

Part III: Clinical Case 4

19

Preoperative Assessment

1. **Frontolateral walls**
   a. Homogenously large and bulky frontolateral walls (Frontal, Direct Dorsal and Overhead Views).
   b. Excess fat at the lower end of the nasal tip (Direct Dorsal and Backward Tilting Views).
   c. Dissociation between the bulky lower third and upper two thirds (Backward Tilting Views).
   d. The alae nasi are over shadowed by the bulbous tip. They are almost not seen. The right ala nasi is naturally larger than the left (Frontal and Direct Dorsal Views).
2. **Medial Wall**
   Mobile tip (Lateral Smiling Views).
3. **Bony pyramid**
   a. Wide base of the boney pyramid (Direct Dorsal and Backward Tilting Views).
   b. Small osteocartilaginous hump caused by the natural concovoconvex anatomy of the nasal bones from above downwards (See Anatomy Section).
4. **Alar base**
   Thick and Wide alar base due to thick posterior and long inferior segments of the rim sill folds successively (Backward Tilting, Basal and Nasal Aperture Views).

Aims of Surgery

1. Reduction of the nasal bulk.
2. Abolishing the mobile tip.
3. Reduction of the size of the boney pyramid.
4. Reduction of the bulk and size of the alar base.

Surgical Plan

1. **Frontolateral walls**
   a. DDD including the weak triangle to reduce the bulk and size of the nasal tip and midvault.
   b. Cephalic trim of lateral crurae to reduce the size of the frontolateral walls.
2. **Medial Wall**
   Division of the Depressor Septi muscle.
3. **Bony pyramid**
   a. Excision of the osteocartilaginous hump.
   b. Osteotomies and medialization of the lateral bony walls to reduce the size of the bony pyramid.
4. **Alar base**
   Resection of the inferior and posterior segments of the rim sill folds.

Surgical Procedure

As per Surgical Plan.

Post-Operative Analysis

1. **Frontolateral Wall**
   a. A Tip definition improved. The nasal tip is slimmer. The alae nasi came into view to share in nasal aesthetics (Frontal, Direct Dorsal, Overhead and Backward Tilting Views). The superior alar grooves are clearer and longer (Oblique and Frontal Views).
   b. Incomplete defatting of the nasal tip have led to less favorable tip projection (post operative Lateral and Oblique Views).

M. H. A. Shafy, *Atlas of Clinical Cases in Rhinoplasty*,
https://doi.org/10.1007/978-3-031-07504-9_19

c. Tip light reflex is seen as one spot off the nasal tip (Frontal and Backward Tilting Views).

2. **Medial Wall**
   Nil of Note.
3. **Bony Pyramid**
   a. Bony pyramid aesthetics improved: the nasal dorsum is straight and the sidewalls are smooth and narrow (all views except the Basal Views).
   b. Dorsal light reflex is seen as an uninterrupted line off the nasal dorsum (Direct Dorsal Views).
4. **Alar Base**
   a. The superior alar grooves now clear off fat, become deeper, longer and visible (Direct Dorsal, Oblique and Lateral Views).
   b. Posterior alar groove aesthetics improved. The angle of the alae nasi with the upper lip is wider. Aesthetics of the alae nasi is better.
   c. On reducing the alar base, removal of the posterior segments of the rim sill folds was omitted.
   d. Removing the inferior segments alone and approximating the alar margins to the nasal sills have resulted in unpleasant, laterally angulated nasal apertures and residual bulky alar base (see illustrations in the pre and post operative Left Nasal Aperture Views). Surprisingly most patients do not show displeasure of this deformity. Very few patients tend to look at their nose from below i.e. basal view.
   e. Marginal light reflexes were only seen at the inferior alar margins (Nasal Aperture Views).

Commentary

a. Generally, the patient was happy with the overall outcome, as the main issue in her mind was the bulky nose.
b. The nasal air flow is not compromised by the reduced size of the alar base.
c. Defatting of the frontolateral walls resulted in the full integration of the lower third with the upper two thirds of the nose.
d. Although the main objective of the surgery was achieved i.e. patient satisfaction by the overall reduction of the bulk and size of the nose, yet two misjudgments took place; the incomplete defatting of nasal tip and omitting resection of the posterior segments of the rim sill folds.

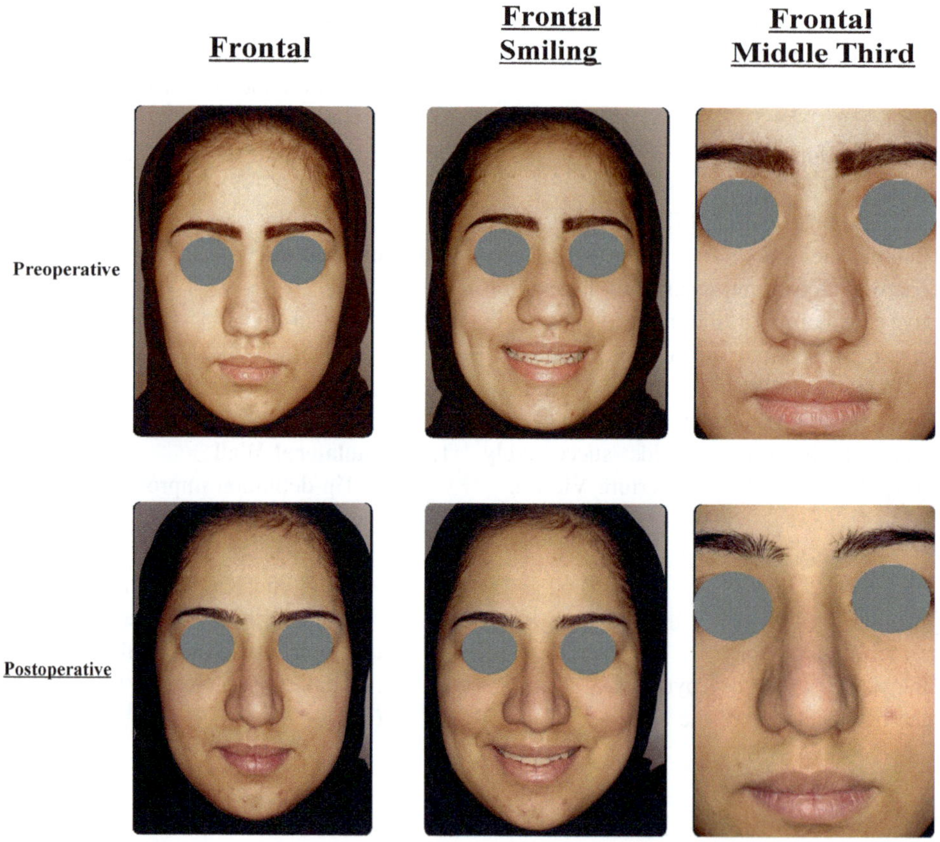

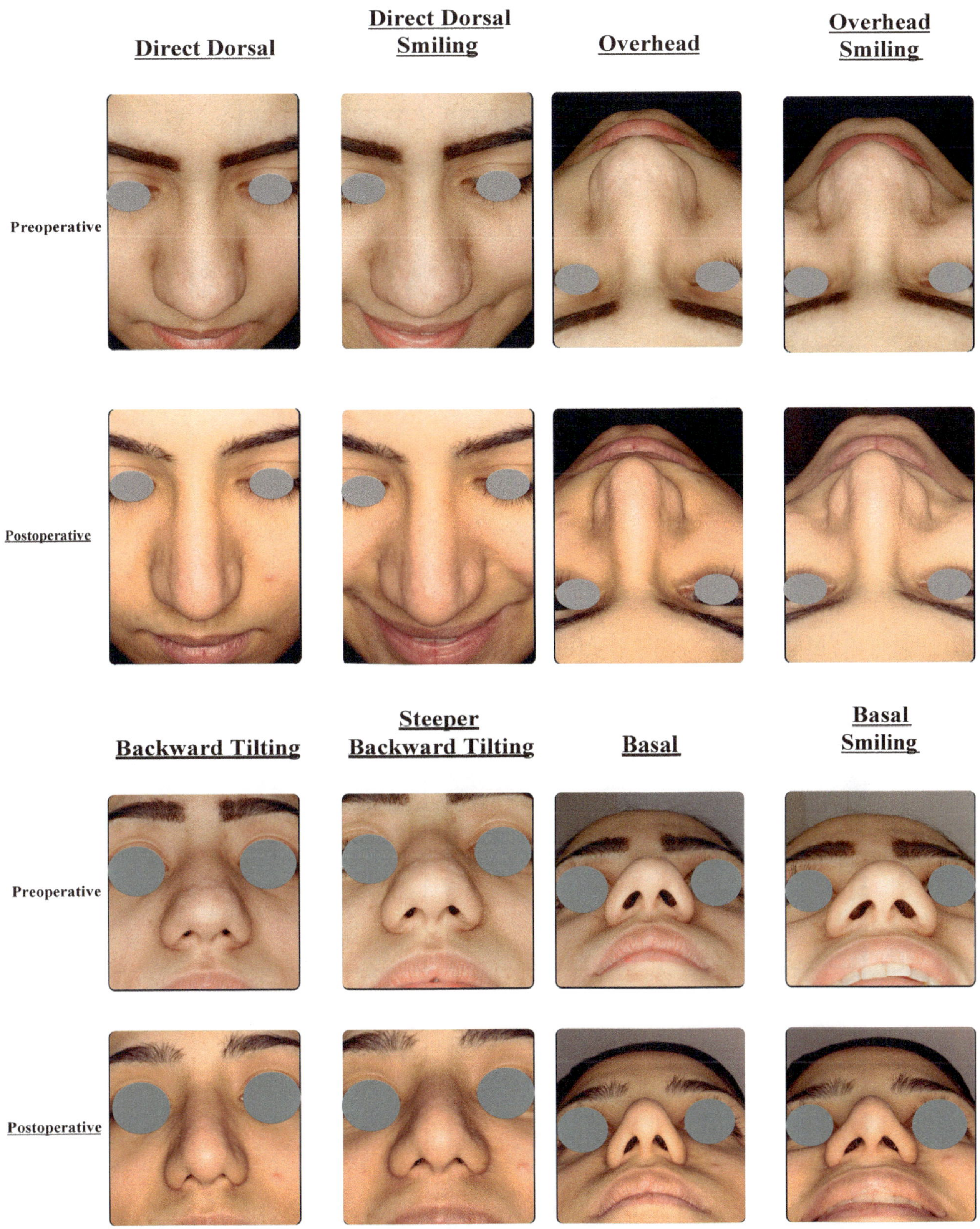

Direct Dorsal
Direct Dorsal Smiling
Overhead
Overhead Smiling
Preoperative
Postoperative
Backward Tilting
Steeper Backward Tilting
Basal
Basal Smiling
Preoperative
Postoperative

Right Nasal Aperture | **Right Nasal Aperture Rim Sill Test** | **Left Nasal Aperture Rim Sill Test** | **Left Nasal Aperture**

Preoperative

Postoperative

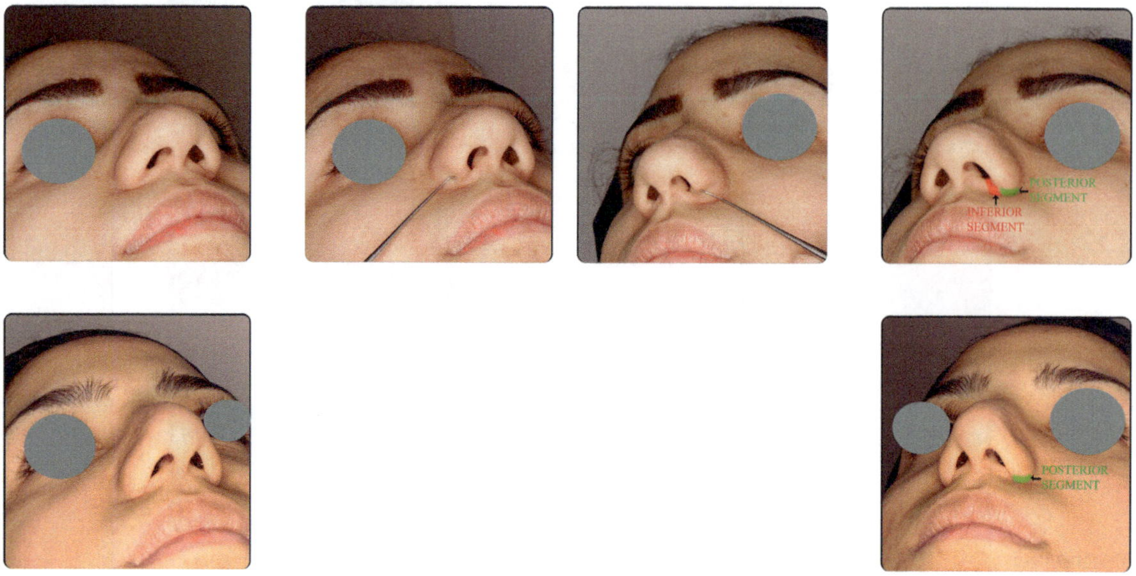

Right Oblique Mid Cheek Full Face | **Left Oblique Mid Cheek Full Face** | **Right Oblique Mid Cheek Middle Third** | **Left Oblique Mid Cheek Middle Third**

Preoperative

Postoperative

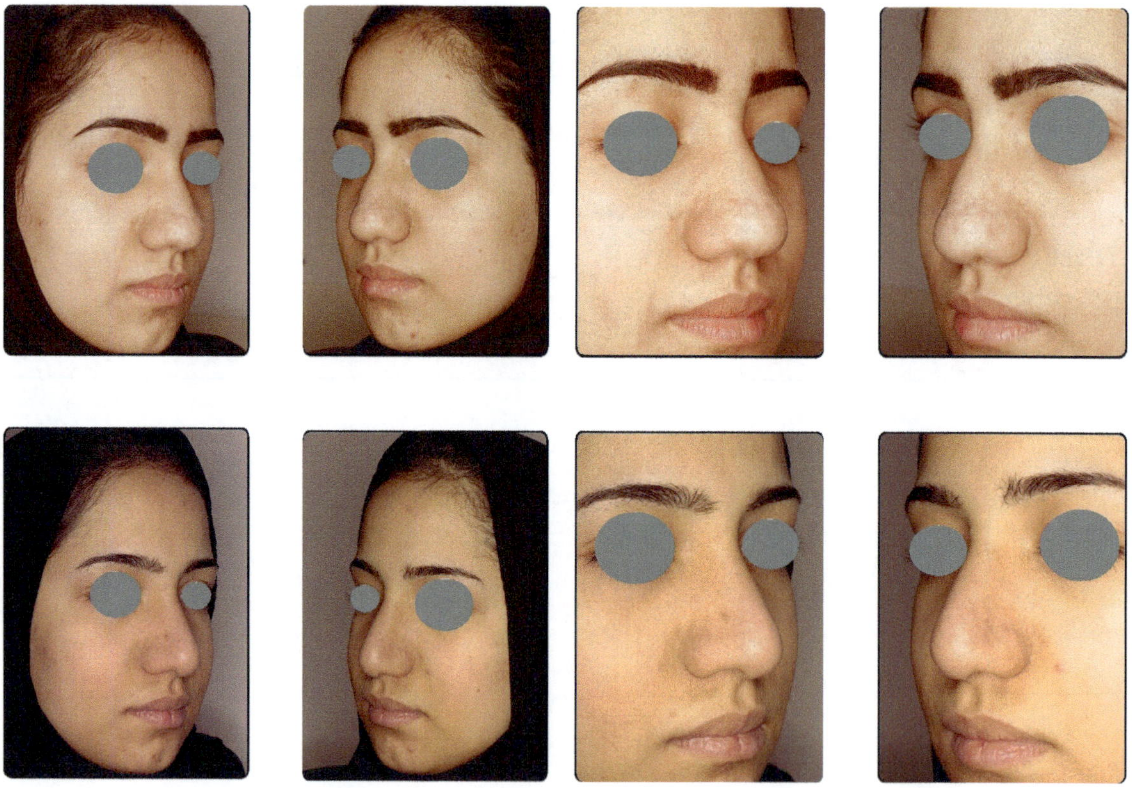

Right Oblique Cheek Margin Full Face

Left Oblique Cheek Margin Full Face

Right Oblique Cheek Margin Middle Third

Left Oblique Cheek Margin Middle Third

Preoperative

Postoperative

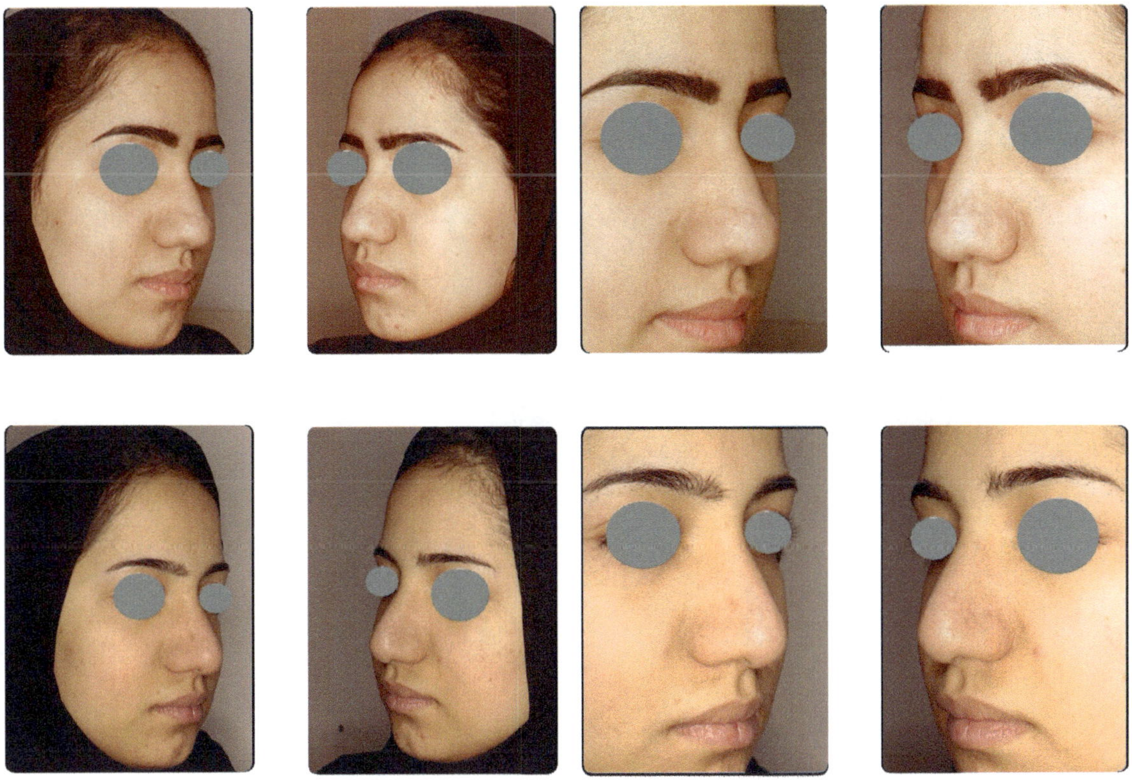

Right Lateral | **Left Lateral** | **Right Lateral Smiling** | **Left Lateral Smiling**

Preoperative

Postoperative

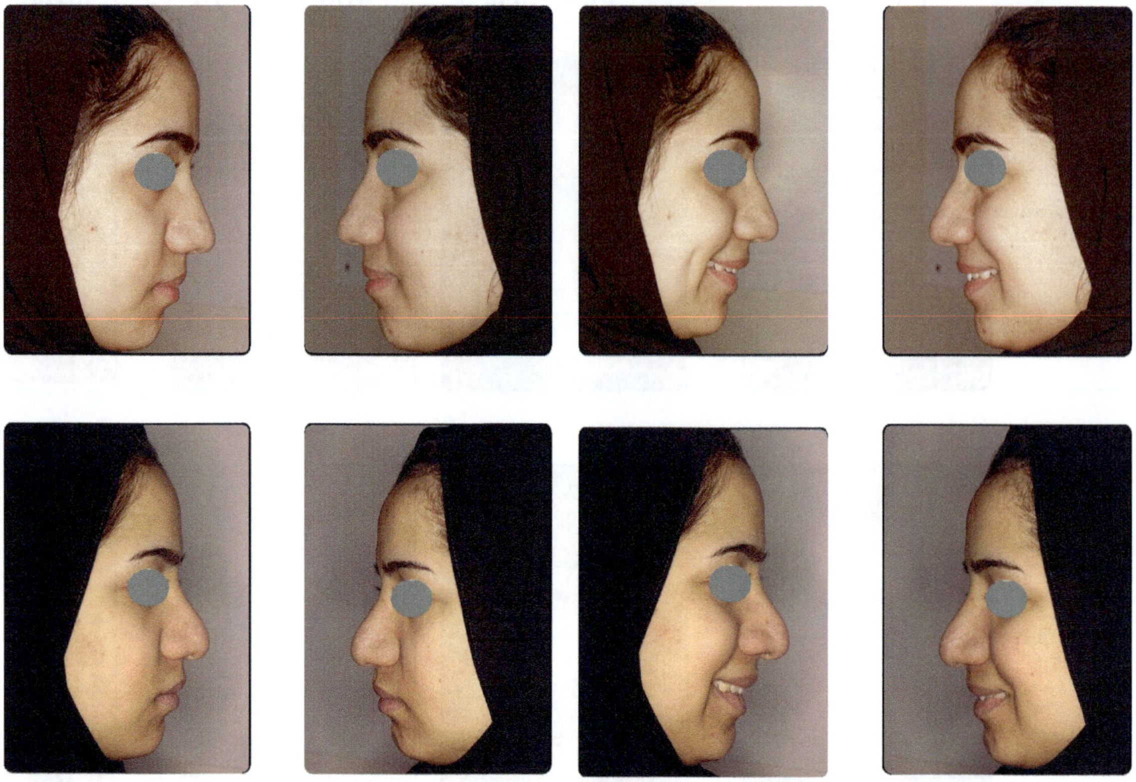

Right Lateral Middle Third | **Left Lateral Middle Third**

Preoperative

Postoperative

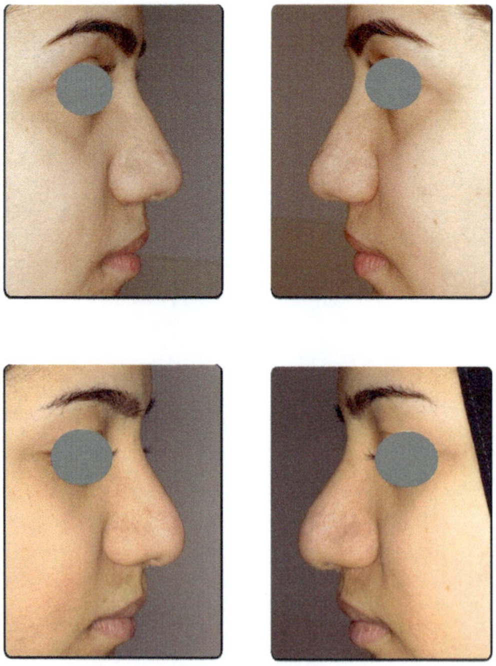

Part III: Clinical Case 5

20

Preoperative Assessment

1. **Frontolateral walls**
   a. The main bulk of the lower third of the nose is caused by the bulky lateral crurae and bulky scroll areas (Frontal Views).
   b. There was dissociation between the lower third and the upper two third. They were semiseparated from each other (Frontal Views).
2. **Medial Wall**
   Nil of note.
3. **Bony pyramid**
   Wide base of the boney pyramid.
4. **Alar base**
   Nil of note.

Aims of Surgery

1. Reduce the bulk of the lower third i.e. the frontolateral walls, including the scroll area.
2. Reduce the width of the boney base.

Surgical Plan

1. **Frontolateral walls**
   a. DDD not including the weak triangle to reduce the bulk of the nasal tip and midvault.
   b. Trimming of the scroll areas, by direct excision of the areas of overlap, to reduce their bulk.
   c. Cephalic trim of lateral crurae to reduce the size of the nasal tip.
2. **Medial Wall**
   Nil of note.
3. **Bony pyramid**
   Bilateral osteotomies and medializations of the lateral bony walls to reduce the size of a bony pyramid.
4. **Alar base**
   Nil of note.

Surgical Procedure

As per Surgical Plan.

Post-Operative Analysis

1. **Frontolateral Wall**
   a. Tip definition: the nasal tip is smaller with thinner and smoother overlying skin. It is more prominent and well identified from the alae nasi on both sides. The alae nasi come into view to become clearly visible and share in nasal aesthetics (Frontal Views).
   b. Tip light reflex is seen as one spot off the nasal tip (Frontal Views).
2. **Medial Wall**
   Nil of Note.
3. **Bony Pyramid**
   Bony pyramid aesthetics: the nasal dorsum is straight and the sidewalls are smooth and narrow.
4. **Alar Base**
   Nil of Note.

Commentary

a. Defatting and trim of the scroll areas have resulted in complete integration between the upper two thirds and the lower third of the nose. The nose appears as one unit.

M. H. A. Shafy, *Atlas of Clinical Cases in Rhinoplasty*,
https://doi.org/10.1007/978-3-031-07504-9_20

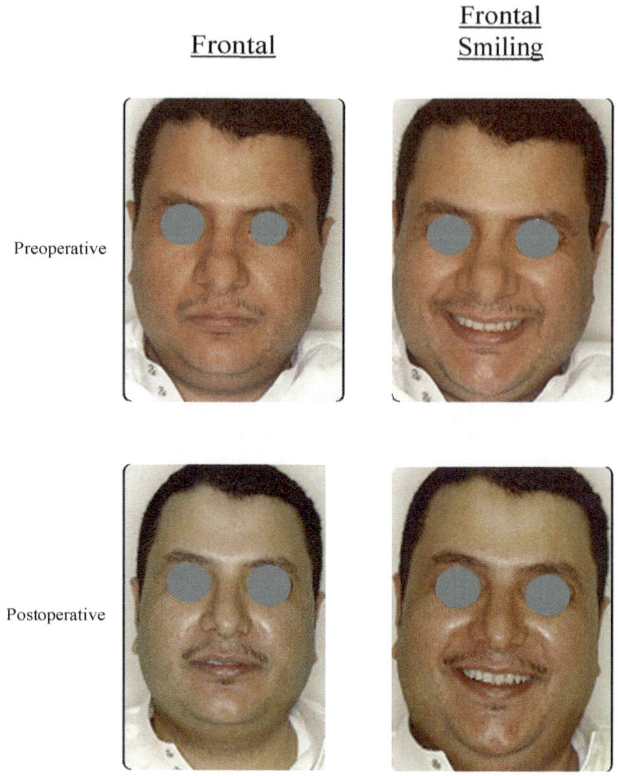
Frontal
Frontal Smiling
Preoperative
Postoperative

Part III: Clinical Case 6

21

Preoperative Assessment

1. **Frontolateral walls**
   a. Bulbous bulky tip, overshadowing the alae nasi on both sides (Frontal, Direct Dorsal, Overhead, Backward Tilting, Basal and Nasal Aperture Views).
   b. There is a dissociation between the bulbous tip and the upper two thirds of the nose (Frontal and Backward Tilting Views).
2. **Medial Wall**
   Nil of note.
3. **Bony pyramid**
   a. Small osteocartilaginous hump due to the natural concavoconvex anatomy of the nasal bones from above downwards (See Anatomy Section) (Backward Tilting, Oblique and Lateral Views).
   b. Wide base of the bony pyramid (Backward Tilting and Direct Dorsal Views).
4. **Alar base**
   a. The nasal apertures are of aesthetically reasonable size. The inferior segments of the rim-sill folds are not long. The posterior segments are not bulky, no flat tire appearance (Backward Tilting and Basal Views). The main bulk of the nose was in the frontolateral walls.
   b. Nasal openings were thick walled and had rounded shape.

Aims of Surgery

1. Reduction of the bulk of the frontolateral walls.
2. Reduction of the size of the bony pyramid.

Surgical Plan

1. **Frontolateral walls**
   a. DDD including the weak triangle to reduce the bulk of the nasaltip and supra tip area.
   b. Cephalic reduction of the lateral crurae to reduce the size.
2. **Medial Wall**
   Nil of note.
3. **Bony pyramid**
   a. Excision of the osteocartilaginous hump.
   b. Osteotomies and medialization of the lateral bony walls.
4. **Alar base**
   Nil of note.

Surgical Procedure

As per Surgical Plan.

Post-Operative Analysis

1. **Frontolateral Walls**
   a. Tip definition improved, the tip is slimmer, the alae nasi came into view to share in nasal aesthetics (Frontal, Direct Dorsal, Overhead, Backward Tilting, Basal and Nasal Aperture Views).
   b. Tip light reflex is seen as one spot off the nasal tip (Frontal and Backward Tilting Views).
2. **Medial Wall**
   Nil of Note.

M. H. A. Shafy, *Atlas of Clinical Cases in Rhinoplasty*,
https://doi.org/10.1007/978-3-031-07504-9_21

3. **Bony Pyramid**
   a. Bony pyramid aesthetics improved: the nasal dorsum is straight and the sidewalls are smooth and narrow (all views except the Basal Views).
   b. Dorsal light reflex is seen as an uninterrupted line off the nasal dorsum (Direct Dorsal Views).
4. **Alar Base**
   a. The superior alar grooves now clear off fat, become deeper, longer and visible (Direct Dorsal, Oblique and Lateral Views).
   b. Posterior alar groove aesthetics improved. The angle of the alae nasi with the upper lip is wider. Aesthetics of the alae nasi is better.
   c. Alae nasi aesthetics improved. They are pulled medially become better seen, smaller and share in nasal aesthetics (Nasal Aperture, Oblique and Lateral Views).
   d. Nasal aperture aesthetics: defatting alone of the frontolateral enhances aesthetics of the nasal openings without affecting their size. They become more elegantly oval in shape posterior to the nicely defined tip (Basal View).
   e. Marginal light reflexes are clearly seen at the inferior alar margins (Nasal Aperture Views).

Commentary

a. The rounded, bulky nasal tip has been a concern to the nasal appearance all his adult life. Simple reduction in the size of the boney pyramid and the bulk of the nasal tip have achieved that goal for him and had a positive aesthetic effect to the nose and the face.
b. The lower third of the nose including the nasal tip is now integrated with the upper two thirds of the nose and they look as one unit (Frontal, Direct Dorsal and Backward Tilting Views).
c. The skeletal structure of this gentleman's nose is quite small as compared to the size of his face and head. Having better defined tip and nasal dorsum resulted in a better aesthetic match with the face.

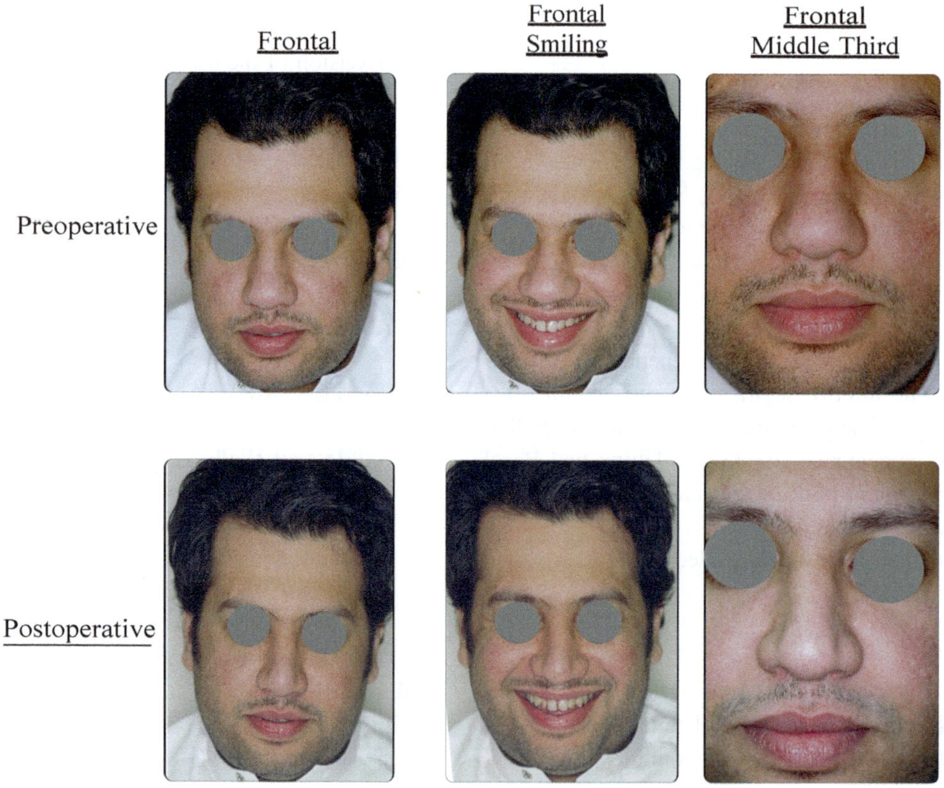

Direct Dorsal | Direct Dorsal Smiling | Overhead

Preoperative

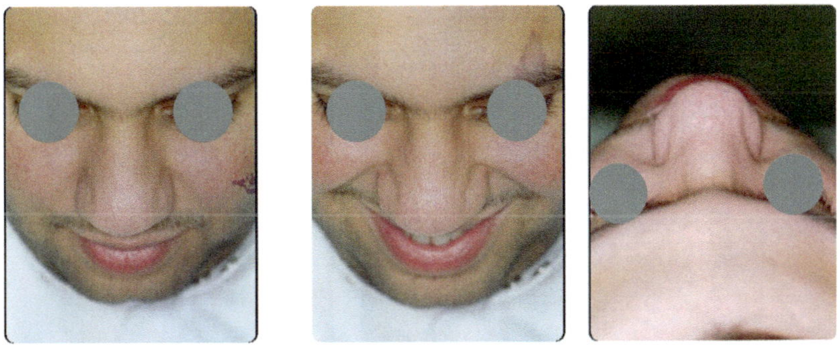

Postoperative

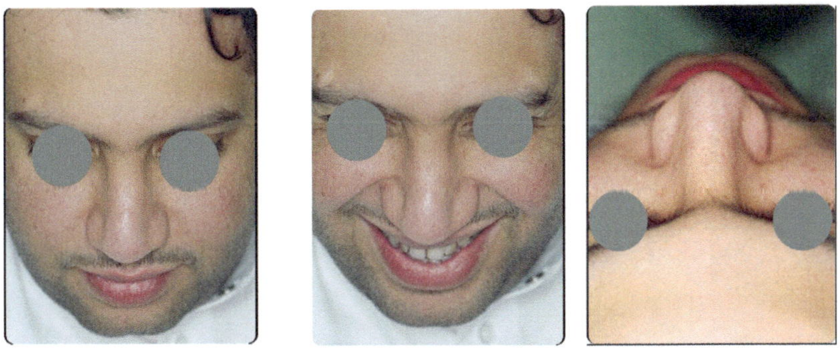

Backward Tilting | Steeper Backward Tilting | Basal | Basal Smiling

Preoperative

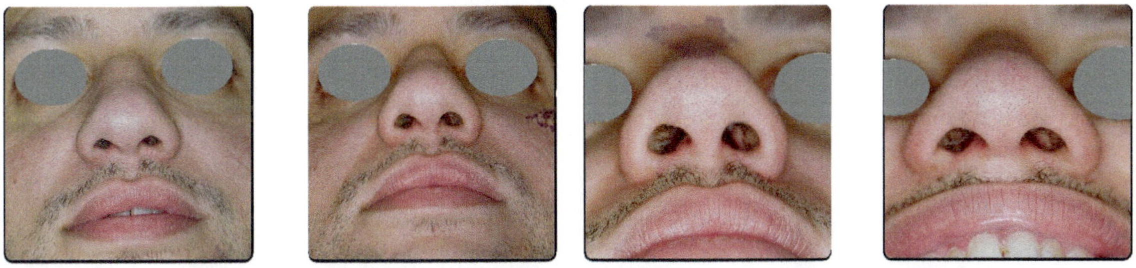

Postoperative

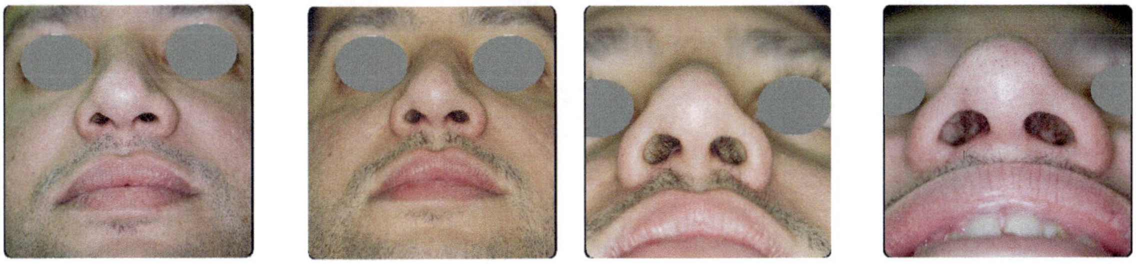

Better nasal tip definition postoperatively

Right Nasal Aperture | Right Nasal Aperture Rim Sill Test | Left Nasal Aperture Rim Sill Test | Left Nasal Aperture

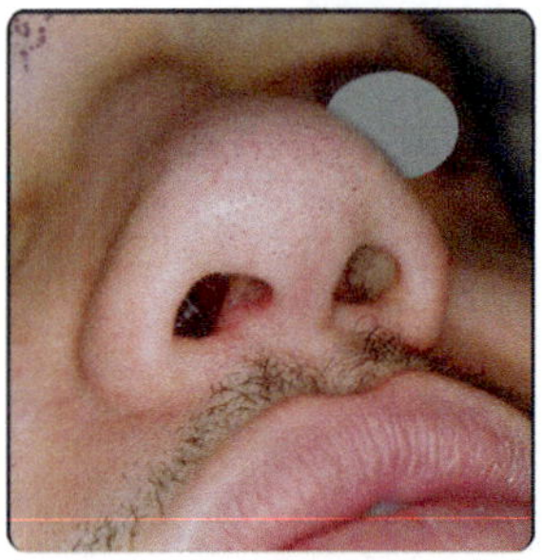

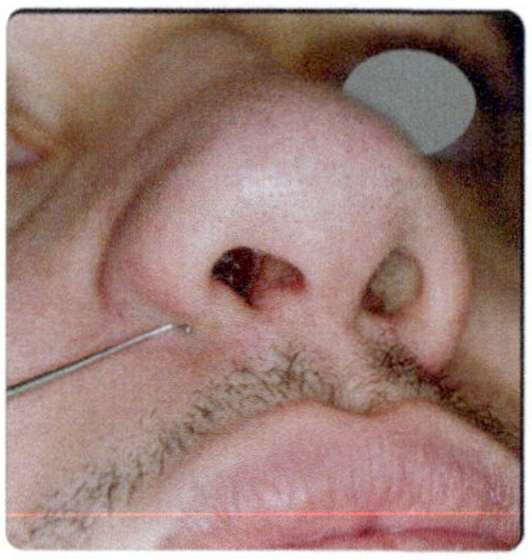

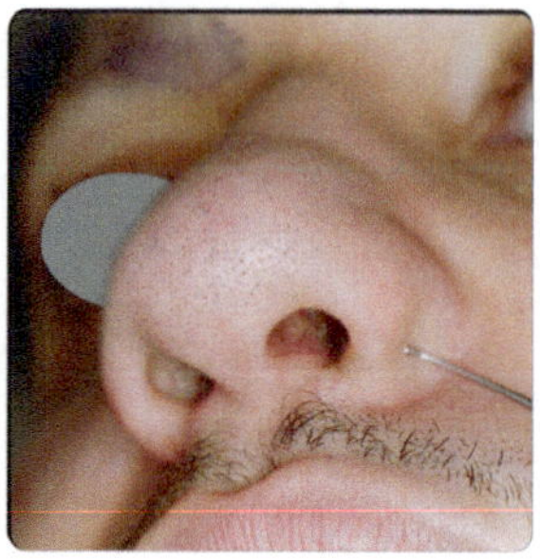

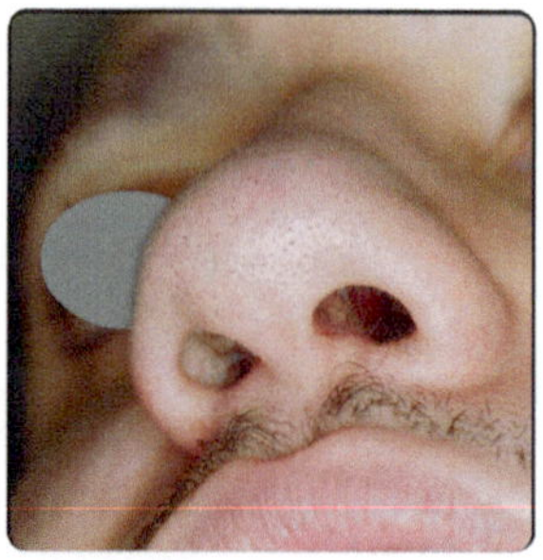

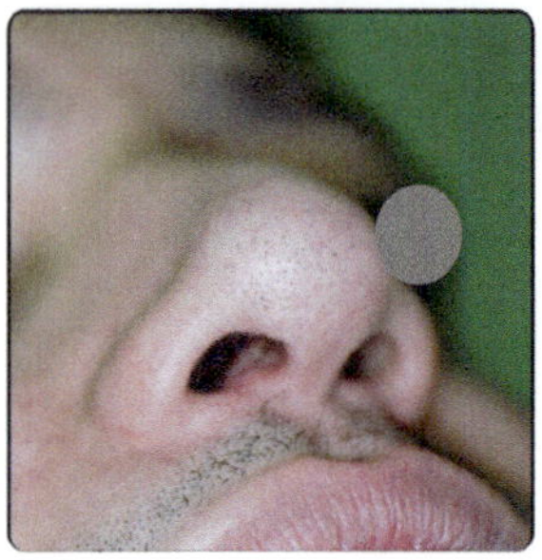

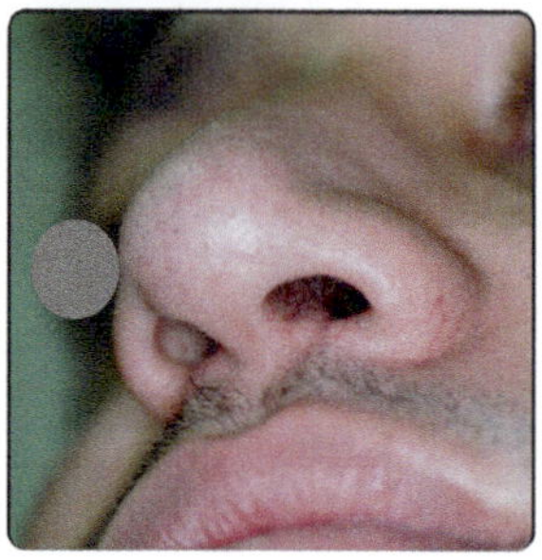

Right Oblique Mid Cheek Full Face | Left Oblique Mid Cheek Full Face | Right Oblique Mid Cheek Middle Third | Left Oblique Mid Cheek Middle Third

Preoperative

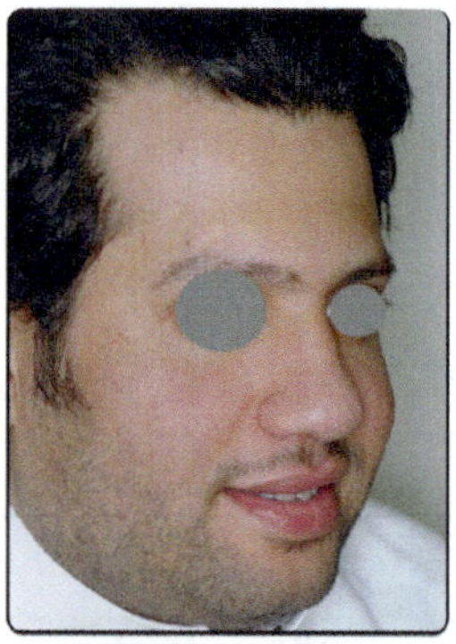

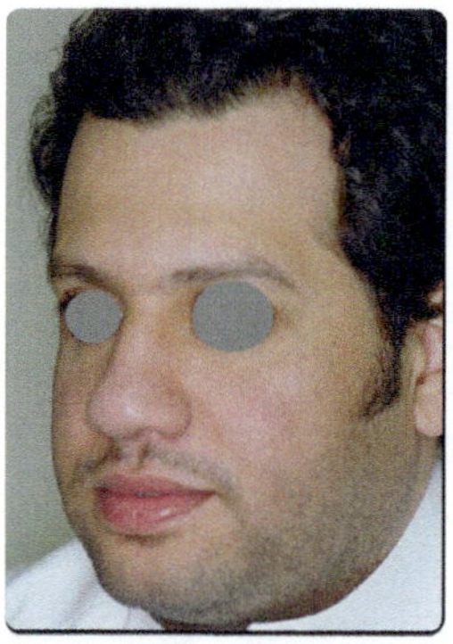

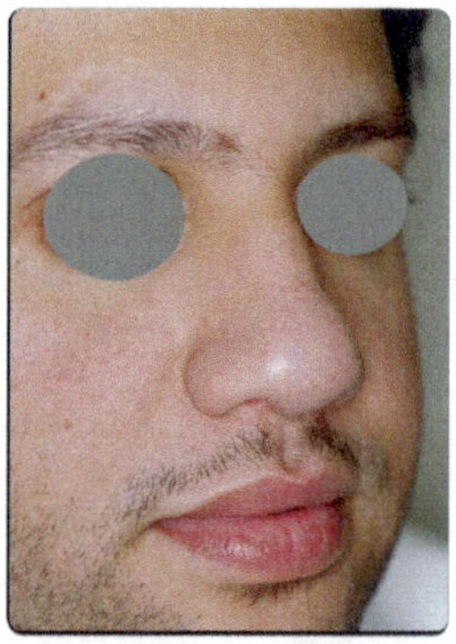

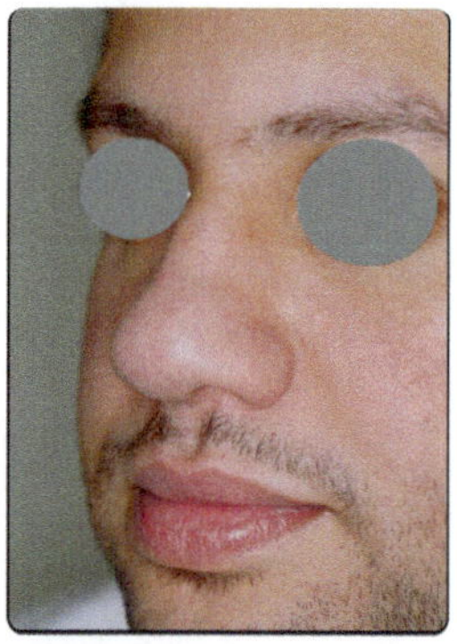

Postoperative

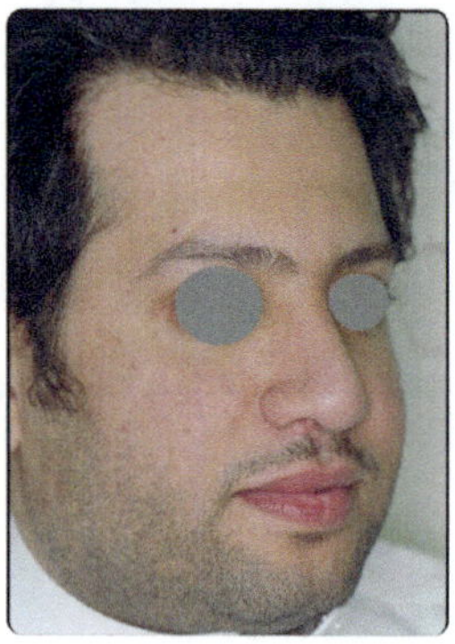

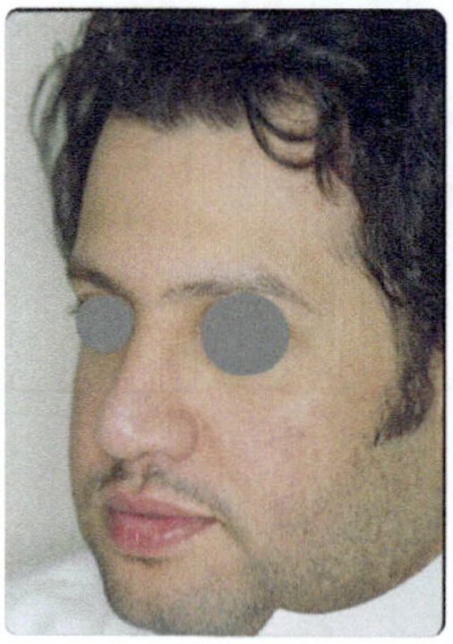

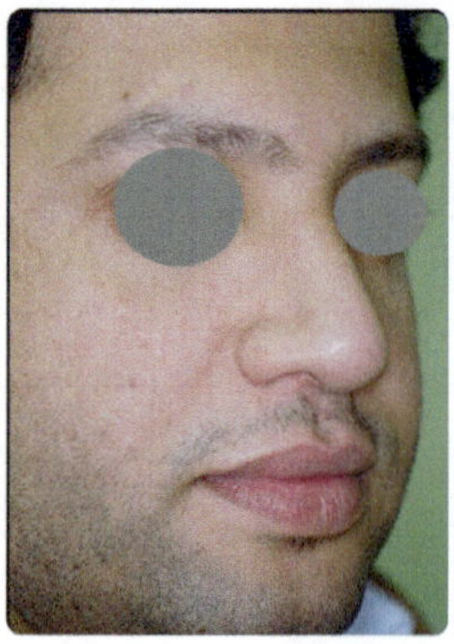

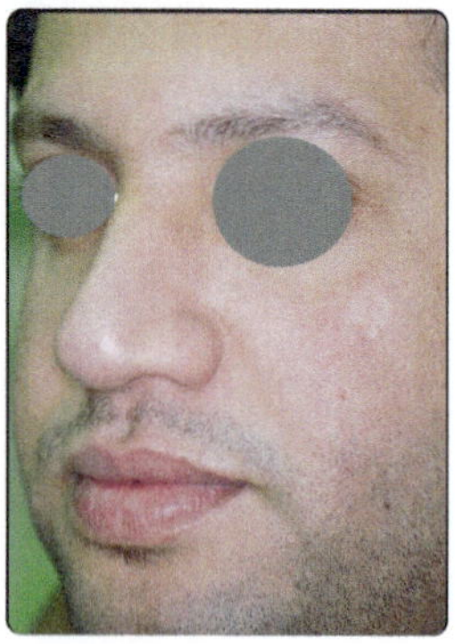

Right Oblique Cheek Margin Full Face | **Left Oblique Cheek Margin Full Face** | **Right Oblique Cheek Margin Middle Third** | **Left Oblique Cheek Margin Middle Third**

Preoperative

Postoperative

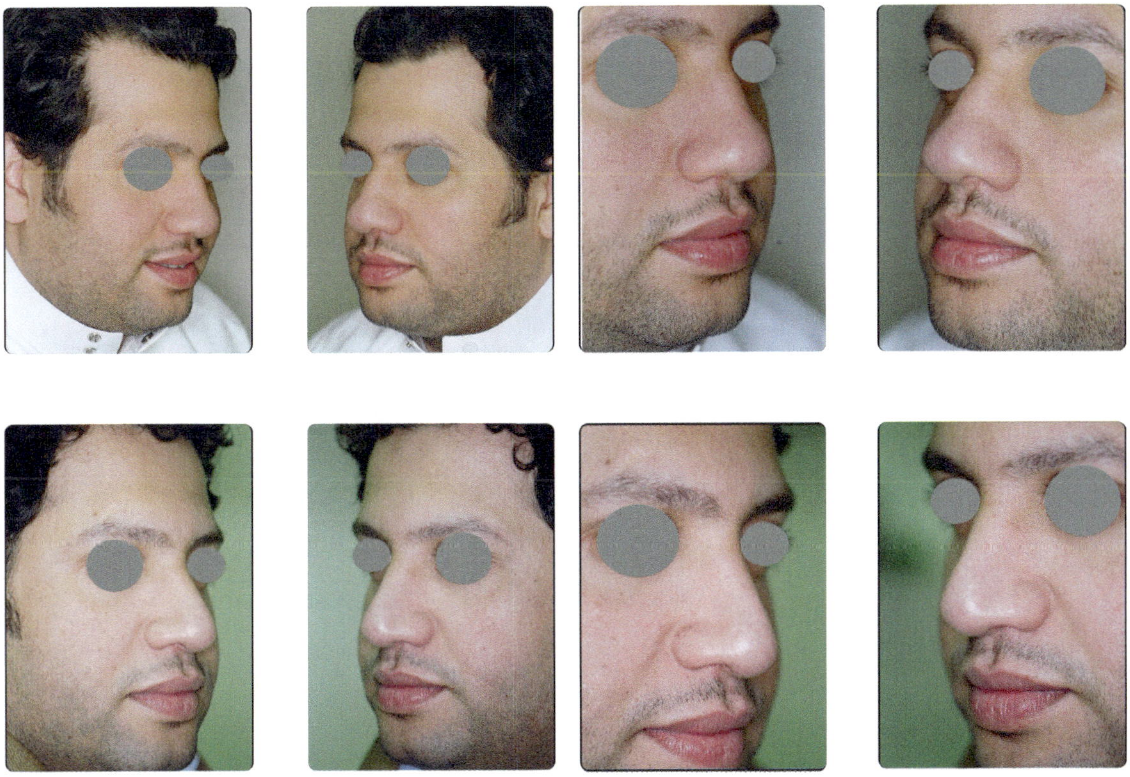

Right Lateral | Left Lateral | Right Lateral Smiling | Left Lateral Smiling

Preoperative

Postoperative

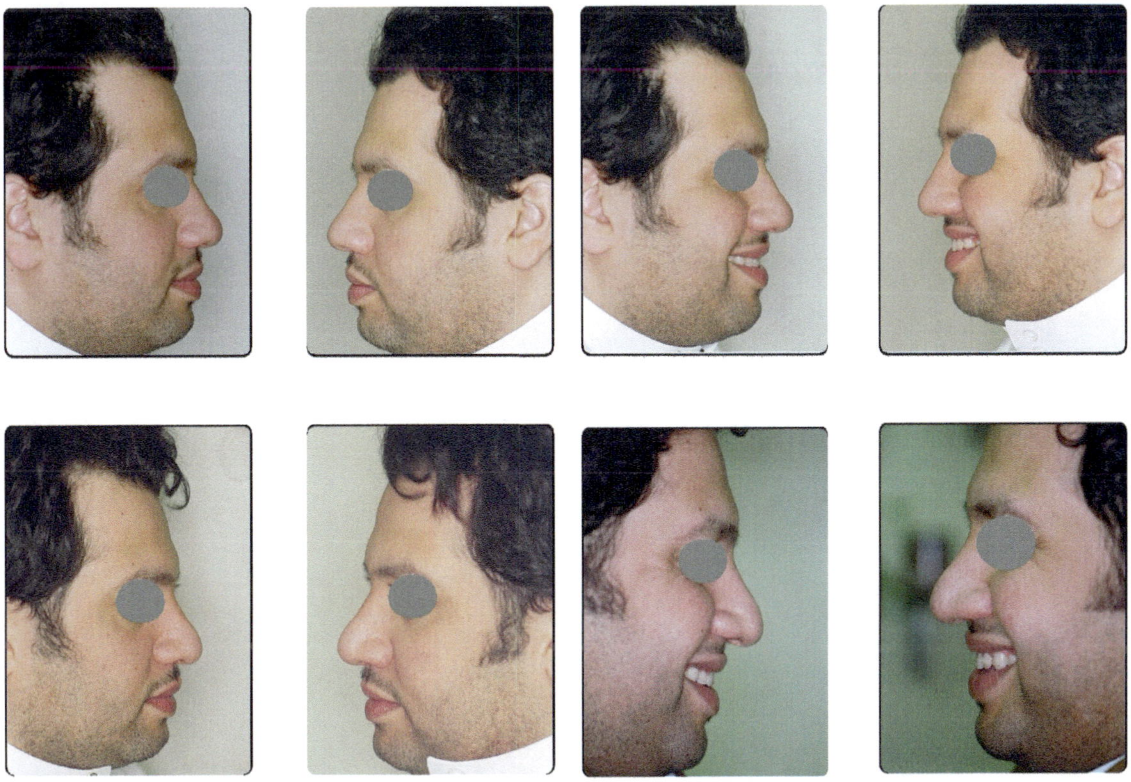

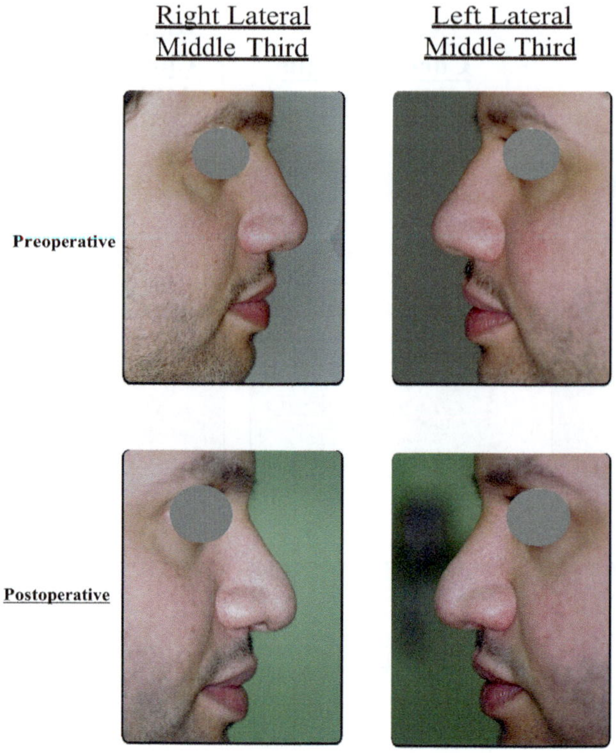
Right Lateral Middle Third
Left Lateral Middle Third
Preoperative
Postoperative

Part III: Clinical Case 7

22

Preoperative Assessment

1. **Frontolateral walls**
   Bulky and large with broad tip. The alae nasi were hardly seen (Frontal, Direct Dorsal and Overhead Views).
2. **Medial Wall**
   Mobile tip (Lateral Smiling Views).
3. **Bony pyramid**
   a. Small osteocartilaginous hump (Lateral and Oblique Views).
   b. Wide base of the boney pyramid (Direct Dorsal and Backward Tilting Views).
4. **Alar base**
   Wide alar base. The nasal openings were wide with transverse long axes.

Aims of Surgery

Reduction of the overall bulk and size of the nose:

a. Reduction of the bulk and size of the tip.
b. Reduction of the size of the bony pyramid.
c. Reduction of the alar base size and bulk.

Surgical Plan

1. **Frontolateral walls**
   a. DDD including the weak triangle to reduce the bulk and size of the tip and supratip area.
   b. Cephalic trim of the lateral crurae to reduce the size.
2. **Medial Wall**
   Division of the Depressor Septi muscles.
3. **Bony pyramid**
   a. Excision of the osteocartilaginous hump.
   b. Osteotomies and medialization of the lateral bony walls to reduce the size of the bony pyramid.
4. **Alar base**
   Bilateral resection of the inferior and posterior segments of the rim sill folds.

Surgical Procedure

a. As per Surgical Plan.
b. A supra tip depression appeared after the procedure. This was dealt with by a supra tip graft using trimming of the lateral crurae.

Post-Operative Analysis

1. **Frontolateral Wall**
   a. Tip definition improved i.e. slimmer and prominently well identified with thinner skin. The alae nasi came into view to share in nasal aesthetics (Frontal, Direct Dorsal, Overhead, Backward Tilting and Basal Views). Note the clear light reflex of nasal tip (Backward Tilting Views).
   b. Tip projection: The nasal tip at the same level of the nasal dorsum with good aesthetic angle. This is coupled with good aesthetic nasolabial angle (lateral and oblique views).
   c. Tip light reflex is clear as one spot off the nasal tip (Frontal and Backward Tilting Views).
2. **Medial Wall**
   Nil of Note.
3. **Bony Pyramid**
   a. Bony pyramid aesthetics improved. The nasal dorsum is straight and the sidewalls are smooth and narrow (all views except the Basal Views).
   b. Dorsal light reflex is seen as a regular one line off the nasal dorsum (Direct Dorsal Views).
4. **Alar Base**
   a. The superior alar grooves now clear off fat, become deeper, longer and visible (Direct Dorsal, Oblique and Lateral Views).
   b. Posterior alar groove aesthetics improved after excising the posterior segment of the rim-sill fold. Flat tire appearance is no longer present (Backward Tilting, Basal and Nasal Aperture Views).

M. H. A. Shafy, *Atlas of Clinical Cases in Rhinoplasty*,
https://doi.org/10.1007/978-3-031-07504-9_22

c. Alae nasi aesthetics improved. They are pulled medially widening the posterior alar groove angles. They are better seen and smaller in size.

d. Nasal aperture aesthetics improved after defatting and excision of the rim sill folds:
   i. The size of the nasal openings are smaller.
   ii. The shape of nasal openings transformed from thick heavy wide and round opening with transverse long axes to thin delicate small oval openings with anterior long axes. (Basal, Backward Tilting and Nasal Aperture Views).

e. Marginal light reflexes are clearly seen at:
   i. Inferior alar margins (Nasal Aperture Views).
   ii. Nasal sill bands (Oblique Views).
   iii. Lateral crural prominences (Lateral Views).

Commentary

a. As he wished for, this gentleman's nose maintained its image and his own nasal print in a smaller scale.

b. The heavy bulky appearance and the large size problems were overcome. His nose looks naturally smaller and more delicately suiting the rest of his other facial features.

Frontal | Frontal Smiling | Frontal Middle Third

Preoperative

Postoperative

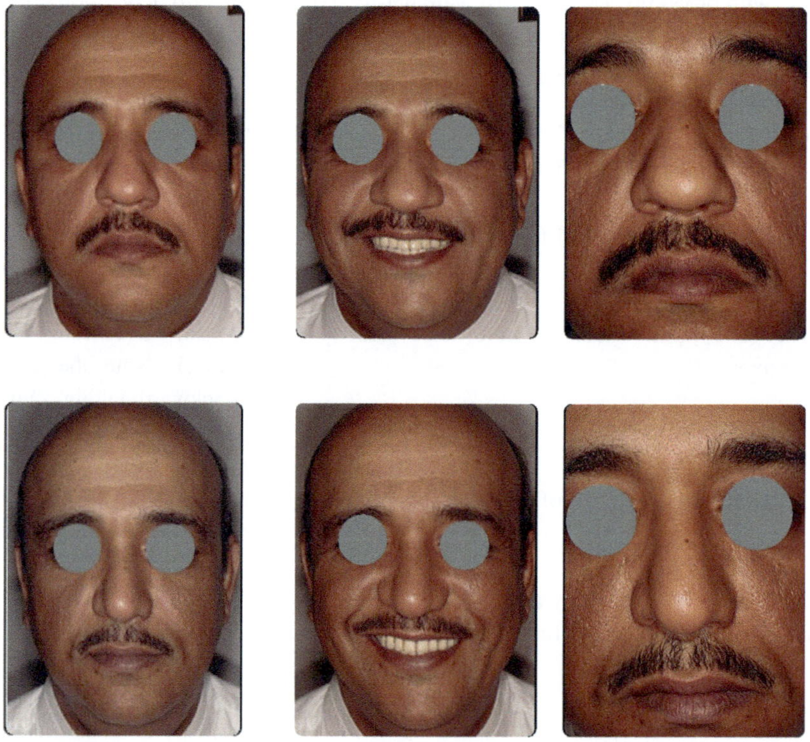

Direct Dorsal | Direct Dorsal Smiling | Overhead | Overhead Smiling

Preoperative

Postoperative

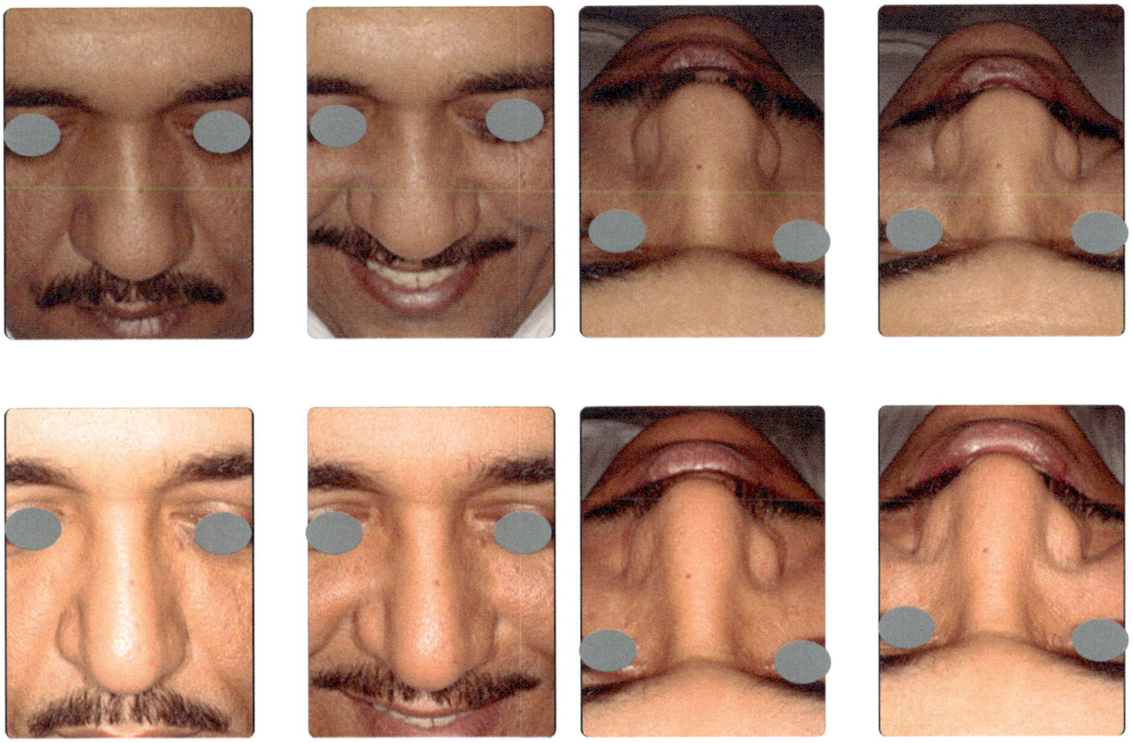

Backward Tilting | Steeper Backward Tilting | Basal | Basal Smiling

Preoperative

Postoperative

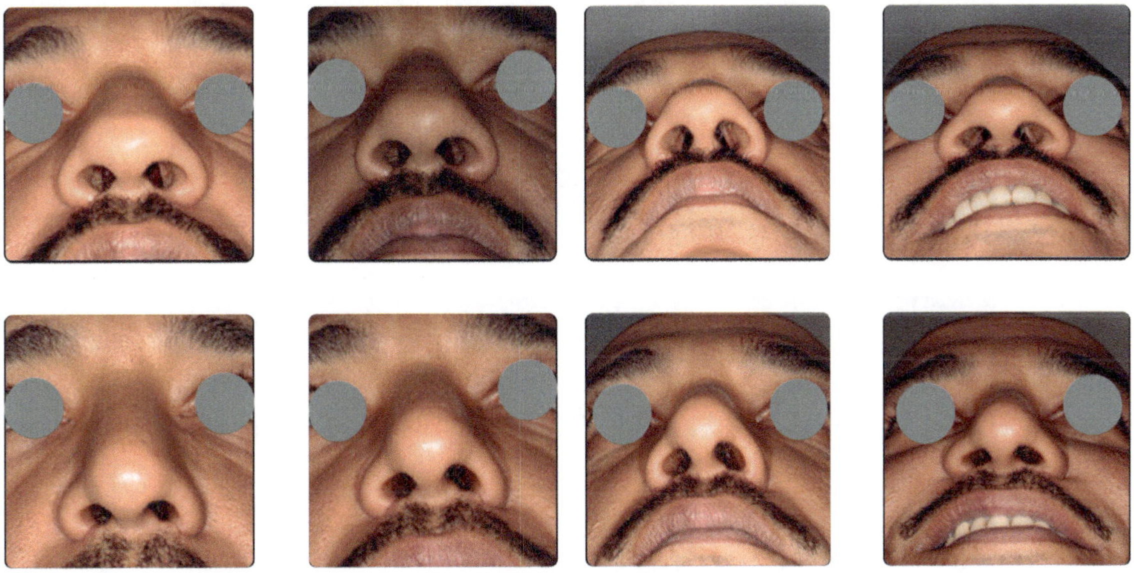

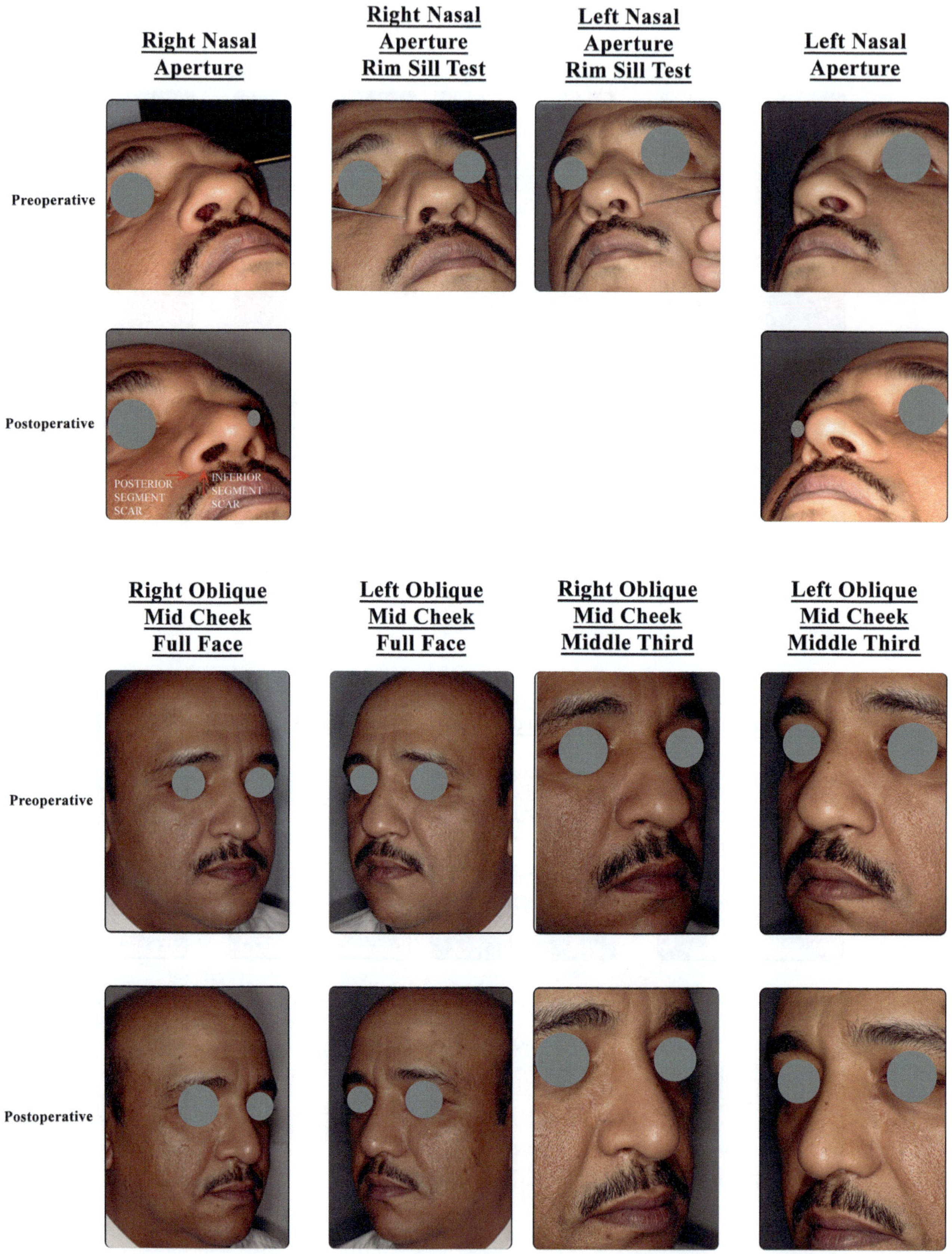
Right Nasal Aperture
Right Nasal Aperture Rim Sill Test
Left Nasal Aperture Rim Sill Test
Left Nasal Aperture
Preoperative
Postoperative
POSTERIOR SEGMENT SCAR
INFERIOR SEGMENT SCAR
Right Oblique Mid Cheek Full Face
Left Oblique Mid Cheek Full Face
Right Oblique Mid Cheek Middle Third
Left Oblique Mid Cheek Middle Third
Preoperative
Postoperative

Right Oblique Cheek Margin Full Face	Left Oblique Cheek Margin Full Face	Right Oblique Cheek Margin Middle Third	Left Oblique Cheek Margin Middle Third

Preoperative

Postoperative

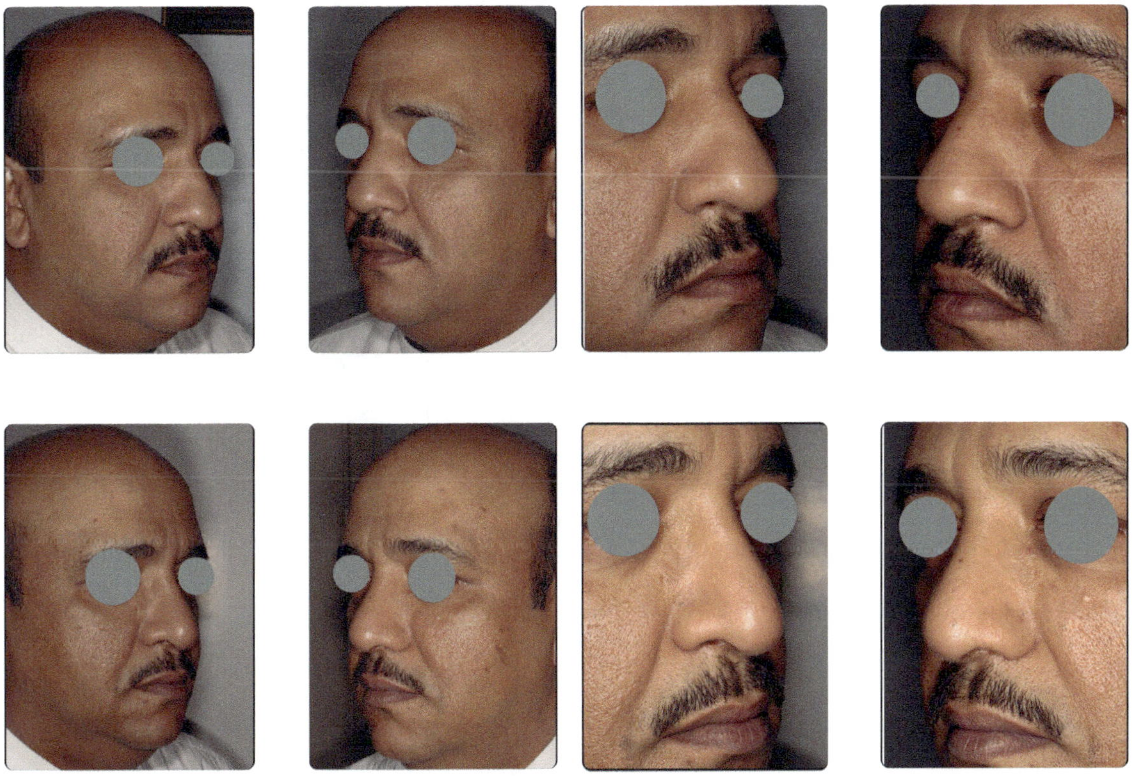

Right Lateral	Left Lateral	Right Lateral Smiling	Left Lateral Smiling

Preoperative

Postoperative

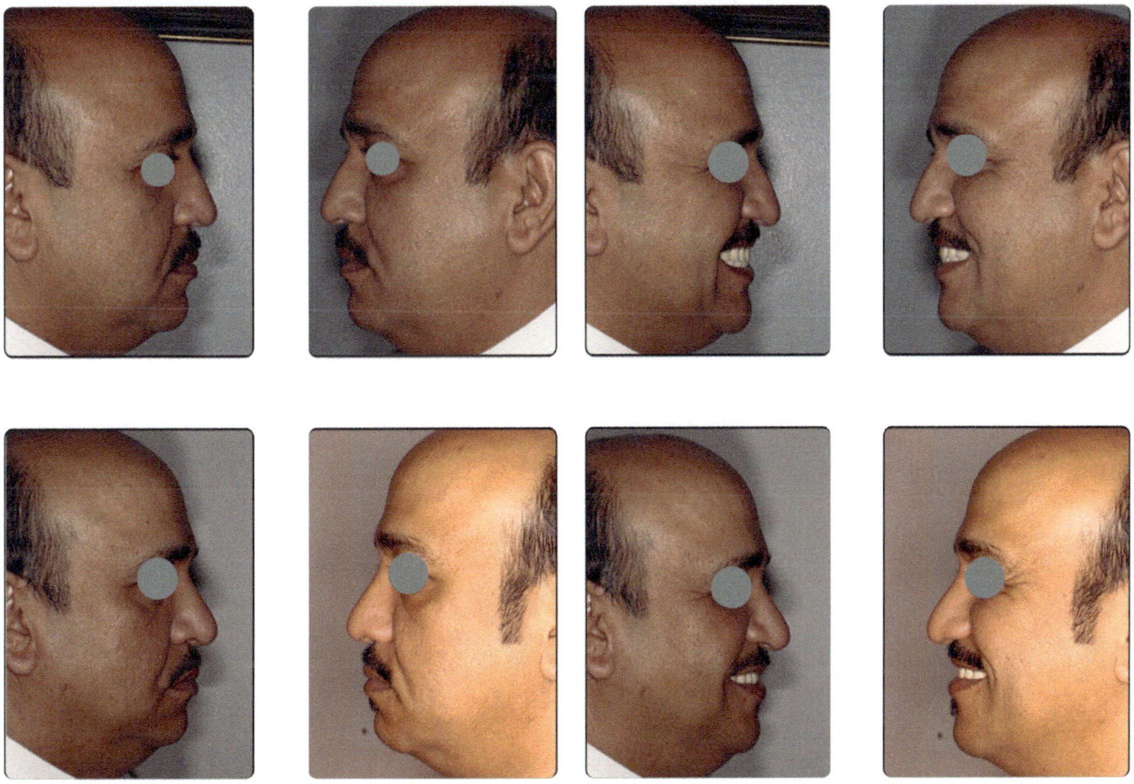

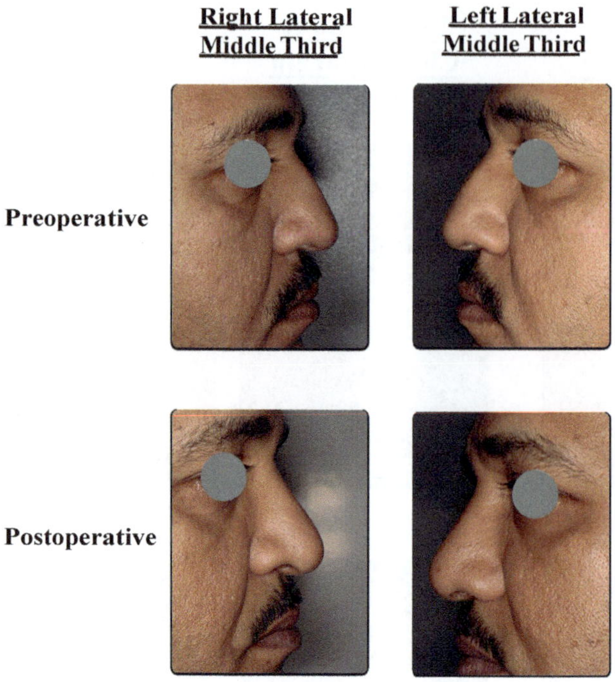
Right Lateral
Middle Third
Left Lateral
Middle Third
Preoperative
Postoperative

Part III: Clinical Case 8

23

Preoperative Assessment

1. **Frontolateral walls**
   a. Bulky, bulbous tip completely overshadowing the alae nasi (Frontal, Direct Dorsal and Overhead Views).
   b. Bifid tip (Frontal, Backward Tilting and Basal Views).
2. **Medial Wall**
   Mobile tip (Lateral Smiling Views).
3. **Bony pyramid**
   a. Wide base of the boney pyramid (Frontal, Direct Dorsal and Backward Tilting Views).
   b. Bilateral maxillary asymmetry, the right maxilla is high and low and the left is low and wid with a smaller frontal process (Backward Tilting Views).
   c. Interrupted light reflex (Direct Dorsal Views).
4. **Alar base**
   a. The nasal openings are small but unaesthetically rounded and thick walled (Backward Tilting, Basal and Nasal Aperture Views).
   b. The posterior alar groove has acute nasolabial angle i.e. flat tire appearance (Backward Tilting, Basal and Nasal Aperture Views).

Aims of Surgery

1. Reduce the bulk of the frontolateral walls.
2. Abolish the mobility of the nasal tip.
3. Reduce the width of the base of the boney pyramid.

Surgical Plan

1. **Frontolateral walls**
   a. DDD including the weak triangle to reduce the bulk of nasal tip and midvault.
   b. Bilateral cephalic trim of the lateral crurae to reduce the size of the nasal tip.
2. **Medial Wall**
   Division of the Depressor Septi muscles.
3. **Bony pyramid**
   Osteotomies and medialization of the lateral bony walls to reduce the width of the bony pyramid.
4. **Alar base**
   Nil of note.

Surgical Procedure

a. As per Surgical Plan.
b. Division of the Depressor Septi muscles was performed intranasally.
c. Dorsal graft using septal cartilage.

Post-Operative Analysis

1. **Frontolateral Wall**
   a. Tip definition improved i.e. slimmer and prominently well identified with thinner overlying skin. The alae nasi come into view to share in nasal aesthetics (Frontal, Direct Dorsal, Overhead, Backward Tilting and Basal Views).
   b. Tip projection: The nasal tip at the same level of the nasal dorsum with good aesthetic angle. This is coupled with good aesthetic nasolabial angle (lateral and oblique views).
   c. Tip light reflex as one spot off the nasal tip (backward tilting and frontal views).
2. **Medial Wall**
   Nil of Note.
3. **Bony Pyramid**
   a. Bony pyramid aesthetics improved: the nasal dorsum is straight and the sidewalls are smooth and narrow (all views except the Basal Views).
   b. Dorsal light reflex is seen as an uninterrupted line off the nasal dorsum (Direct Dorsal Views).

M. H. A. Shafy, *Atlas of Clinical Cases in Rhinoplasty*,
https://doi.org/10.1007/978-3-031-07504-9_23

4. **Alar Base**
   a. The superior alar groove aesthetics improved: now clear off fat, become deeper, longer and visible (Direct Dorsal, Oblique and Lateral Views).
   b. Posterior alar groove aesthetics improved by defatting. Flat tire appearance is no longer present (Backward Tilting, Basal and Nasal Aperture Views).
   c. Aesthetic of the alae nasi improved. They are pulled medially by defatting, become better seen and look larger.
   d. Nasal aperture aesthetics improved by defatting alone without the change in their size. They were transformed from round thick walled heavy looking openings to oval thin walled delicate openings with anteriorly directed long axes.
   e. Marginal light reflexes are clearly seen at:
      a. Inferior alar margins (Nasal Aperture Views).
      b. Nasal sill bands (Oblique Views).
      c. Lateral crural prominences (Lateral Views).

Commentary

a. Small noses are very challenging. Any small deformity, natural or iatrogenic, is exaggerated and appears as a large one and vice versa any positive aesthetic, addition, appears, attractively nice.
b. The post operative photographs were taken only seven days post-operatively.
c. This lady had a small, short, but bulky nose. Visually, the nose seemed to be made up of two dissociated parts; the upper two thirds and the lower third. There was no smooth continuity between the two parts (Frontal and Backward Tilting).
d. The upper third is made up of a low, wide based boney pyramid covered by thin skin. This is followed by the rapid increase in the skin thickness over the lower half of the midvault and the nasal tip, i.e. the bulky part occupies almost 50% of the whole nose.
e. Although the nasal dorsum did not appear low preoperatively, yet after osteotomies it was low compared to the lower third of the nose. A septal cartilaginous graft was necessary to augment it. As the boney pyramid was very short, osteotomies and medialization of its lateral walls were not sufficient to proportionately elevate the nasal dorsum.
f. The location of the right osteotomy was farther away from the mid line than the left due to bilateral maxillary asymmetry (refer to the frontal and backward tilting views).
g. No tip grafts and no direct crural stitching. The nose maintained its natural soft feeling and the normal physiological role.
h. Postoperatively the nose appears as one continuous unit that is slimmer and longer. The naso-facial relationship has greatly improved with better overall facial appearance (Frontal Direct Dorsal and Overhead Views).

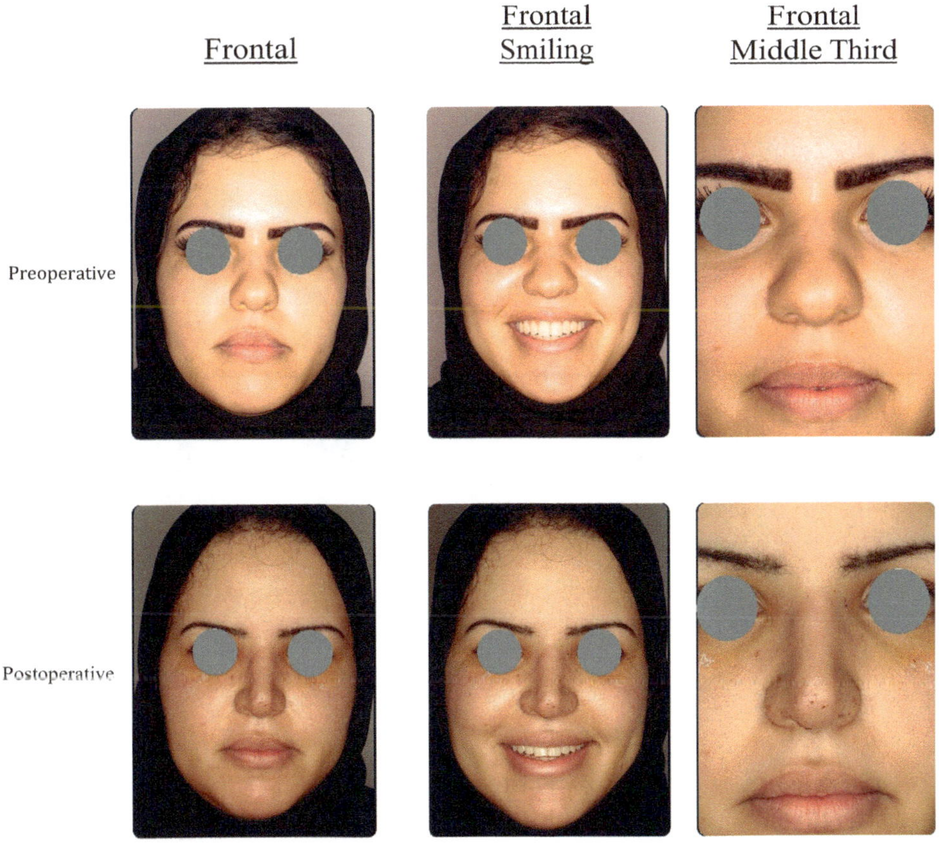
Frontal
Frontal Smiling
Frontal Middle Third
Preoperative
Postoperative

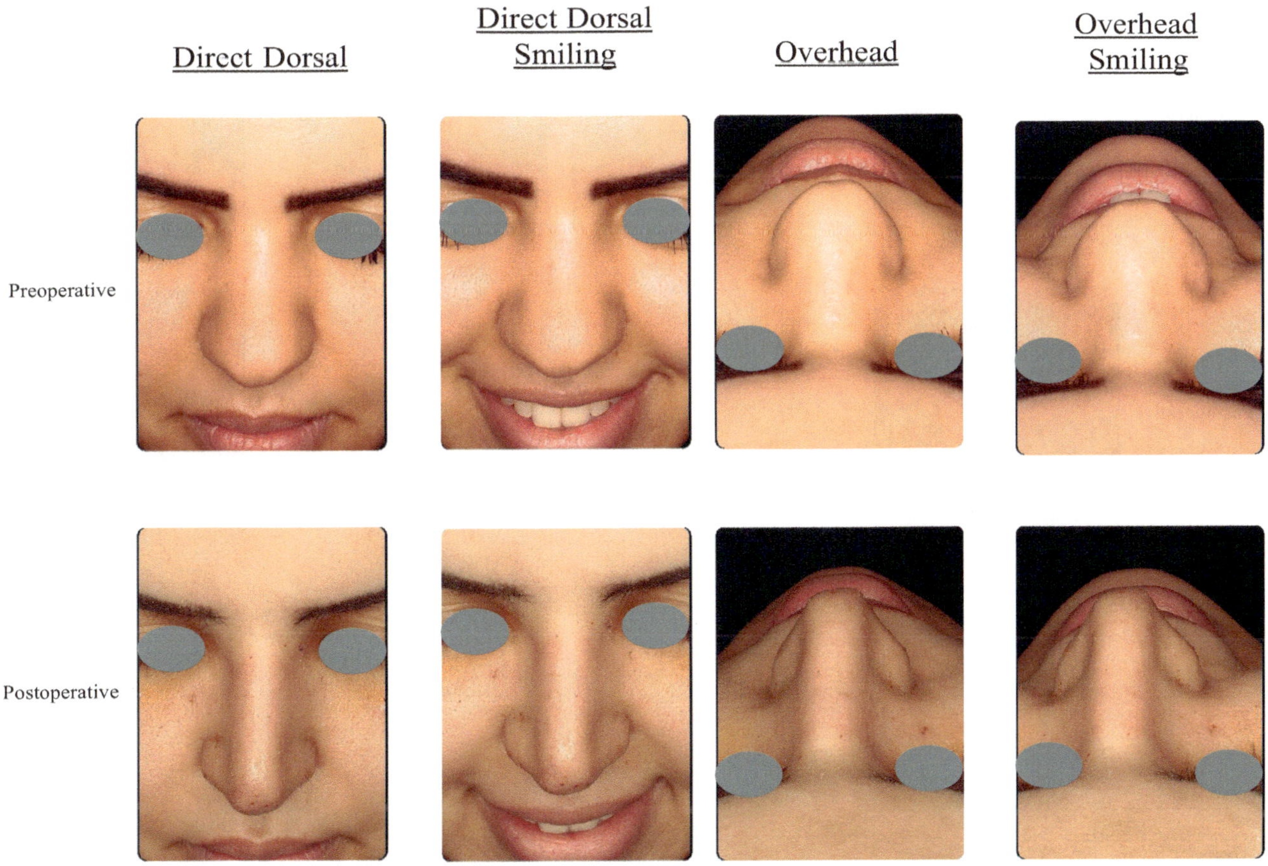
Direct Dorsal
Direct Dorsal Smiling
Overhead
Overhead Smiling
Preoperative
Postoperative

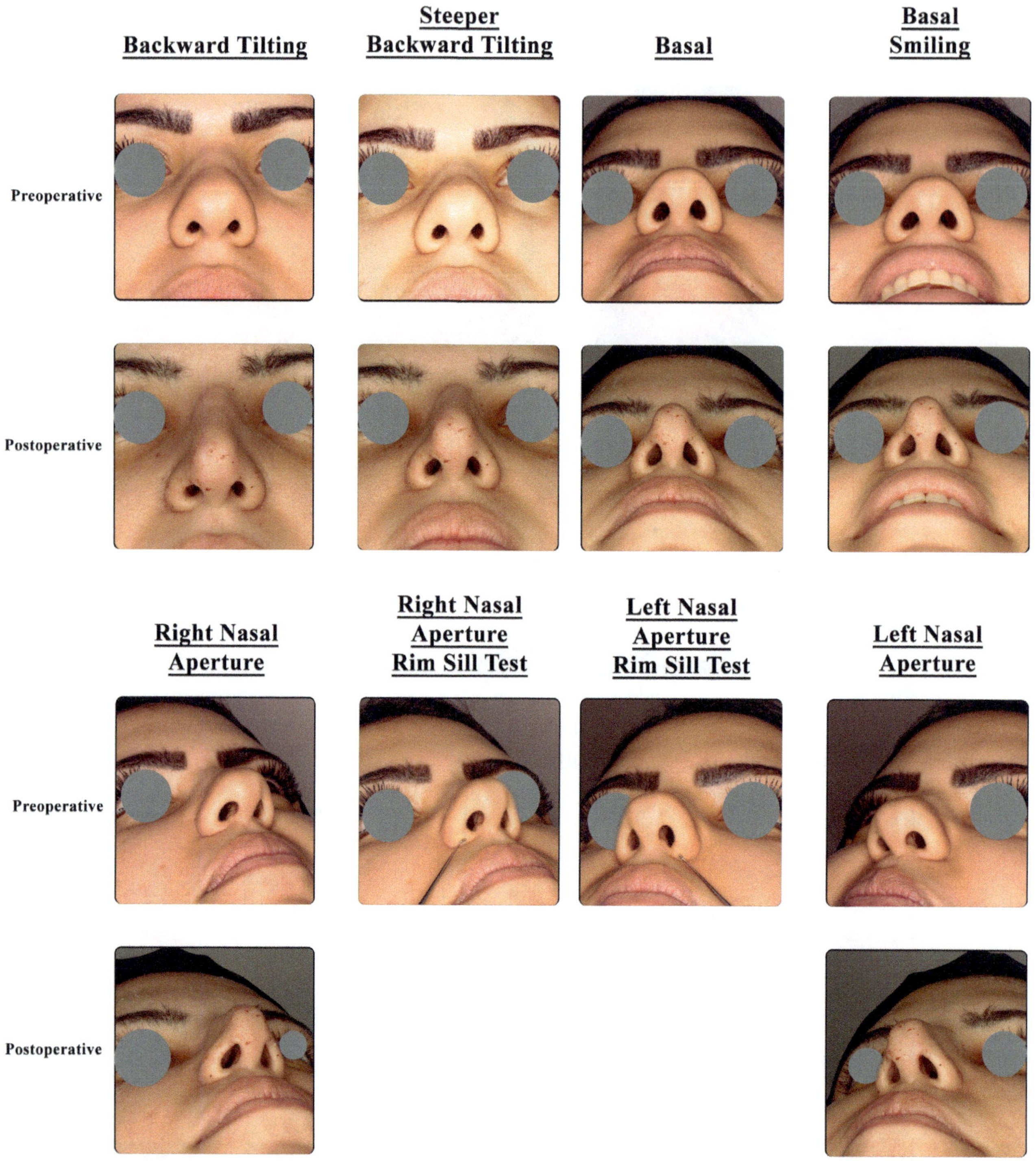
Backward Tilting
Steeper Backward Tilting
Basal
Basal Smiling
Preoperative
Postoperative
Right Nasal Aperture
Right Nasal Aperture Rim Sill Test
Left Nasal Aperture Rim Sill Test
Left Nasal Aperture
Preoperative
Postoperative

Right Oblique Mid Cheek Full Face	Left Oblique Mid Cheek Full Face	Right Oblique Mid Cheek Middle Third	Left Oblique Mid Cheek Middle Third

Preoperative

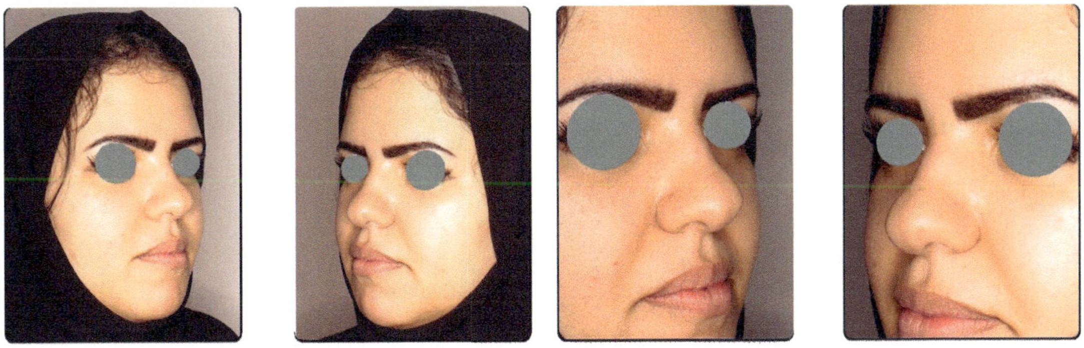

Postoperative

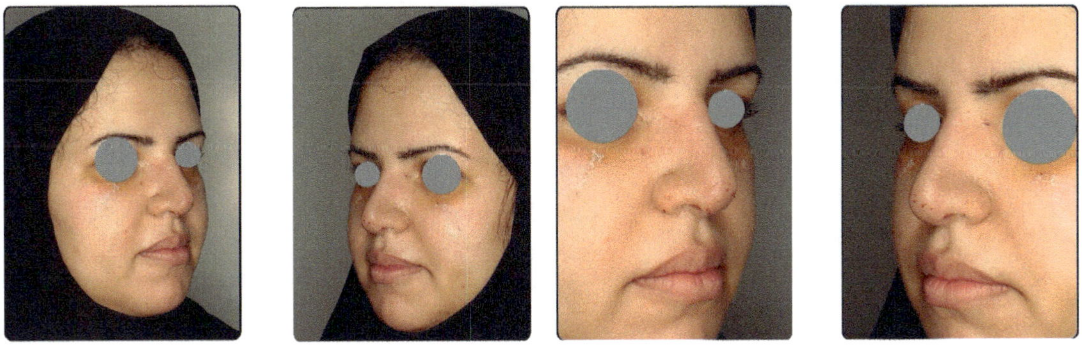

Right Oblique Cheek Margin Full Face	Left Oblique Cheek Margin Full Face	Right Oblique Cheek Margin Middle Third	Left Oblique Cheek Margin Middle Third

Preoperative

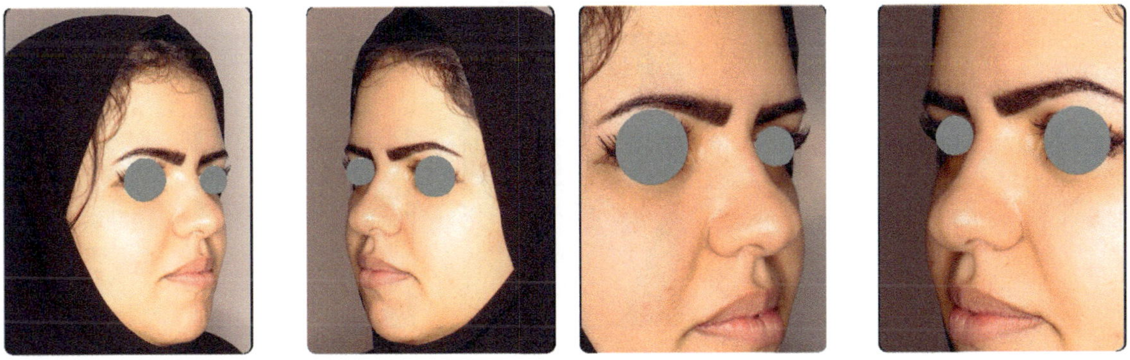

Postoperative

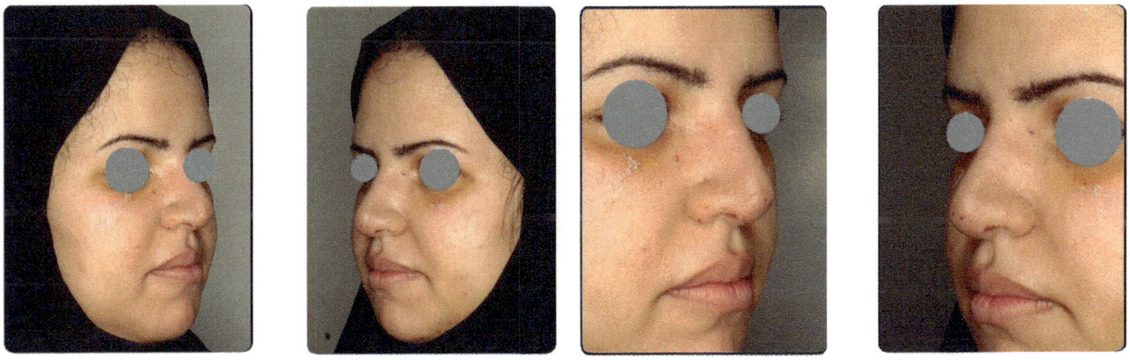

Right Lateral | **Left Lateral** | **Right Lateral Smiling** | **Left Lateral Smiling**

Preoperative

Postoperative

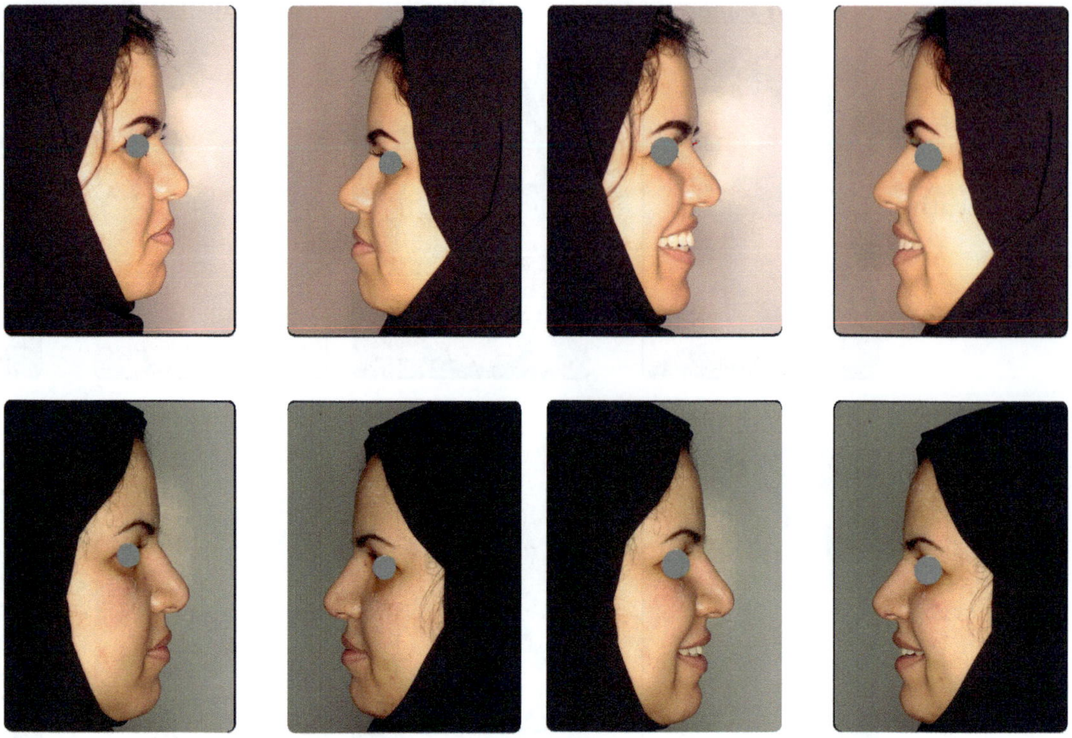

Right Lateral Middle Third | Left Lateral Middle Third

Preoperative

Postoperative

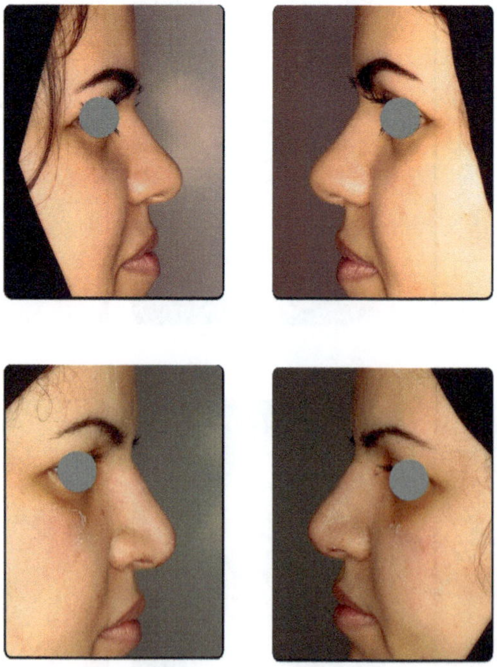

24 Part III: Clinical Case 9

Preoperative Assessment

1. **Frontolateral walls**
   a. Bulky and large nasal tip as compared to the small size of the nose (Frontal, Direct Dorsal, Overhead, and Backward Tilting Views).
   b. The bulky tip overshadows the alae nasi (Frontal, Direct Dorsal and Overhead Views).
   c. The lower third of the nose is disproportionally large. In the lateral view it occupies the lower half of the nose. In the frontal view, however, its size and bulk is overwhelming.
   d. Relatively large rounded face (Frontal Views).
2. **Medial Wall**
   Nil of note.
3. **Bony pyramid**
   a. The bony pyramid is short and low. The boney pyramid occupies the upper 1/5th of the nose rather than the usual 1/3rd (Frontal Views).
   b. The dorsum, made by the bony pyramid and mid vault, is quite low compared to the lower half of the nose made by the frontolateral walls.
4. **Alar base**
   a. Wide alar base due to long inferior segments of rim-sill folds. This results in wide nasal openings (Backward Tilting, Basal, and Nasal Aperture Views).
   b. Thick alar base due to thick posterior segments of the rim-sill folds. The angles between the alae nasi and the upper lip are acute. This results in the flat tire appearance (Backward Tilting, Basal and Nasal Aperture Views).
   c. The right ala nasi is naturally larger than the left (Frontal Views).

Aims of Surgery

1. Reduce the bulk and size of the frontolateral walls, to make it proportionate with the rest of the nose.
2. Elevation of the nasal dorsum.
3. Reduction of the size and bulk of the alar base.

Surgical Plan

1. **Frontolateral walls**
   a. DDD including the weak triangle to reduce the bulk of nasal tip and midvault.
   b. Cephalic trim of the lateral crurae to reduce the size of the fronto lateral walls.
2. **Medial Wall**
   Nil of note.
3. **Bony pyramid**
   a. Osteotomies and medialization of the lateral bony walls.
   b. Dorsal augmentation using septal graft.
4. **Alar base**
   Bilateral excision of the inferior and posterior segments of rim-sill folds to reduce the length and balk of the alar base successively (see illustrations in the right nasal aperture views).

Surgical Procedure

a. As per Surgical Plan.
b. A double layer of osteocartilaginous graft was used to augment the nasal dorsum. The boney septum was used for the deeper layer, while the cartilaginous septum was used for the superficial layer. The latter was scored longitudinally to give it a rounded appearance simulating the natural dorsum.
c. A noticeable depression appeared just above the right lateral crus area during surgery. Trimmings of the lateral crurae were used as a graft to fill this depression. This depression was noticed retrospectively in the preoperative frontal and overhead views.

M. H. A. Shafy, *Atlas of Clinical Cases in Rhinoplasty*,
https://doi.org/10.1007/978-3-031-07504-9_24

Post-Operative Analysis

1. **Frontolateral Wall**
   a. Tip definition improved: the tip is slimmer with thinner skin. It is well defined from the surrounding alae nasi on both sides. The alae nasi came into view to share in nasal aesthetics (Frontal, Direct Dorsal, Overhead, Backward Tilting, Basal and Nasal Aperture Views).
   b. Tip projection: nasal tip is high at the end of nasal dorsum with good aesthetic angle coupled with aesthetic nasolabial angle (Lateral and Oblique Views).
   c. Tip light reflex is seen as one spot off the nasal tip (Frontal and Backward Tilting Views).
2. **Medial Wall**
   Nil of Note.
3. **Bony Pyramid**
   a. Bony pyramid aesthetics: the nasal dorsum is high, straight and the sidewalls are smooth and narrow (all views except the Basal Views).
   b. Dorsal light reflex is seen as an uninterrupted line off the nasal dorsum (Direct Dorsal Views).
4. **Alar Base**
   a. The superior alar groove aesthetics improved, after defatting, they are deeper and longer (Oblique, Lateral, Direct Dorsal and Overhead Views).
   b. Posterior alar groove aesthetics improved by defatting as well as excising the posterior segments of the rim-sill folds. The flat tire appearance is no longer present (Backward Tilting, Basal and Nasal Aperture Views).
   c. The inferior segments of the rim sill folds were surprising short, i.e. only 2 mm long. It was the thickness of the posterior segments that mainly contributed to the bulky alar base.
   d. Alae nasi aesthetics improved. They are pulled medially, better seen and of smaller size.
   e. Nasal aperture aesthetic improved by defatting and excision of the rim-sill folds:
      i. The size of apertures are smaller.
      ii. The shape of the nasal apertures transformed from wide rounded with transverse axes to small triangular with long anterior axes (Backward Tilting, Basal, and Nasal Aperture Views).
   f. Marginal light reflexes are clearly seen at:
      i. Inferior alar margins (Nasal Aperture Views).
      ii. Nasal sill bands are too small to be seen in Oblique views.
      iii. Lateral crural prominences only partly seen in the right lateral views.

Commentary

a. Three of the four areas of Rhinoplasty areas were addressed i.e. frontolateral walls, bony pyramid and alar base.
b. The "drum stick" appearance of the nose totally disappeared. The lower third is intergrated with the upper two thirds in an attractive double empathy.
c. No tip grafts and no direct crural stitching. The nasal tip and columella maintained their natural softness and normal physiological roles.

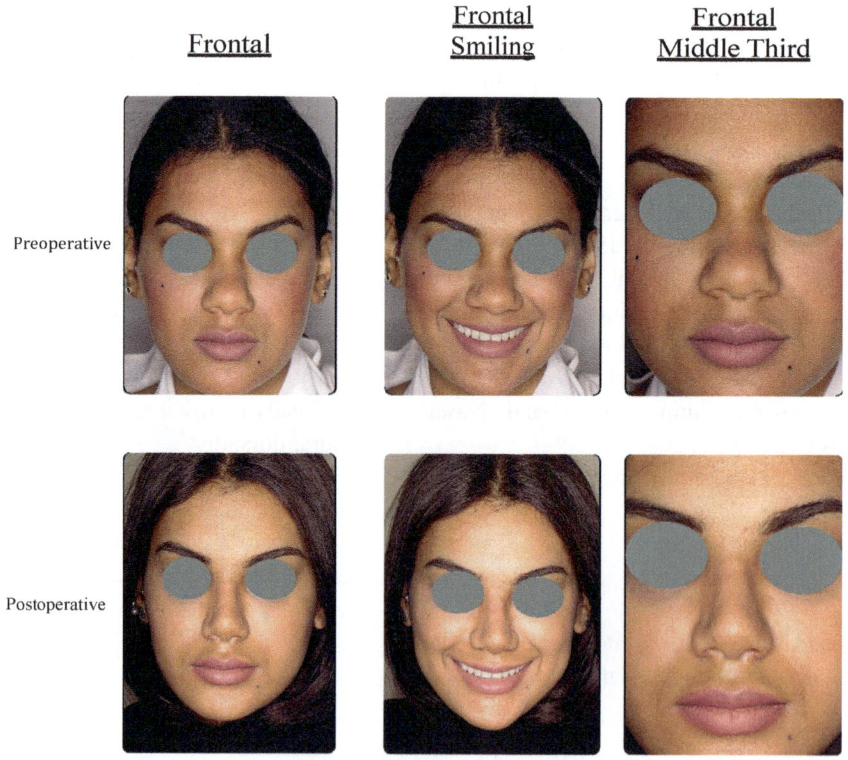

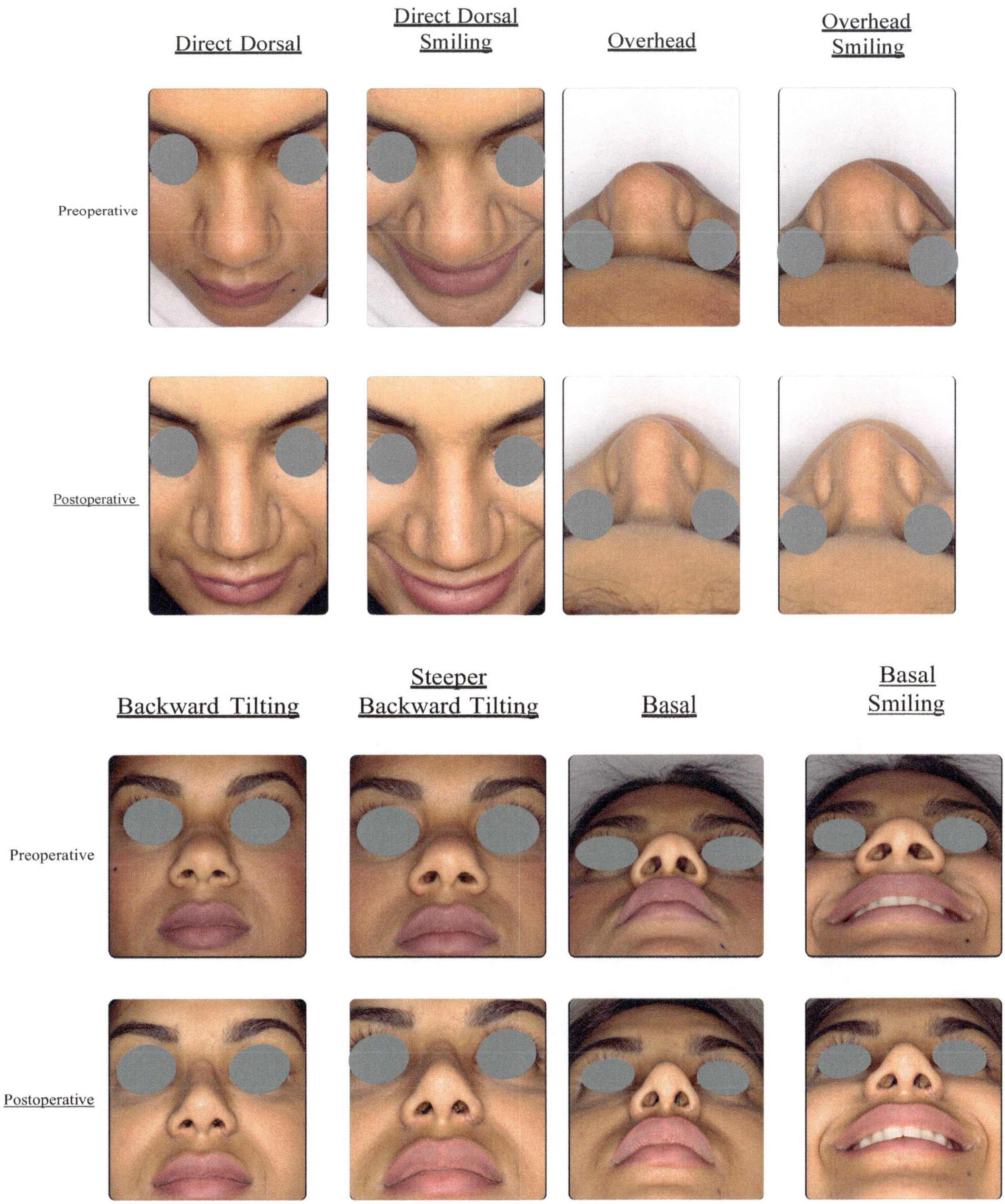

Direct Dorsal
Direct Dorsal Smiling
Overhead
Overhead Smiling
Preoperative
Postoperative
Backward Tilting
Steeper Backward Tilting
Basal
Basal Smiling
Preoperative
Postoperative

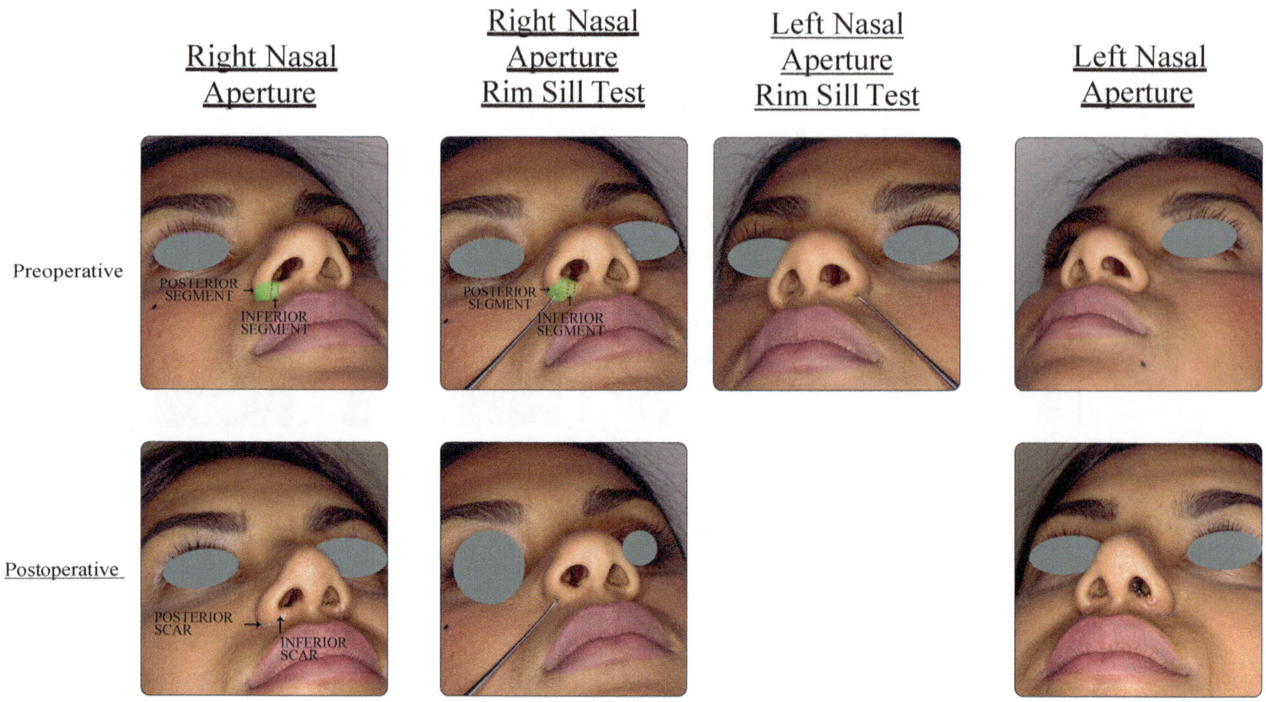
Right Nasal Aperture
Right Nasal Aperture Rim Sill Test
Left Nasal Aperture Rim Sill Test
Left Nasal Aperture
Preoperative
POSTERIOR SEGMENT
INFERIOR SEGMENT
POSTERIOR SEGMENT
INFERIOR SEGMENT
Postoperative
POSTERIOR SCAR
INFERIOR SCAR

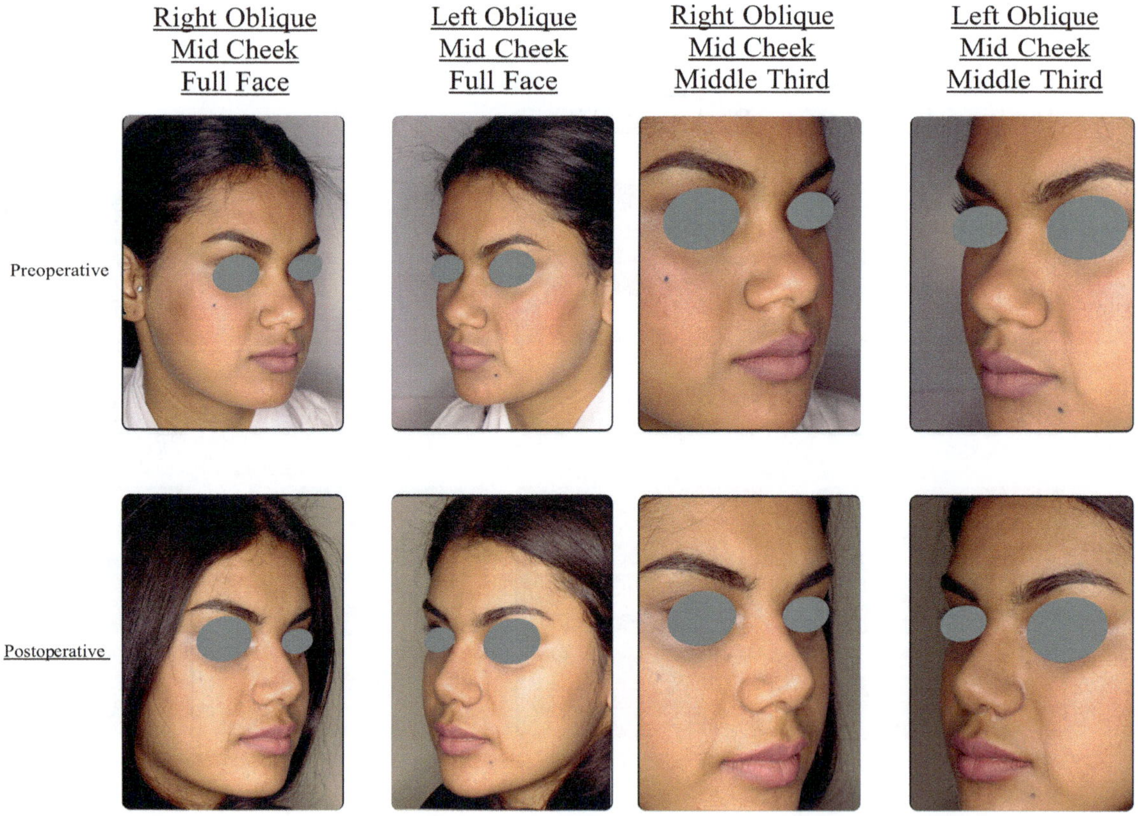
Right Oblique Mid Cheek Full Face
Left Oblique Mid Cheek Full Face
Right Oblique Mid Cheek Middle Third
Left Oblique Mid Cheek Middle Third
Preoperative
Postoperative

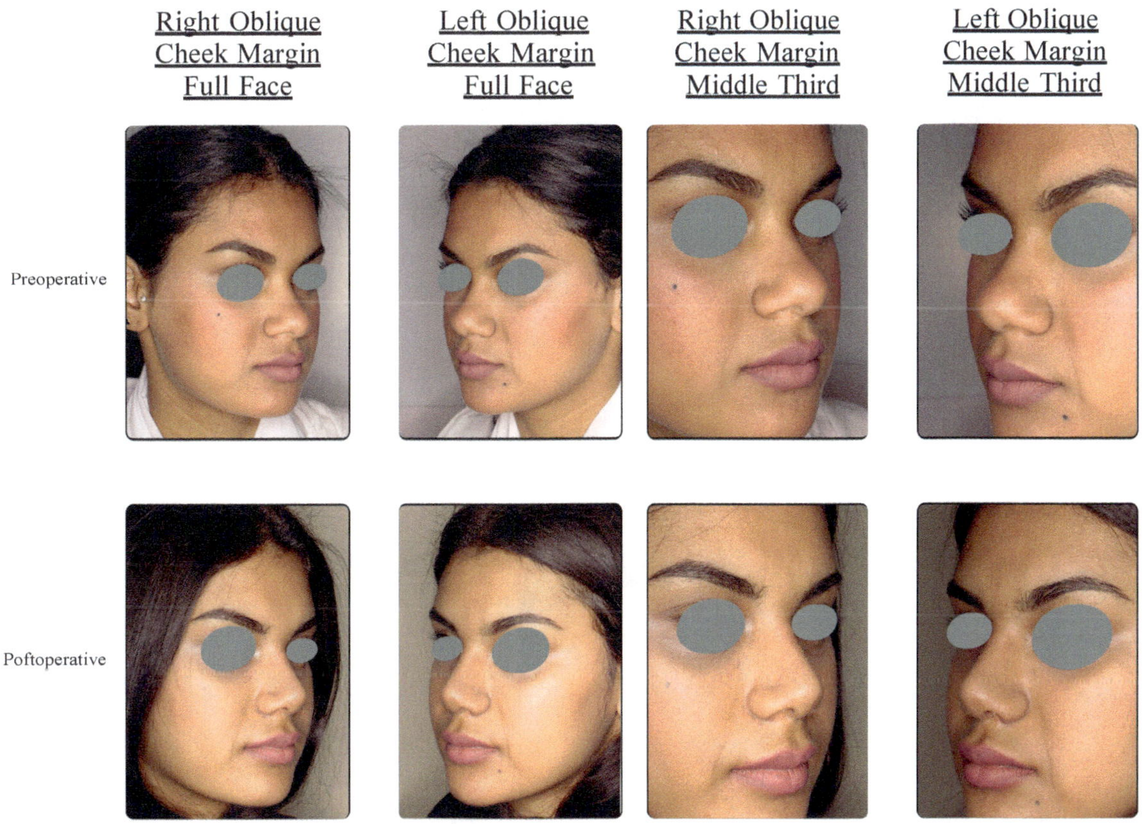
Right Oblique Cheek Margin Full Face
Left Oblique Cheek Margin Full Face
Right Oblique Cheek Margin Middle Third
Left Oblique Cheek Margin Middle Third
Preoperative
Poftoperative

Right Lateral | Left Lateral | Right Lateral Smiling | Left Lateral Smiling

Preoperative

Postoperative

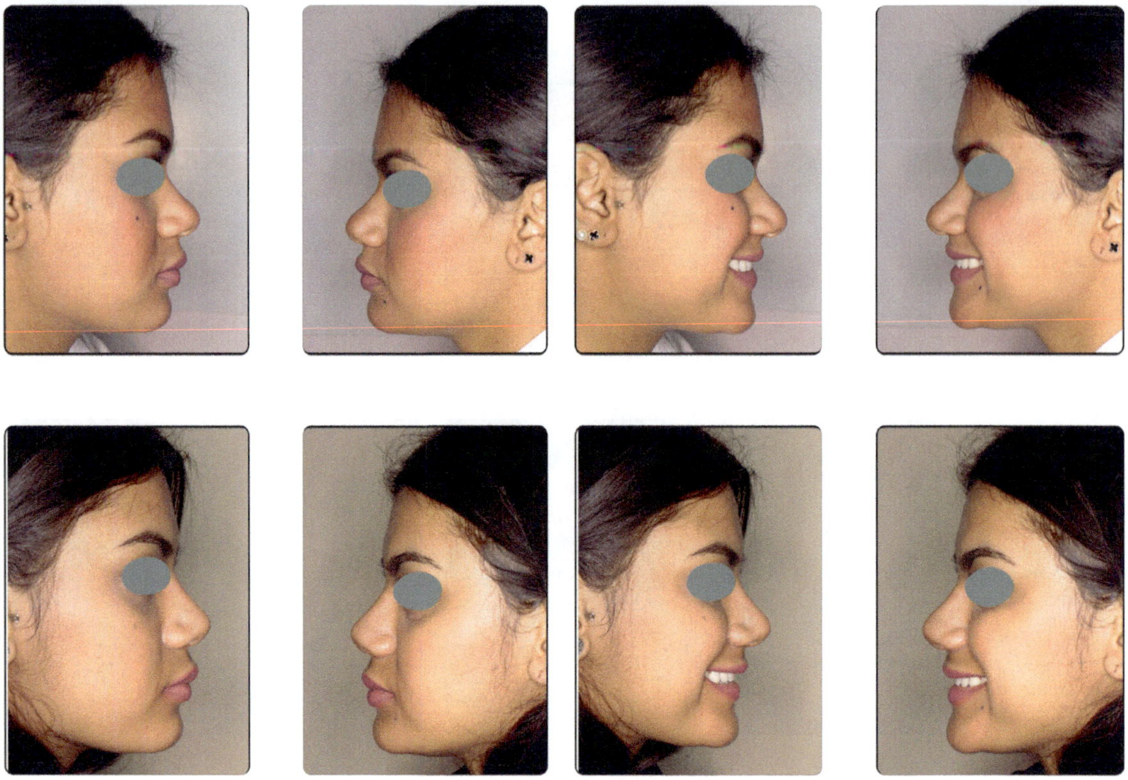

Right Lateral Middle Third | Left Lateral Middle Third

Preoperative

Postoperative

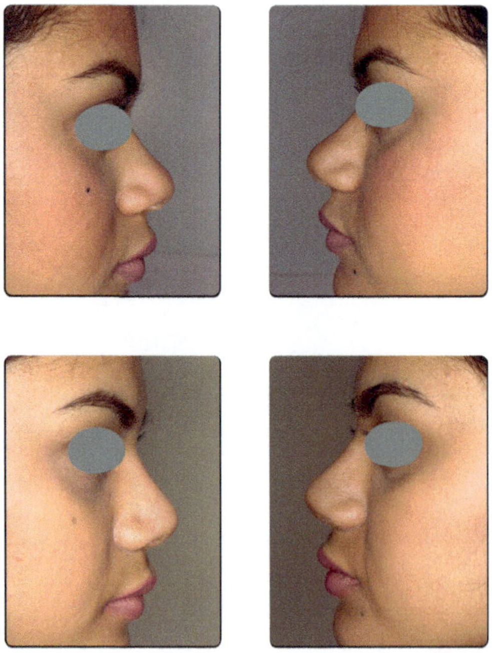

Part III: Clinical Case 10

25

Preoperative Assessment

1. **Frontolateral walls**
   Bulbous bulky tip partially overshadowing the alae nasi (Frontal, Direct Dorsal and Overhead Views).
2. **Medial Wall**
   a. Hanging columella (lateral views).
   b. Right caudal septal deviation (Right Nasal Aperture View).
3. **Bony pyramid**
   a. Osteocartilaginous hump (Oblique and Lateral views).
   b. Slight right sided oblique bony pyramid due to maxillary asymmetry. The right cheek is wide and low and the left cheek is narrow and high (Backward Tilting Views).
4. **Alar base**
   Nil of note.

Aims of Surgery

1. Overall reduction of the bulk of the lower third nose.
2. Excision of the osteo-cartilagenous hump.
3. Abolishing the hanging columella.

Surgical Plan

1. **Frontolateral walls**
   a. D.D.D. including the weak triangle to reduce the bulk of the nasal tip and midvault.
   b. Cephalic trim of lateral crurae to reduce the size of the frontao lateral walls.
2. **Medial Wall**
   a. Septoplasty.
   b. Trim 2 mm of the caudal septum.
3. **Bony pyramid**
   a. Excision of osteocartilaginous hump.
   b. Kazanjian maneuver to the left i.e. cross fracture of the bony pyramid after osteotomies (see Surgery of Bony Pyramid in the Text).
4. **Alar base**
   Nil of note.

Surgical Procedure

a. As per surgical plan.
b. The nasal hump was mostly cartilaginous.

Post-Operative Analysis

1. **Frontolateral Wall**
   a. Tip definition improved i.e. the tip is slimmer and prominently well identified with thinner overlying skin. The alae nasi come into view to share in nasal aesthetics (Frontal, Direct Dorsal, Overhead, Backward Tilting and Basal Views).
   b. Tip projection: the nasal tip is at the same level of the nasal dorsum with good aesthetic angle. This is coupled with good aesthetic nasolabial angle (lateral and oblique views).
   c. Tip light reflex is seen as one spot off the nasal tip (Frontal and Backward Tilting Views).
2. **Medial Wall**
   Caudal septal deviation is corrected (Right Nasal Aperture View).
3. **Bony Pyramid**
   a. Bony pyramid aesthetics improved: the nasal dorsum is straight, centralized in the midline and the sidewalls are smooth and narrow (all views except the Basal Views).

M. H. A. Shafy, *Atlas of Clinical Cases in Rhinoplasty*,
https://doi.org/10.1007/978-3-031-07504-9_25

b. Dorsal light reflex is seen as an uninterrupted line off the nasal dorsum (Direct Dorsal Views).

4. **Alar Base**
   a. Superior alar groove aesthetics improved by defatting. The grooves become longer and deeper (Oblique, Lateral and Direct Dorsal grooves).
   b. Alae nasi aesthetics improved. They are better seen and more attractive looking (Nasal Aperture, Oblique and Lateral Views).
   c. Marginal light reflexes are clearly seen at:
      i. Inferior alar margins (Nasal Aperture Views).
      ii. Nasal sill bands (Oblique Views).
      iii. Lateral crural prominences (Lateral Views).

Commentary

a. Post-operative photographs were taken only two weeks after the surgery. The nasal tip will gradually and proportionately become smaller.
b. Post-operatively the nose receded nicely back to the face and integrated smoothly with the cheeks, mouth and eyes.

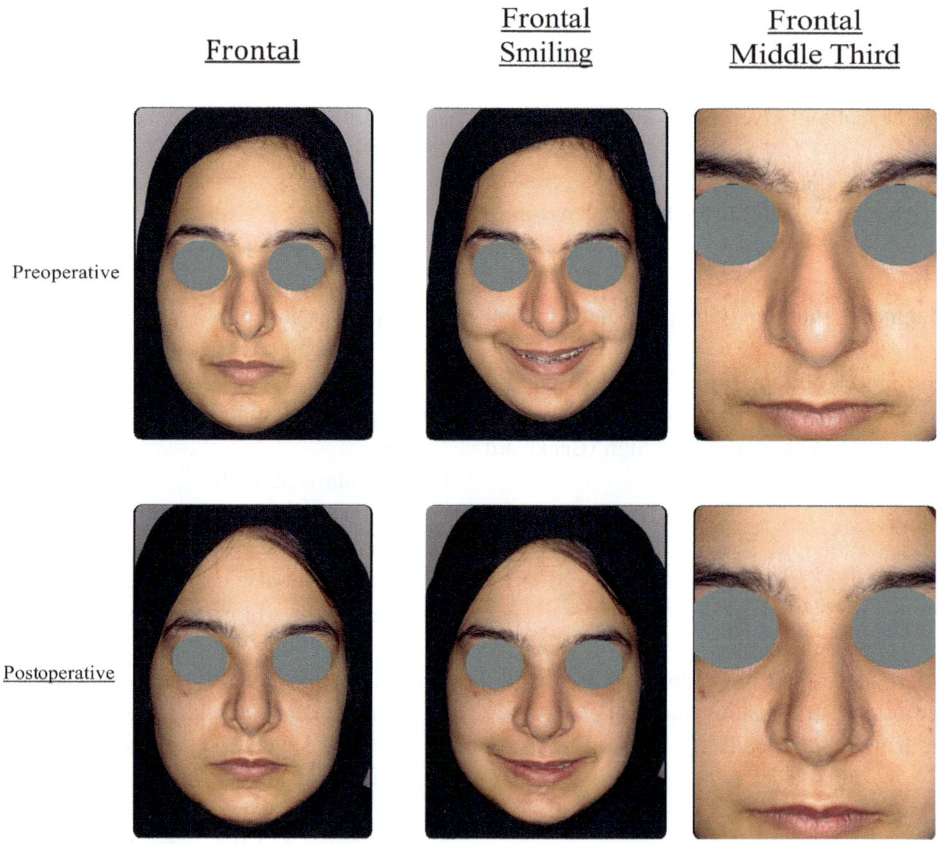

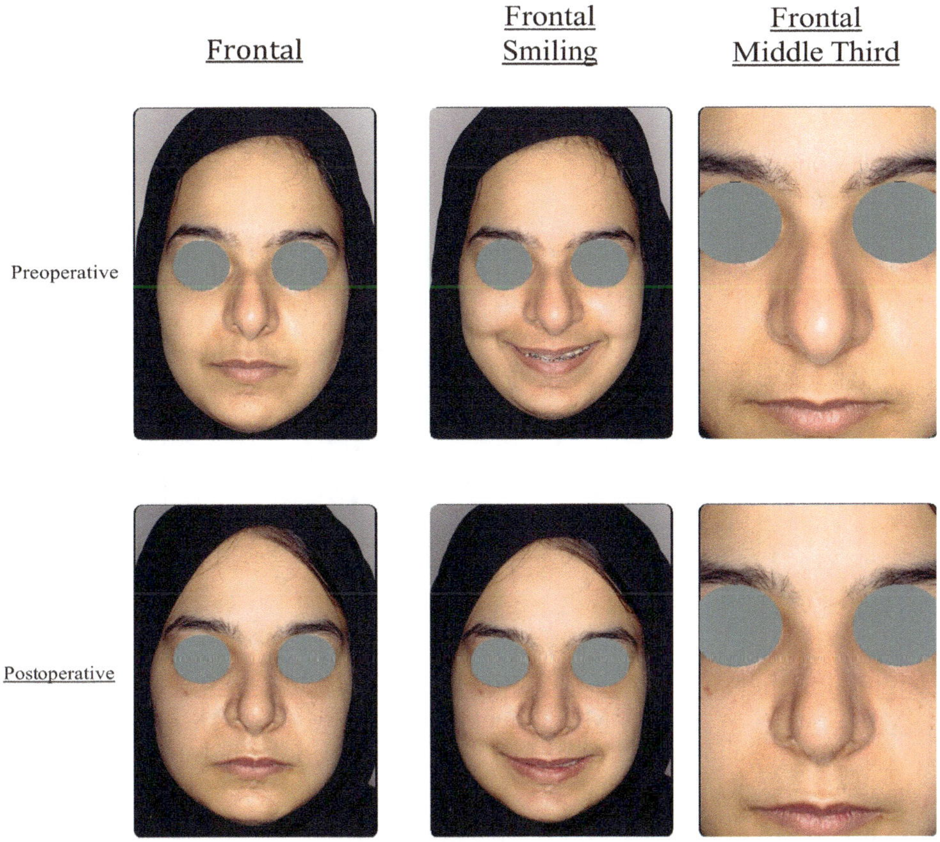
Frontal
Frontal Smiling
Frontal Middle Third
Preoperative
Postoperative

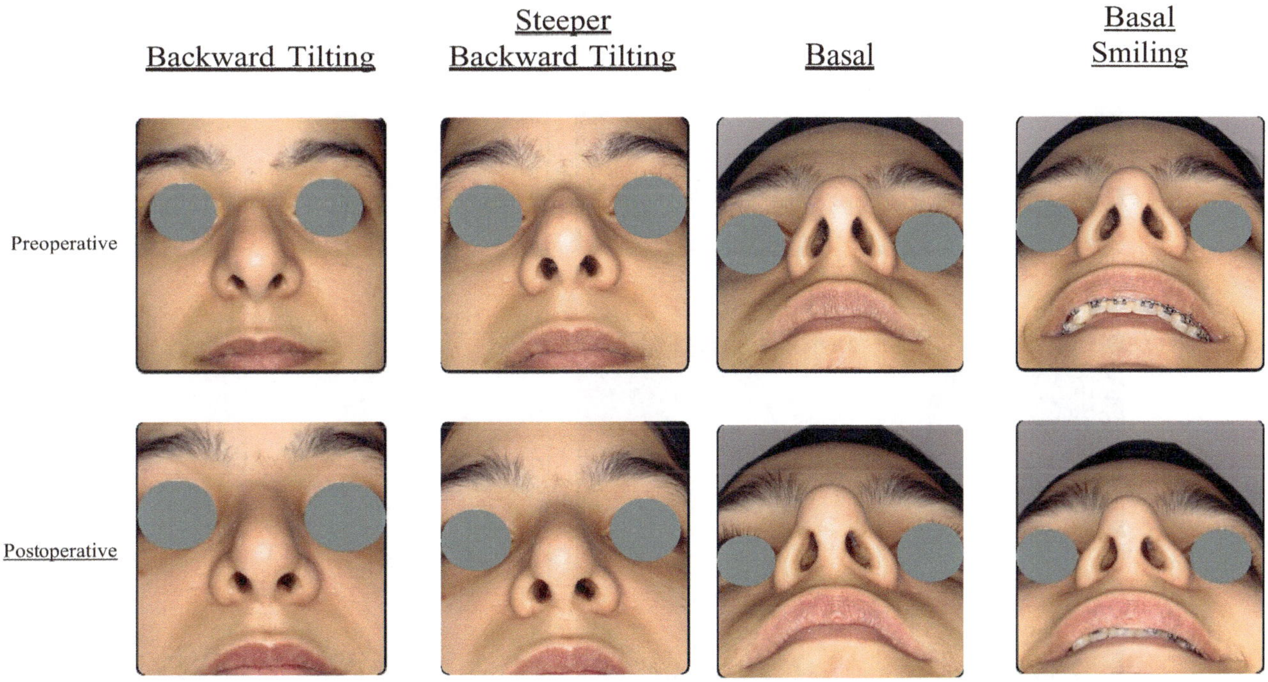
Backward Tilting
Steeper Backward Tilting
Basal
Basal Smiling
Preoperative
Postoperative

Right Nasal Aperture | Left Nasal Aperture

Preoperative

Postoperative

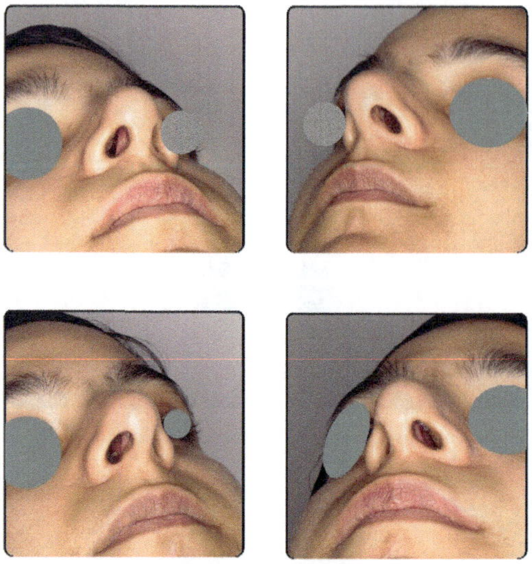

Right Oblique Mid Cheek Full Face | Left Oblique Mid Cheek Full Face | Right Oblique Mid Cheek Middle Third | Left Oblique Mid Cheek Middle Third

Preoperative

Postoperative

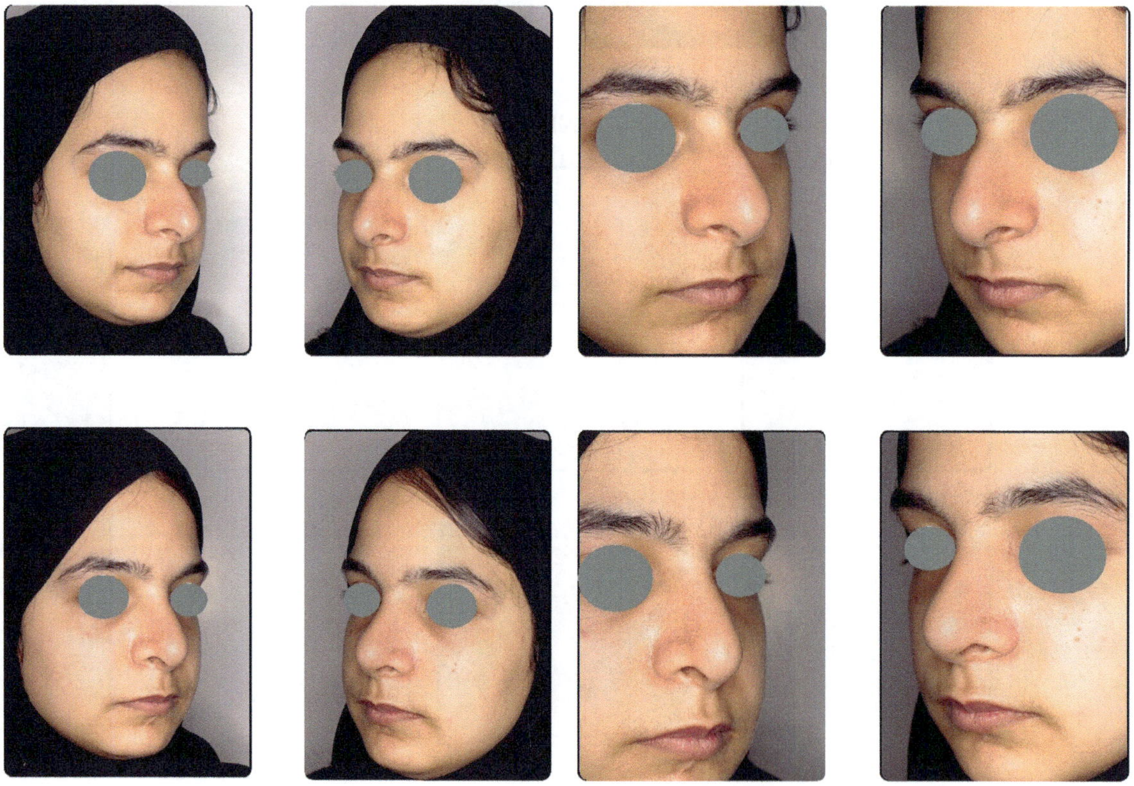

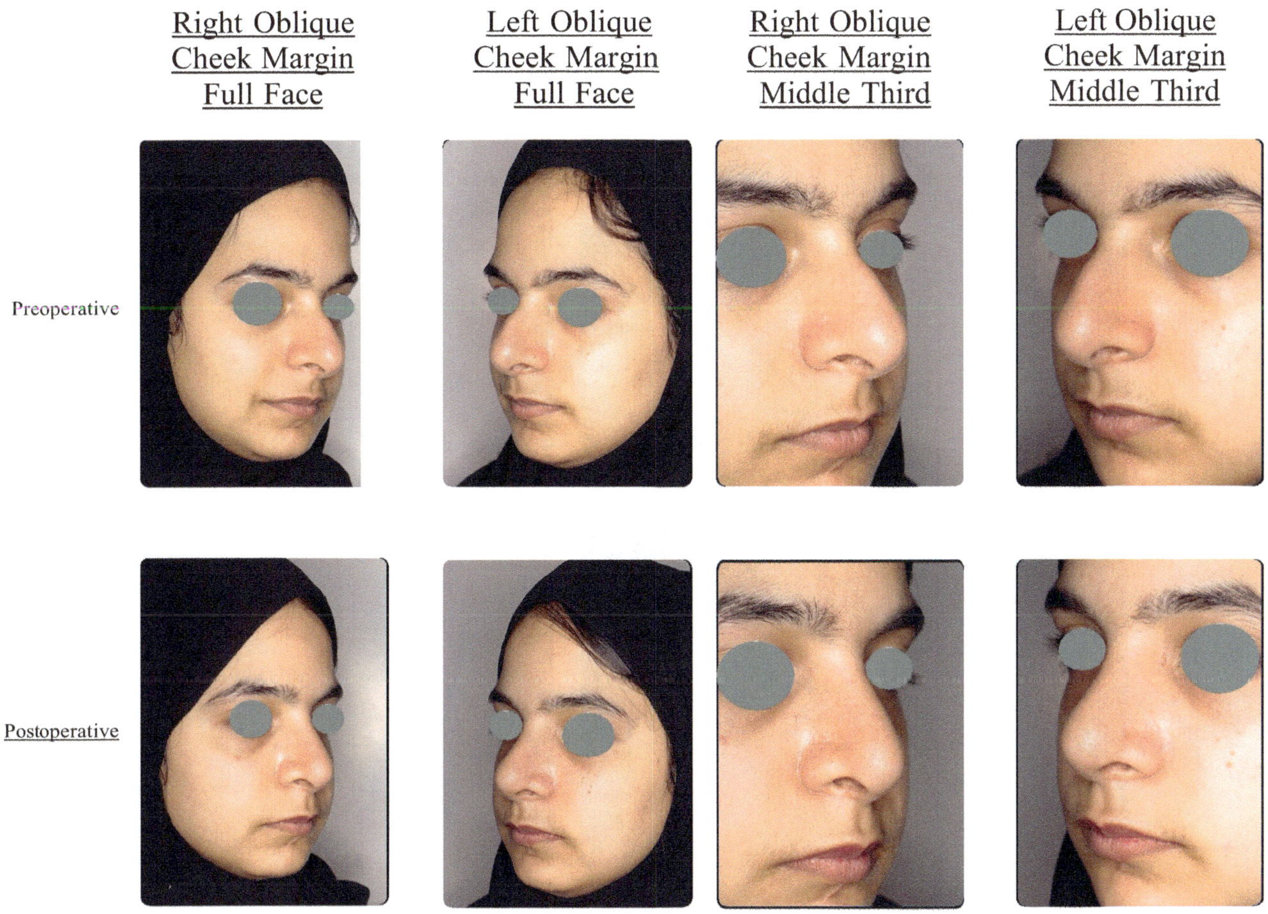
Right Oblique
Cheek Margin
Full Face
Left Oblique
Cheek Margin
Full Face
Right Oblique
Cheek Margin
Middle Third
Left Oblique
Cheek Margin
Middle Third
Preoperative
Postoperative

Right Lateral | Left Lateral | Right Lateral Smiling | Left Lateral Smiling

Preoperative

Postoperative

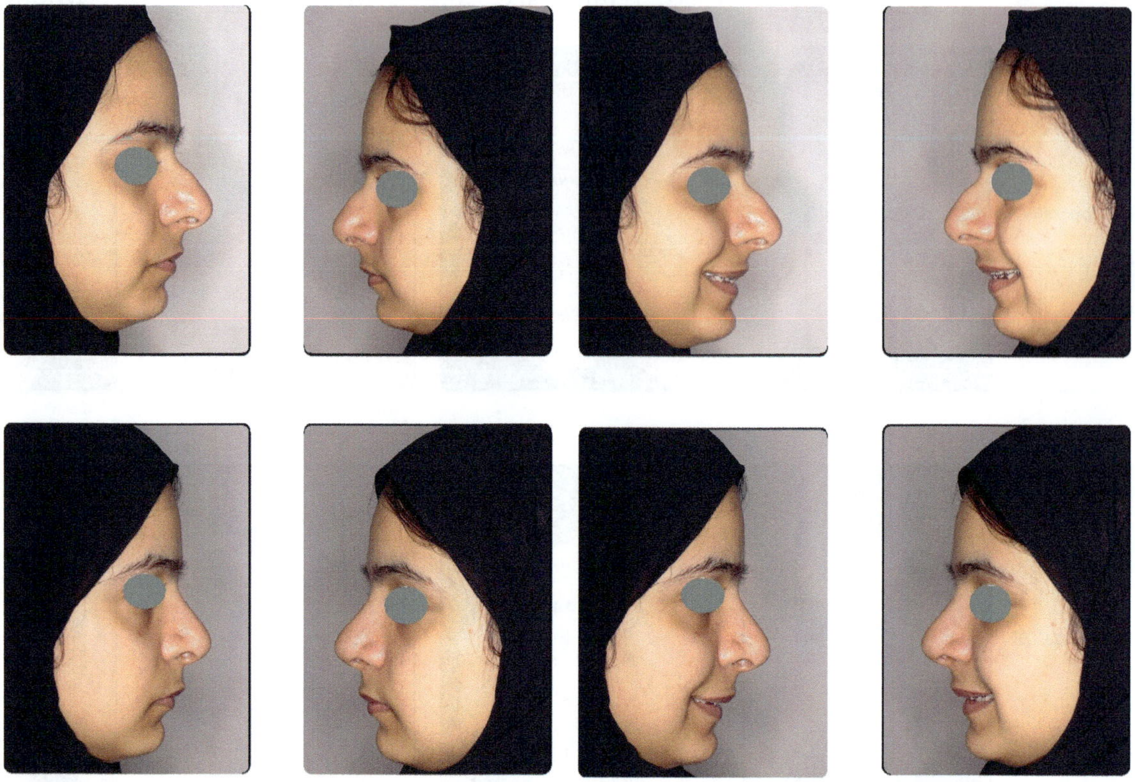

Right Lateral Middle Third | Left Lateral Middle Third

Preoperative

Postoperative

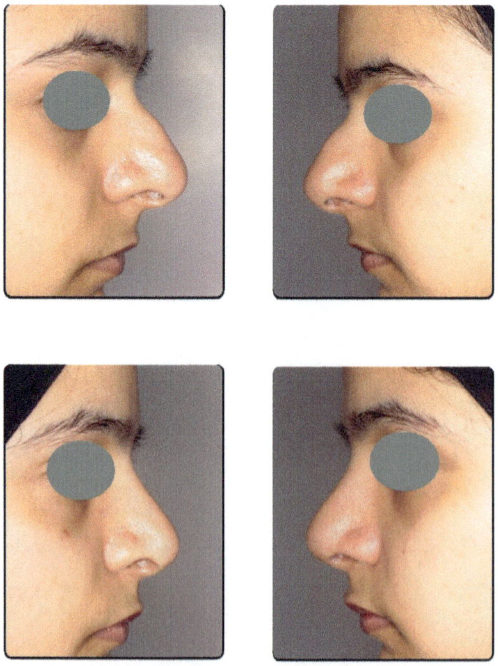

Part III: Clinical Case 11

26

Preoperative Assessment

1. **Frontolateral walls**
   Bulky and large tip that completely overshadowes the alae nasi (Frontal, Direct Dorsal and Overhead Views).
2. **Medial Wall**
   a. Acute nasolabial angle (Lateral Views).
   b. Mobile tip (Lateral Smiling Views).
3. **Bony pyramid**
   a. Wide base of the bony pyramid (Direct Dorsal, Overhead and Backward Tilting Views).
   b. Osteocartilaginous hump (Oblique and Lateral Views).
4. **Alar base**
   Nasal apertures are thick walled, rounded and the alae nasi have acute angles with the upper lip i.e. flat tire appearance (Backward Tilting, Basal, and Nasal Aperture Views).

Aims of Surgery

1. Reduction of the bulk of the nasal tip.
2. Abolish the mobility of the tip as well as improving the nasolabial angle.
3. Reduction of the size of the bony pyramid and excision of the hump.

Surgical Plan

1. **Frontolateral walls**
   a. DDD including the weak triangle to reduce the bulk of the fronto lateral walls, including the nasal tip.
   b. Cephalic trim of the lateral crurae to reduce the tip size.
2. **Medial Wall**
   a. Partial trim of the membranous septum including all three layers (the two vestibular skin layers and the intervening loose connective tissue layer).
   b. Division of the Depressor Septi muscles.
3. **Bony pyramid**
   a. Excision of the osteocartilaginous hump.
   b. Osteotomies and medialization of the bony lateral walls to reduce the size of the bony pyramid.
4. **Alar base**
   Nil of note.

Surgical Procedure

As per Surgical Plan.

Post-Operative Analysis

1. **Frontolateral Wall**
   a. Tip definition improved: the tip is slimmer and prominently well identified. The overlying skin is thinner and smoother. The alae nasi come into view to share in nasal aesthetics (Frontal, Direct Dorsal, Overhead, Backward Tilting and Basal Views).
   b. Tip projection: The nasal tip at the same level of the nasal dorsum with good aesthetic angle. This is coupled with good aesthetic nasolabial angle (lateral and oblique views).
   c. Tip light reflex is seen as one spot off the nasal tip (Frontal, Backward Tilting and Basal Views).
2. **Medial Wall**
   a. The nasolabial angle became aesthetically acceptable i.e. 90 degrees.
   b. Mobile tip is abolished.

M. H. A. Shafy, *Atlas of Clinical Cases in Rhinoplasty*,
https://doi.org/10.1007/978-3-031-07504-9_26

3. **Bony Pyramid**
   a. Bony pyramid aesthetics improved: the nasal dorsum is straight and the sidewalls are smooth and narrow (all views except the Basal Views).
   b. Dorsal light reflex is seen as a regular one line off the nasal dorsum (Direct Dorsal Views).
4. **Alar Base**
   a. Superior alar groove aesthetics improved after defatting: after clearing off the fat, the grooves become deeper, longer and visible (Direct Dorsal, Oblique and Lateral Views).
   b. Posterior alar groove aesthetics improved by defatting. The angle between the alae nasi and upper lip are wider as the alae pulled medially.
   c. Alae nasi aesthetics improved. They are pulled medially, better seen and of larger size.
   d. Nasal aperture aesthetics improved: Although they are of the same size yet the aperture shapes changed from tick walled rounded openings to more elegantly thin walled oval openings (Backward Tilting and Basal Views).
   e. Marginal light reflexes are clearly seen at:
      i. Inferior alar margins (Nasal Aperture Views).
      ii. Nasal sill bands (Oblique Views).
      iii. Lateral crural prominences (Lateral Views).

Commentary

a. This young lady's only request was to reduce the size of the nasal hump.
b. A better result was achieved by enhancing the aesthetics of all parts of the nose, i.e. nasal tip, nasolabial angle and mobile tip, rather than only removing the nasal hump.
c. Simple removal of the nasal hump of this lady would have resulted in a long nose that has a bulbous, mobile tip, which is acutely bent over the upper lip. The final result would be an extremely long nose with a large bulky tip that looks like a trumpet.

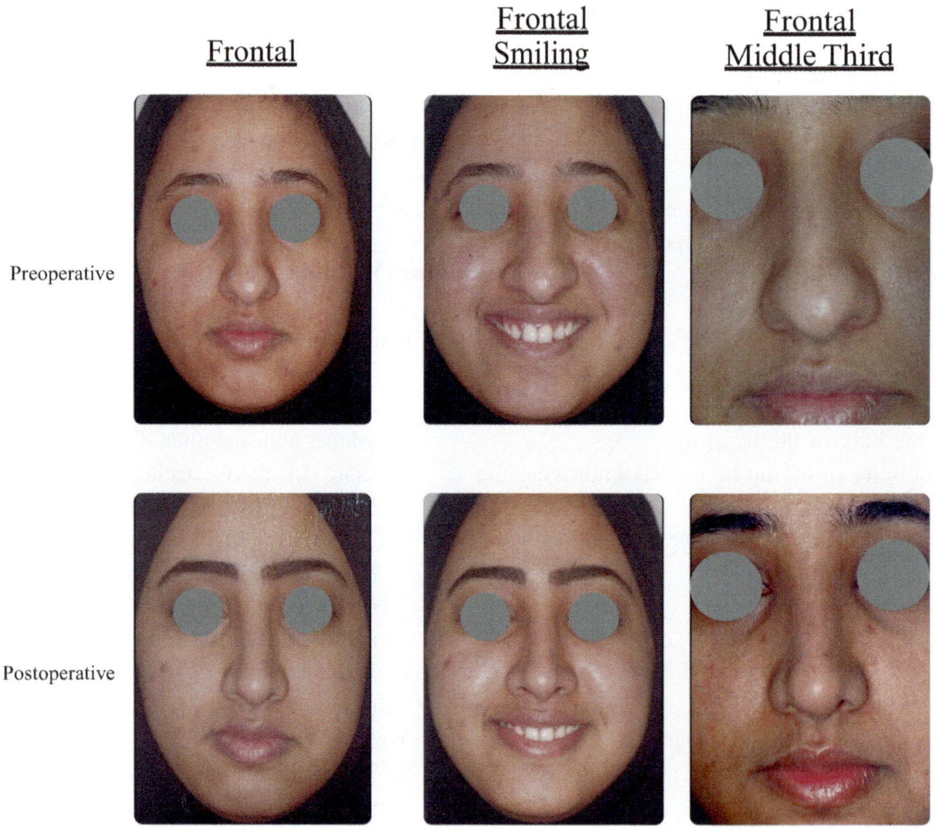

Direct Dorsal | Direct Dorsal **Smiling** | Overhead | Overhead Smiling

Preoperative

Postoperative

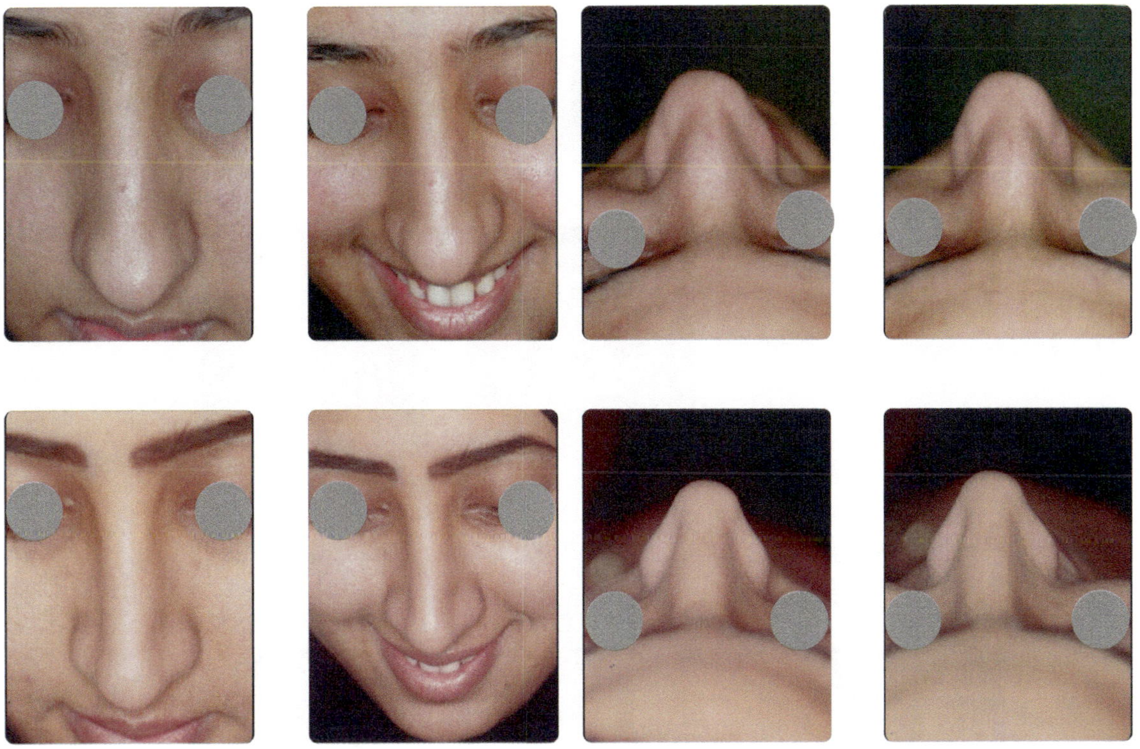

Backward Tilting | Steeper Backward Tilting | Basal | Basal Smiling

Preoperative

Postoperative

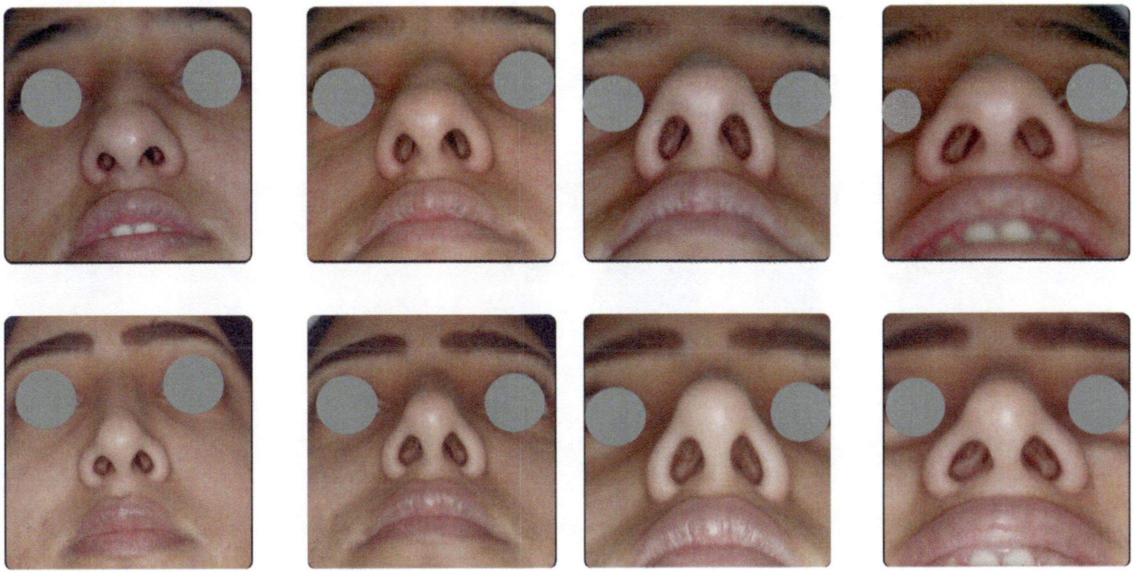

Right Nasal Aperture | Left Nasal Aperture

Preoperative

Postoperative

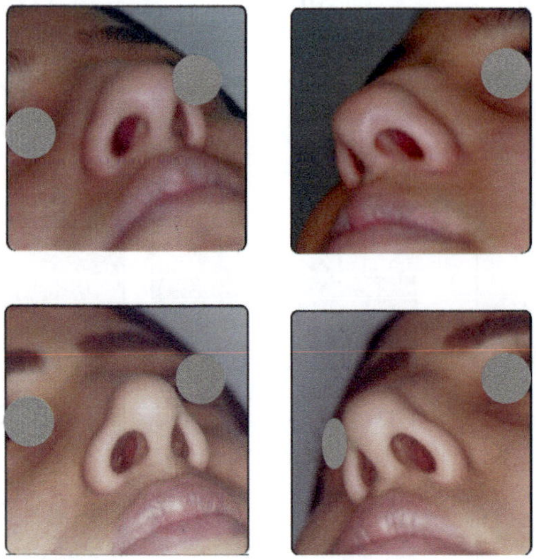

Right Oblique Mid Cheek Full Face | Left Oblique Mid Cheek Full Face | Right Oblique Mid Cheek Middle Third | Left Oblique Mid Cheek Middle Third

Preoperative

Postoperative

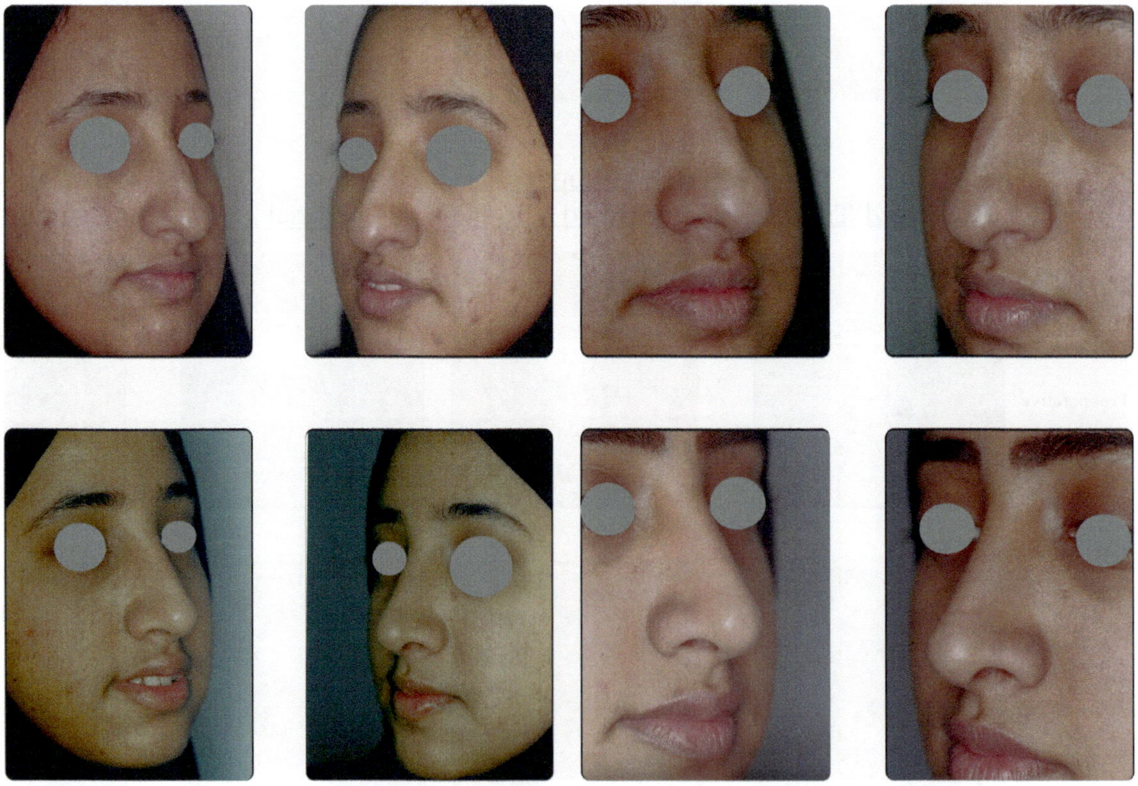

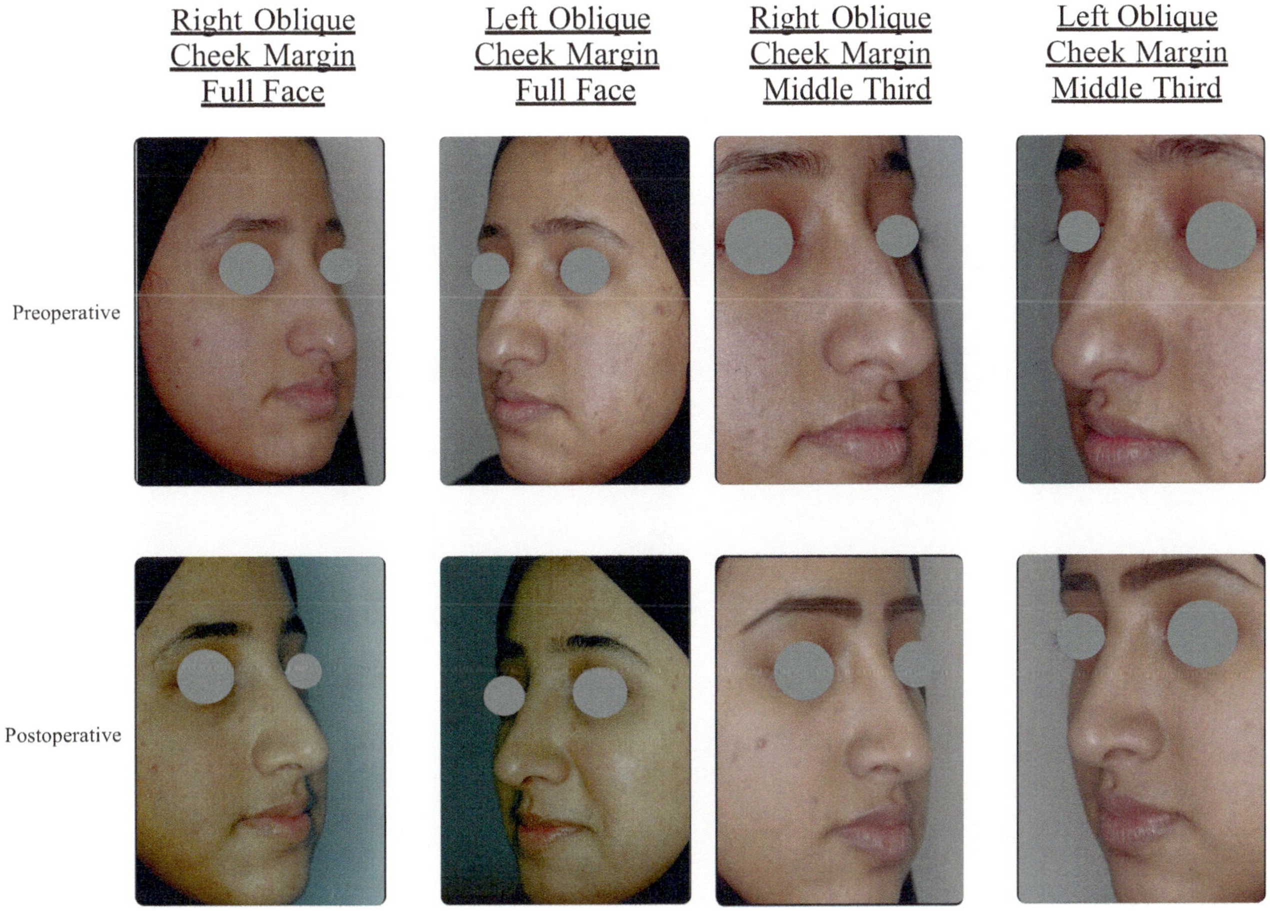
Right Oblique Cheek Margin Full Face
Left Oblique Cheek Margin Full Face
Right Oblique Cheek Margin Middle Third
Left Oblique Cheek Margin Middle Third
Preoperative
Postoperative

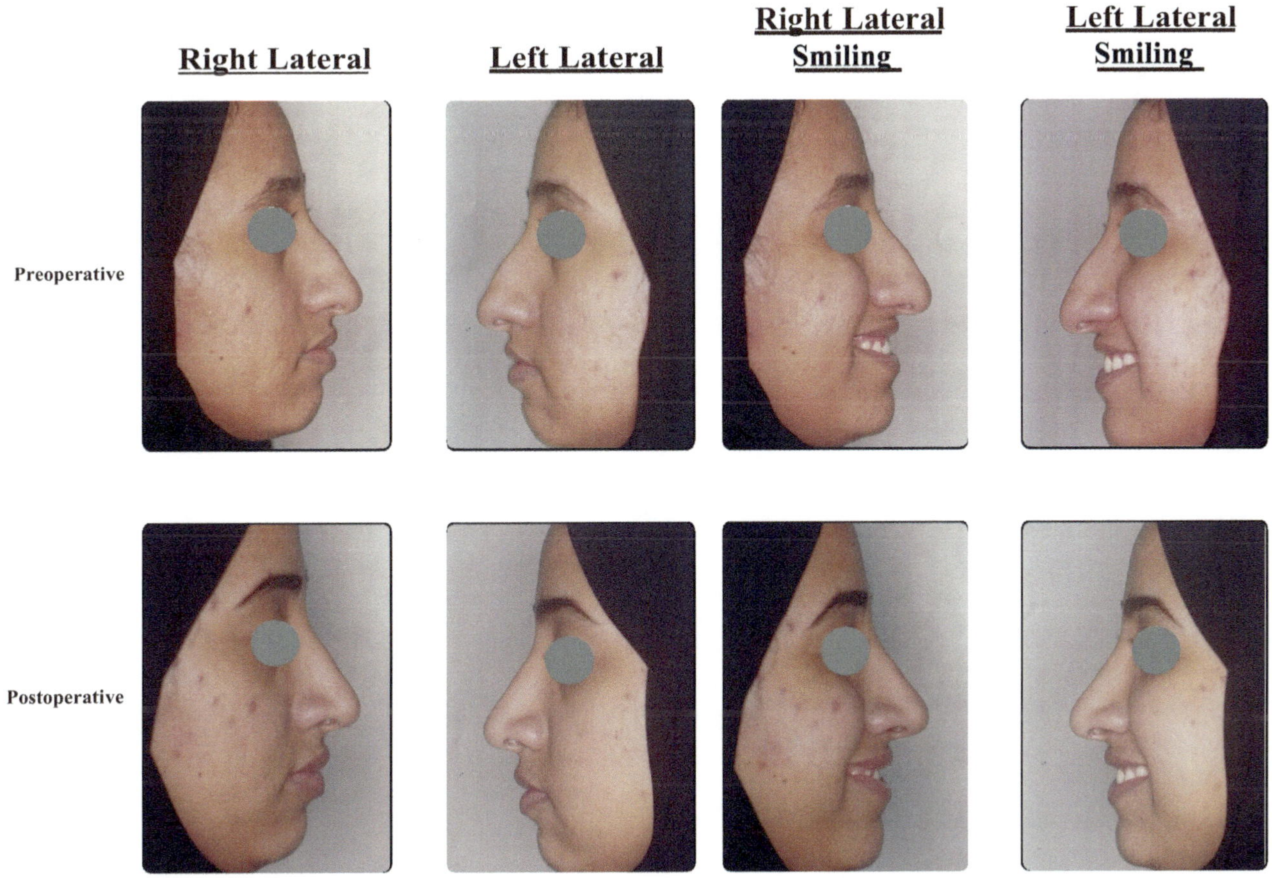
Right Lateral
Left Lateral
Right Lateral Smiling
Left Lateral Smiling
Preoperative
Postoperative

Part III: Clinical Case 12

27

Preoperative Assessment

1. **Frontolateral walls**
   a. Irregularly bulky nasal tip—left side is larger than the right. The alae nasi are hidden behind the bulky tip (Frontal and Direct Dorsal Views).
   b. The main bulk is in the scroll areas (area of the overlap between the lateral crus and upper lateral cartilage).
2. **Medial Wall**
   Nil of Note.
3. **Bony pyramid**
   a. Wide base of the boney pyramid (Direct Dorsal Views).
   b. Small osteocartilaginous hump which overshadowed by the high scroll area overlap of the lateral crurae over the upper lateral cartilage. The small hump is no more than the natural concovoconvex bodies of the nasal bones from above downwards. (see Anatomy Section).
4. **Alar base**
   Nil of note.

Aims of Surgery

1. Reduction of the bulk of the frontolateral wall.
2. Reduction of the size of boney pyramid.

Surgical Plan

1. **Frontolateral walls**
   a. DDD including the weak triangle to reduce the bulk.
   b. Excision of the bulky, left scroll area.
2. **Median Wall**
   Nil of Note.
3. **Bony pyramid**
   a. Excision of the osteocartilaginous hump.
   b. Osteotomies and medialization of the lateral bony walls.
4. **Alar base**
   Nil of note.

Surgical Procedure

As per Surgical Plan.

Post-Operative Analysis

1. **Frontolateral Wall**
   a. Tip definition improved i.e. slimmer and prominently well identified. The alae nasi come into view to share in nasal aesthetics (Frontal, Direct Dorsal, Overhead, Backward Tilting and Basal Views). Note the clear light reflex of the nasal tip as one spot in the backward tilting view.
   b. Tip projection: The nasal tip at the same level of the nasal dorsum with good aesthetic angle. This is coupled with good aesthetic nasolabial angle (lateral and oblique views).
   c. Tip light reflex is seen as one spot off the nasal tip. (Frontal and Backward Tilting Views).
2. **Medial Wall**
   Nil of Note.
3. **Bony Pyramid**
   a. Bony pyramid aesthetics: the nasal dorsum is straight and the sidewalls are smooth and narrow (all views except the Basal Views).
   b. Dorsal light reflex is seen as an uninterrupted line off the nasal dorsum (Direct Dorsal Views).
4. **Alar Base**
   Nil of Note.

Commentary

a. DDD was sufficient to reduce the bulk of the lower third of the nose but did not affect the scroll area. The scroll area was trimmed by direct surgical approach.
b. The slight depression on the left side of the nose was later addressed by local injection.

M. H. A. Shafy, *Atlas of Clinical Cases in Rhinoplasty*,
https://doi.org/10.1007/978-3-031-07504-9_27

Frontal | Frontal Smiling | Frontal Middle Third

Preoperative

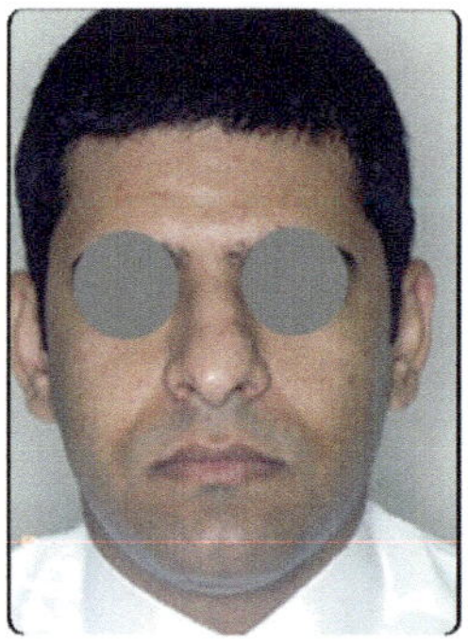
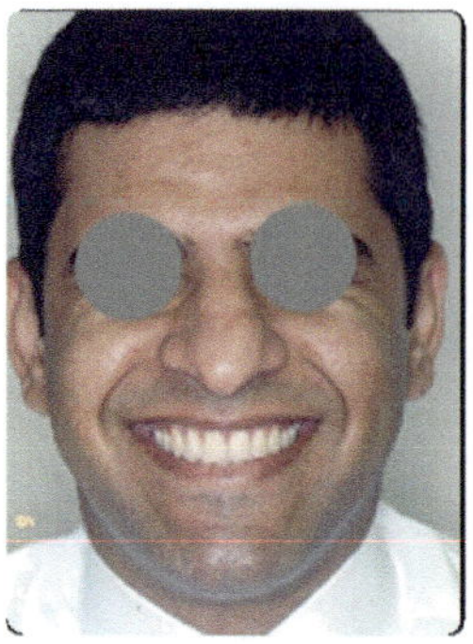
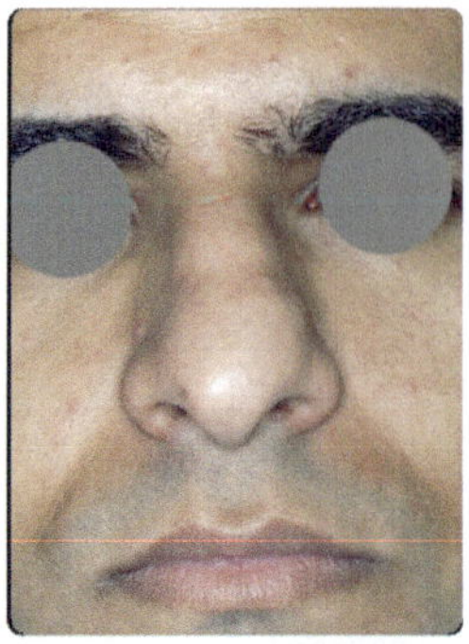

Postoperative

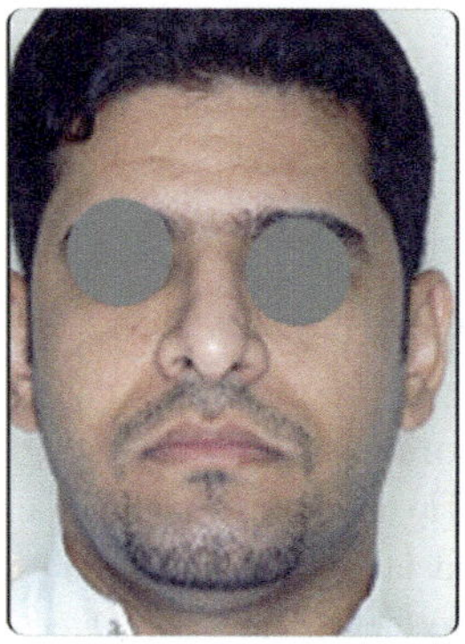
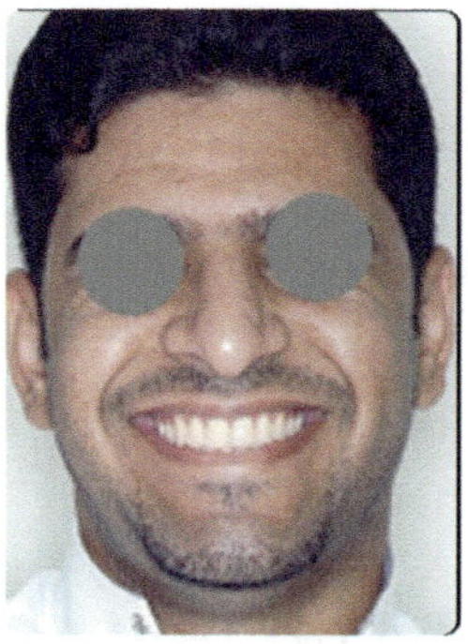
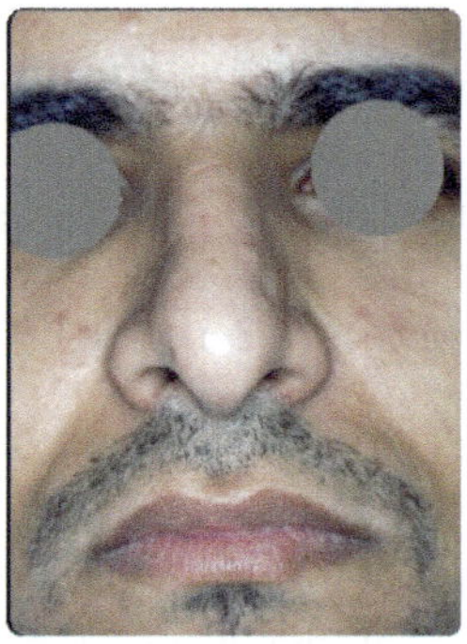

Direct Dorsal

Preoperative

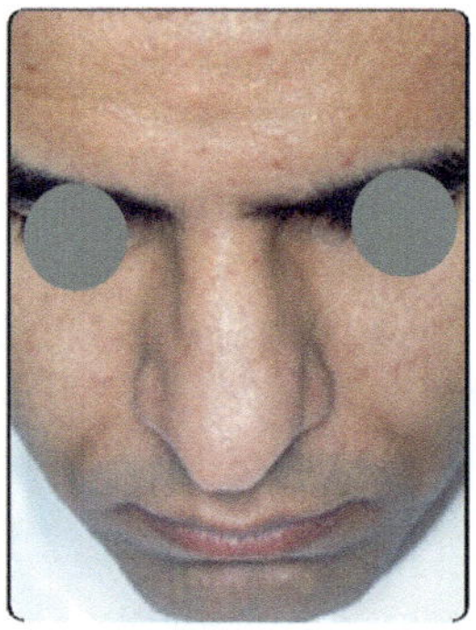

Postoperative

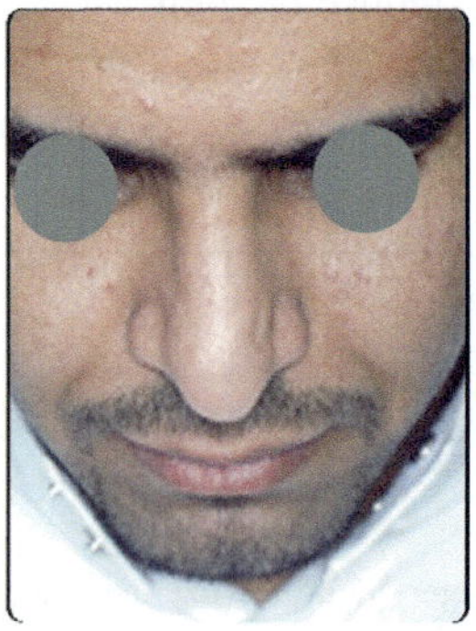

Steeper Backward Tilting | Basal

Preoperative

Postoperative

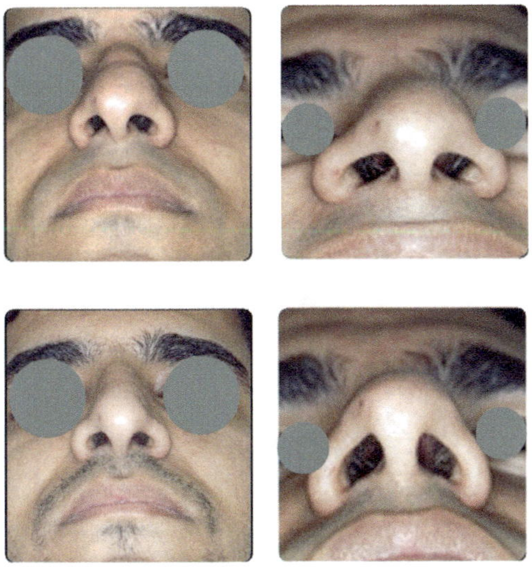

Right Oblique Mid Cheek Full Face | Left Oblique Mid Cheek Full Face

Preoperative

Postoperative

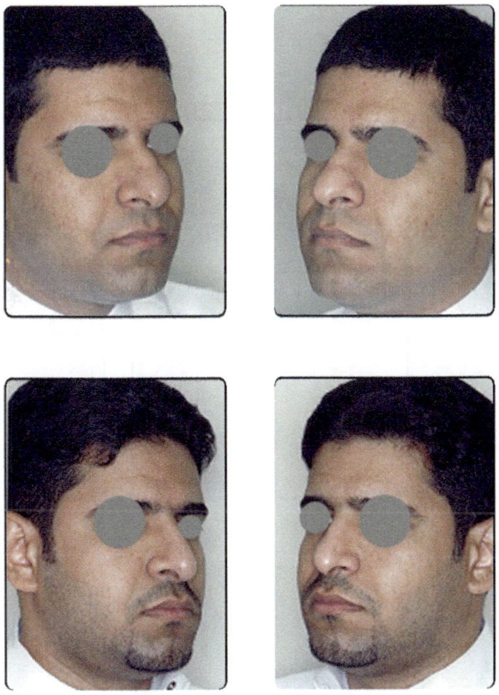

Right Oblique Cheek Margin Full Face

Left Oblique Cheek Margin Full Face

Preoperative

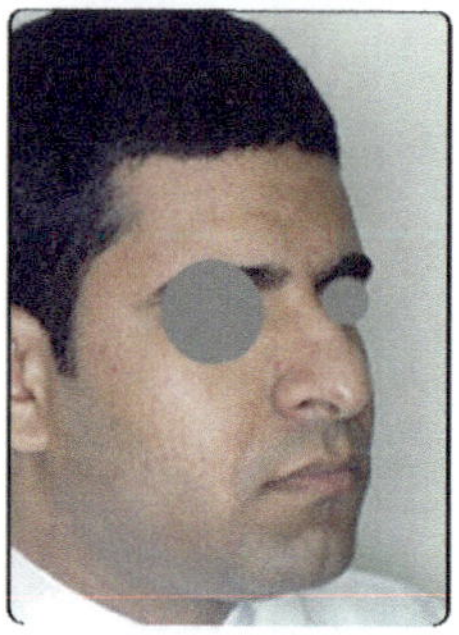

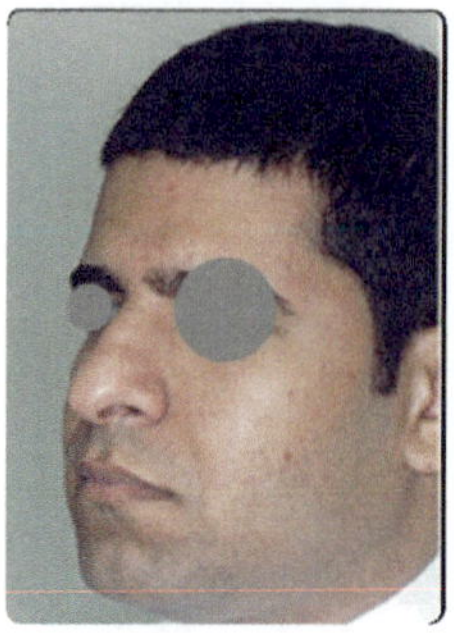

Postoperative

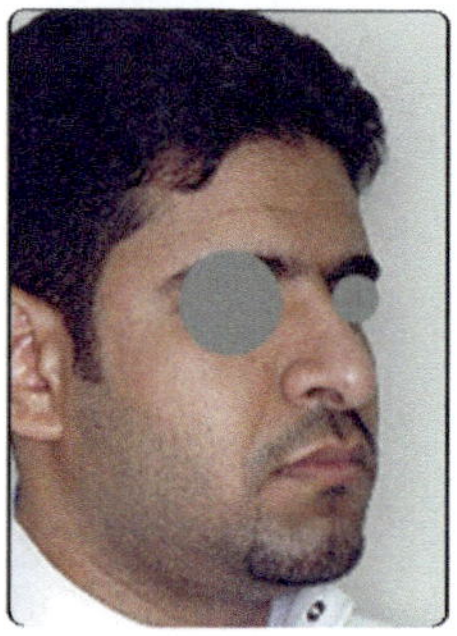

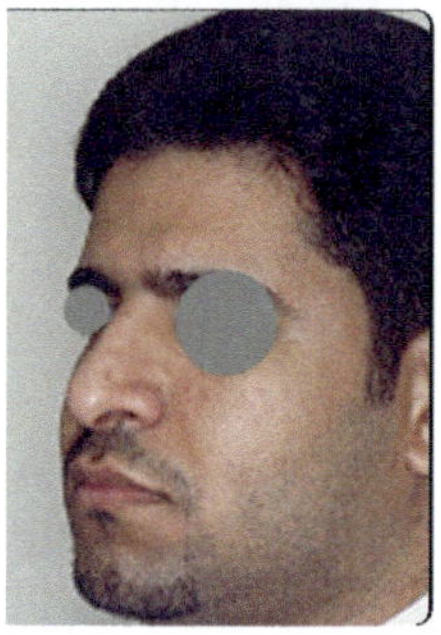

Right Lateral

Left Lateral

Right Lateral Smiling

Left Lateral Smiling

Preoperative

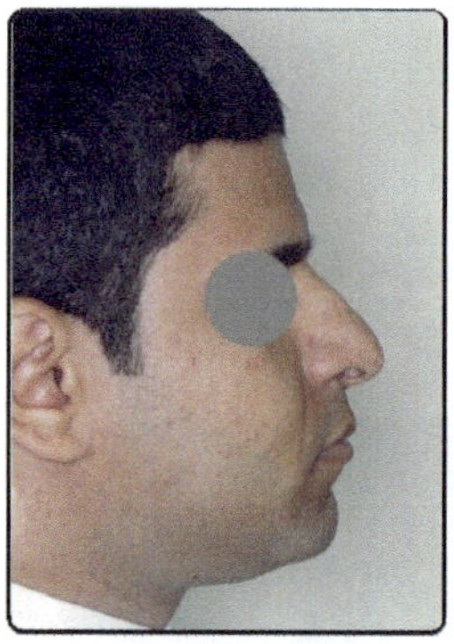

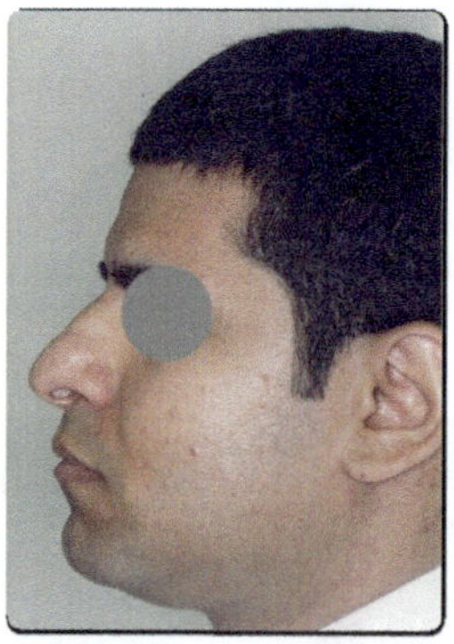

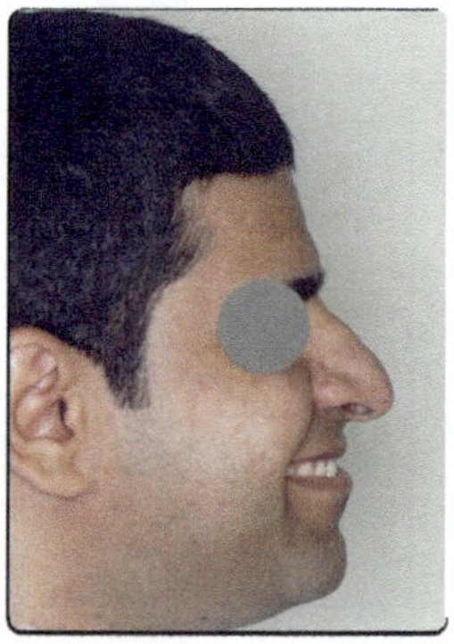

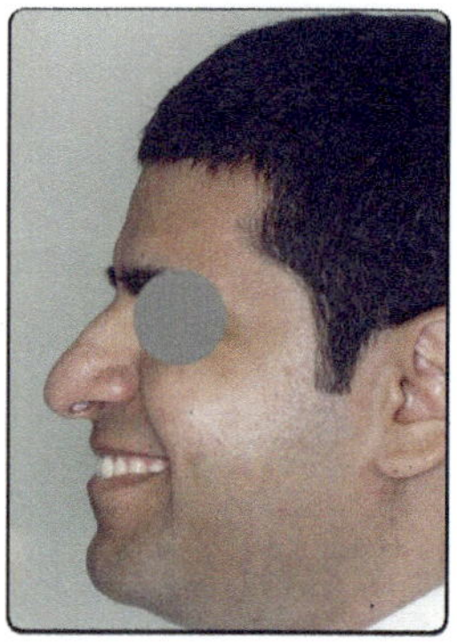

Postoperative

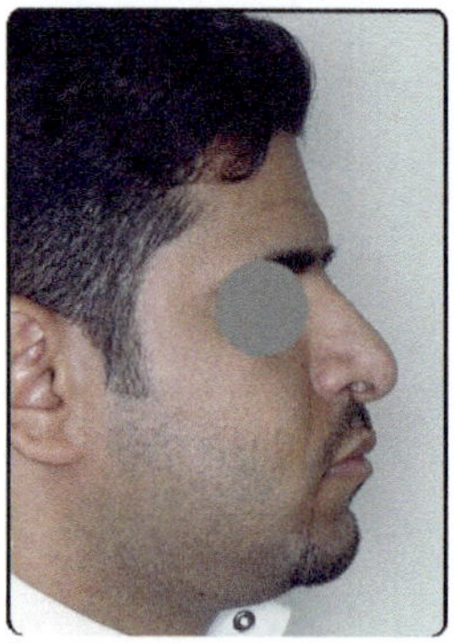

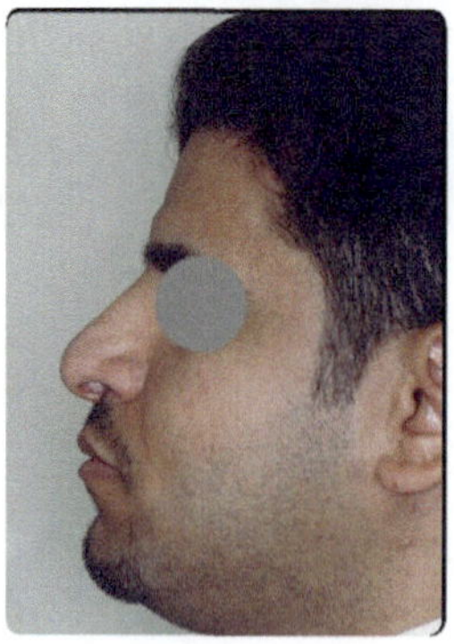

28 Part III: Clinical Case 13

Preoperative Assessment

1. **Frontolateral walls**
   a. Large and bulky nasal tip overshadowing the alae nasi on both sides (Frontal and Direct Dorsal Views).
2. **Medial Wall**
   Mobile tip (Lateral Smiling Views).
3. **Bony pyramid**
   a. Wide base of the boney pyramid (Direct Dorsal and Backward Tilting Views).
   b. The bony pyramid is slightly deviated, but not oblique, to the left side due to bilateral maxillary asymmetry. The left maxilla is wide and law, while the right axilla is narrow and high (Backward Tilting Views).
4. **Alar base**
   a. Thick alar base due to thick posterior segments of the rim-sill folds that are acutely bend over the upper lip giving the impression of a flat tire appearance. This is clearly seen in the illustrations of the right nasall aperture views with rim sill test. (Basal, Nasal Aperture and Backward Tilting Views).
   b. Wide alar base due to long inferior segments of rim-sill folds (Backward Tilting, Basal and Nasal Aperture Views).

Aims of Surgery

1. Reduce the bulk and size of the frontolateral walls.
2. Abolish the mobility of the nasal tip.
3. Reduce the width of the bony pyramid.
4. Reduce the bulk and size of the alar base.

Surgical Plan

1. **Frontolateral walls**
   a. DDD not including the weak triangle to reduce the bulk and size of the nasal tip and avoid supratip depression.
   b. Bilateral cephalic trim of the lateral crurae to reduce the size of the nasal tip.
2. **Medial Wall**
   Division of the depressor septi muscles.
3. **Bony pyramid**
   Bilateral osteotomies and medialization of the bony sidewalls to reduce the width of the bony pyramid.
4. **Alar base**
   Bilateral resection of the posterior and inferior segments of the rim-sill folds. Observe that clearly in illustrations of the left nasal aperture view with rim sill test.

Surgical Procedure

As per Surgical Plan.

Post-Operative Analysis

1. **Frontolateral Wall**
   a. Tip definition improved i.e. the tip is slimmer and prominently well identified. The alae nasi come into view to share in nasal aesthetics (Frontal, Direct Dorsal, Overhead, Backward Tilting and Basal Views).
   b. Tip projection: The nasal tip at the same level of the nasal dorsum with good aesthetic angle. This is coupled with good aesthetic nasolabial angle (lateral and oblique views).
   c. Tip light reflex is seen as one spot off the nasal tip. (Frontal and Backward Tilting Views).
2. **Medial Wall**
   Tip mobility was abolished (Smiling Lateral Views).
3. **Bony Pyramid**
   a. Bony pyramid aesthetics improved: the nasal dorsum is straight and the sidewalls are smooth and narrow (all views except the Basal Views).
   b. Dorsal light reflex is seen as an uninterrupted line off the nasal dorsum (Direct Dorsal Views).

M. H. A. Shafy, *Atlas of Clinical Cases in Rhinoplasty*,
https://doi.org/10.1007/978-3-031-07504-9_28

4. **Alar Base**
   a. Superior alar groove aesthetics improved by defatting. The grooves become longer and deeper (Oblique, Lateral and Direct Dorsal grooves).
   b. Posterior alar groove aesthetics improved by defatting. The alae nasi pulled medially and the angles of the posterior alar groove became wider. (Backward Tilting, Basal and Nasal Aperture Views).
   c. Alae nasi aesthetics improved. They were pulled medially, better seen and of smaller size. (Nasal Aperture and Oblique Views).
   d. Nasal aperture aesthetics improved after defatting and excision of the rim-sill folds:
      i. The size of nasal openings are smaller.
      ii. The shape of nasal apertures transformed from round thick walled openings with transverse axes to oval thin walled openings with anterior axes. The flat tire effects disappeared. (Backward Tilting, Basal and Nasal Aperture Views.
   e. Marginal light reflexes are clearly seen at:
      i. Inferior alar margins (Nasal Aperture Views).
      ii. Nasal sill bands (Oblique Views).
      iii. Lateral crural prominences (Lateral Views).

Commentary

a. Extensive defatting can only be achieved in closed Rhinoplasty to secure the nasal tip blood supply. Dividing the two columellar arteries, by a columellar incision, deprives the tip from good source of blood supply.
b. The lower lateral cartilages are too weak and small to have any effect on nasal aesthetics without thinning the skin by removing the the subdermal fatty layer as well as excising the thick fatty capsules of the middle and lateral crurae i.e. two step defatting procedure. Direct stitching and a columellar strut would have minimal, if any, effect on the patient's tip definition and tip projection and certainly no effect on the size or the bulk of the nose.
c. The subdermal fat as well as the fatty capsules of the middle and lateral crurae were extensive in this young lady. The postoperative reduction in the bulk was dramatic. The overall reduction of the nasal size had completely altered the appearance of her nose and face. The nasal skin became thinner, smoother and more attractive looking.
d. Personality changes: Preoperatively, this young lady was known to be quite rude, displayed an aggressive attitude and always used very strong language. Postoperatively, her first words were, "I can't believe that this is my nose and face!". A few months later, her mother stated that she had a completely different attitude, behavior and language. She is much more refined and lady like.
e. The young lady paid more attention to the health of her skin post-operatively. Previously she couldn't care less about going to a Dermatologist to receive treatment for her face.

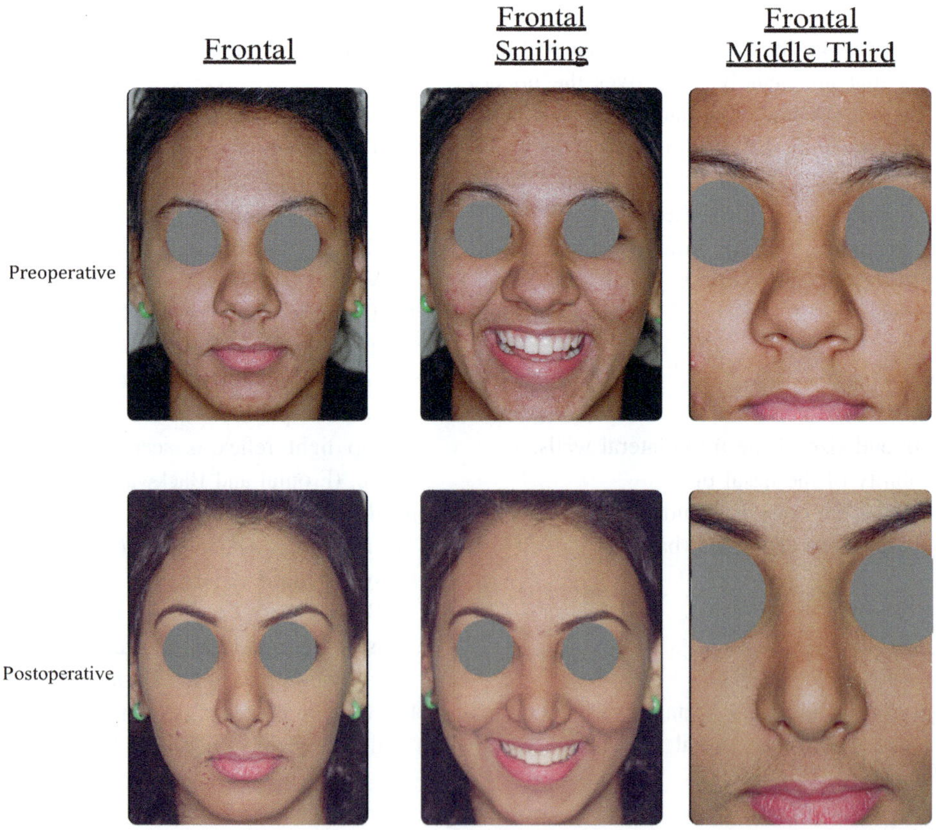

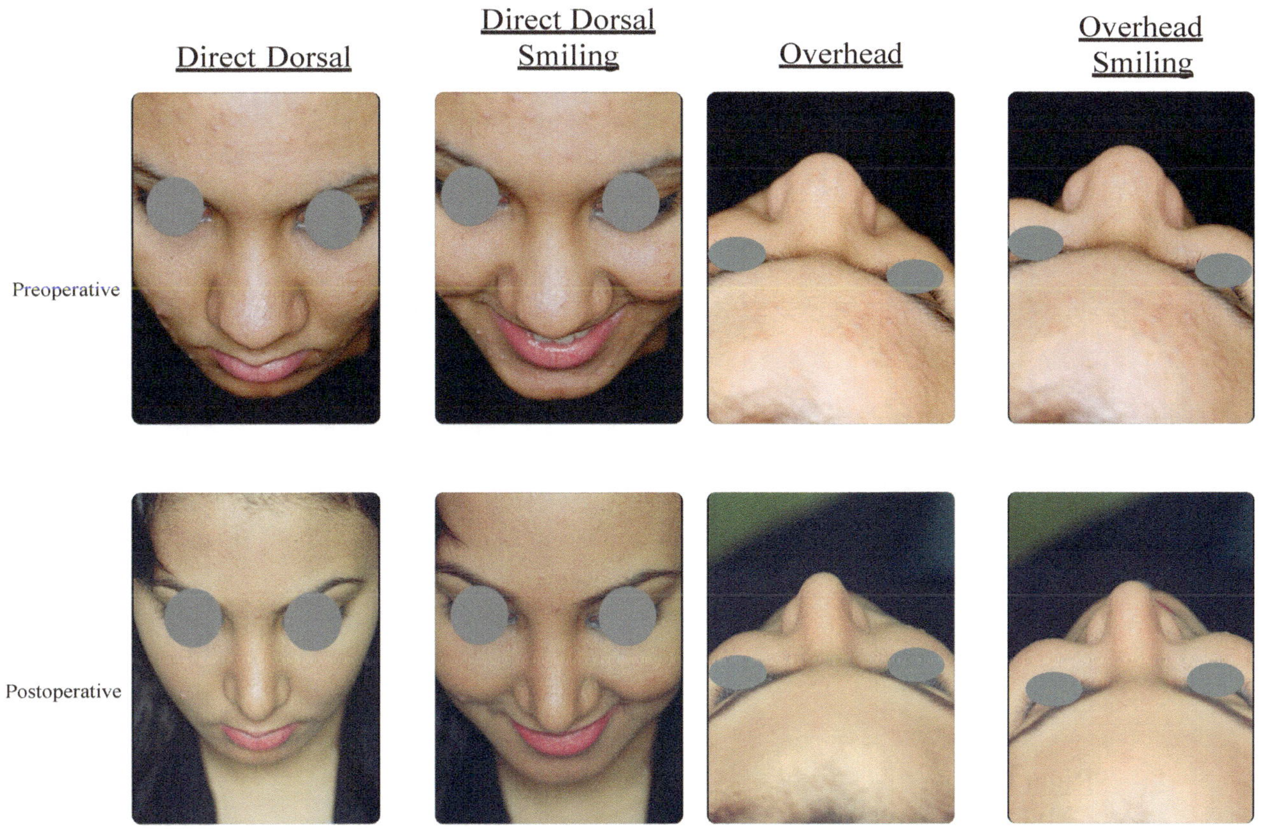
Direct Dorsal
Direct Dorsal Smiling
Overhead
Overhead Smiling
Preoperative
Postoperative

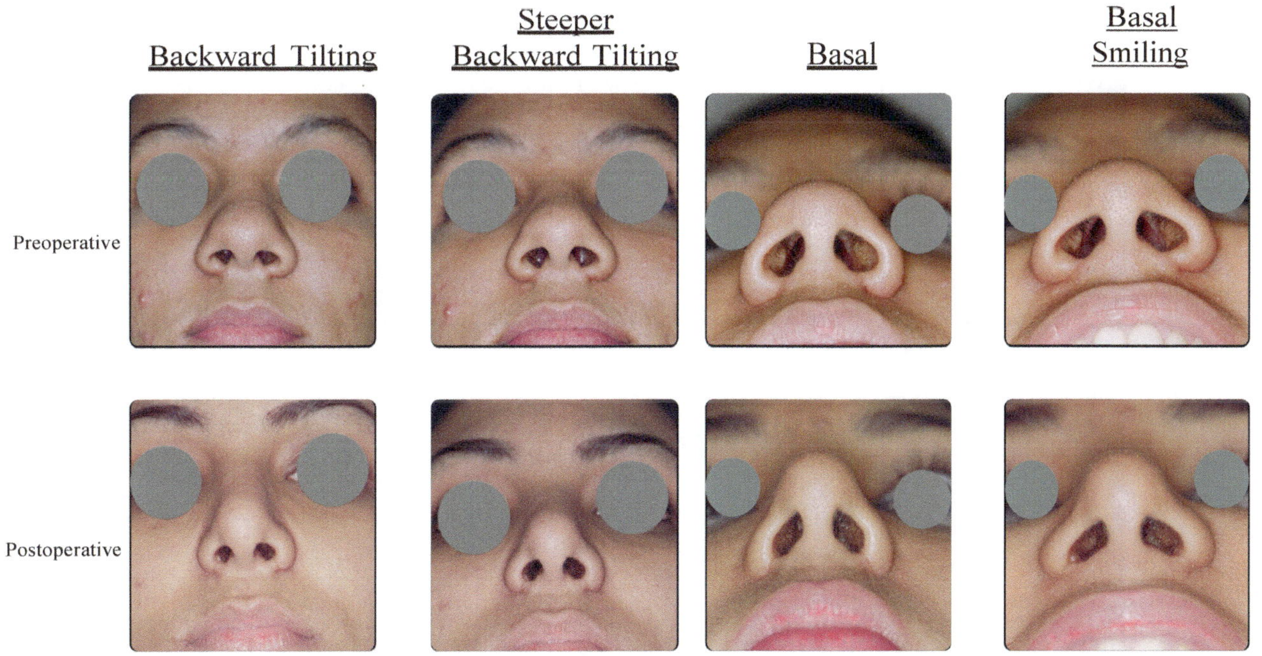
Backward Tilting
Steeper Backward Tilting
Basal
Basal Smiling
Preoperative
Postoperative

Right Nasal Aperture | **Right Nasal Aperture Rim Sill Test** | **Left Nasal Aperture Rim Sill Test** | **Left Nasal Aperture**

Preoperative

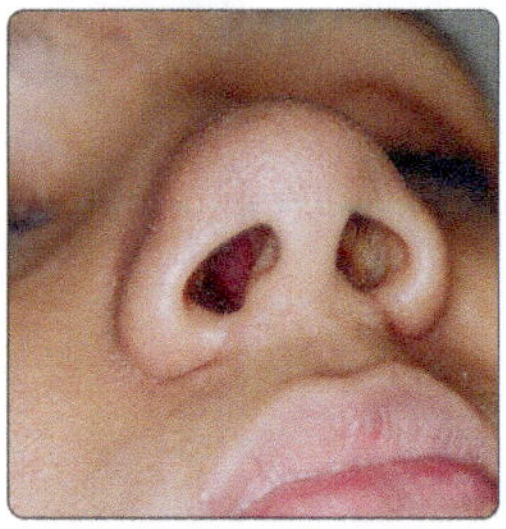
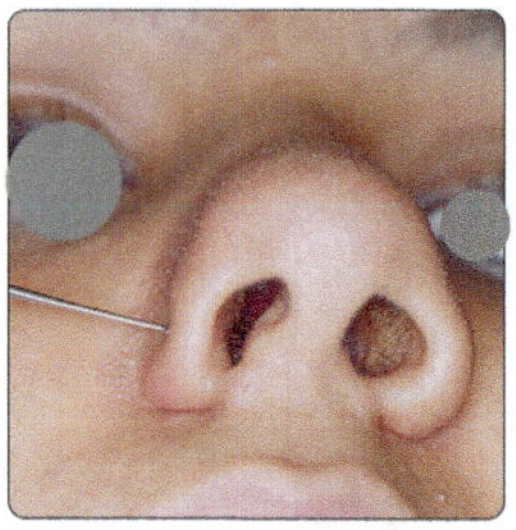
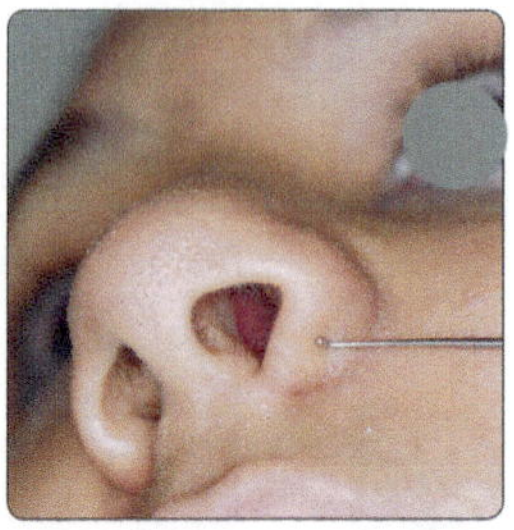
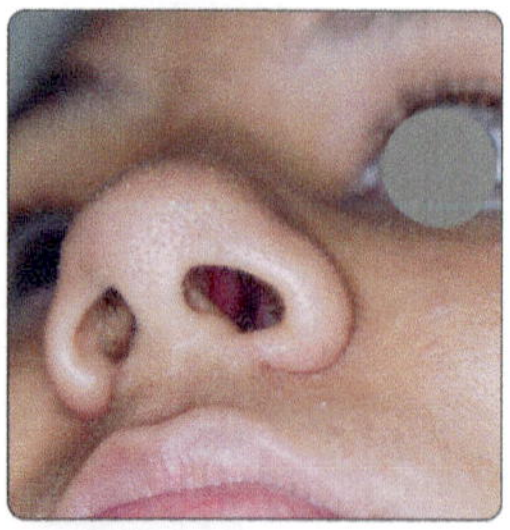

Postoperative

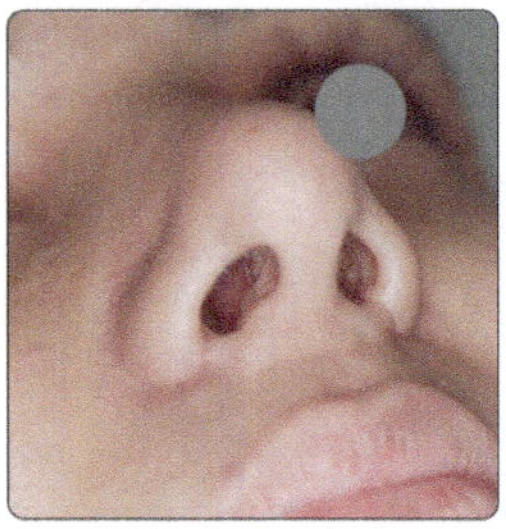
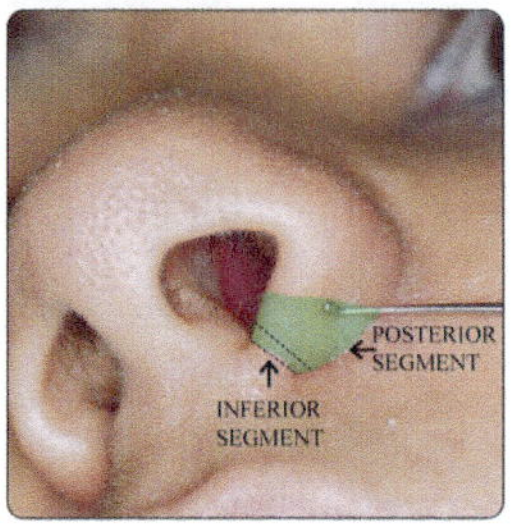

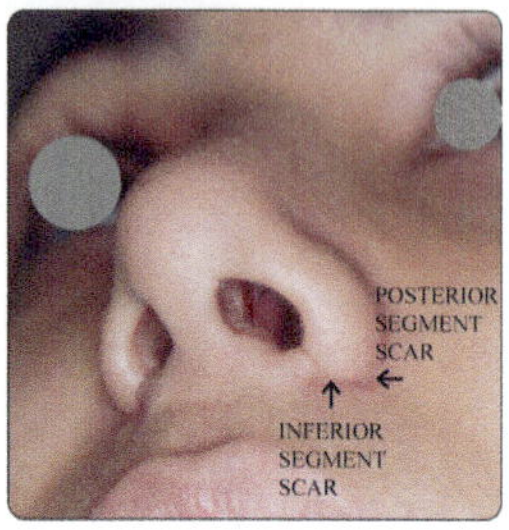

Right Oblique Mid Cheek Full Face | Left Oblique Mid Cheek Full Face | Right Oblique Mid Cheek Middle Third | Left Oblique Mid Cheek Middle Third

Preoperative

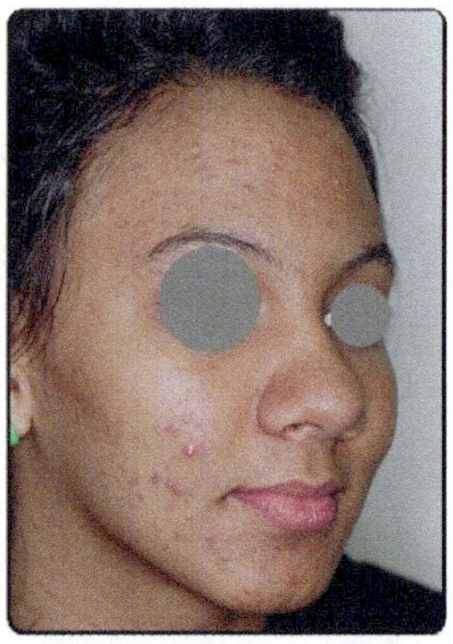
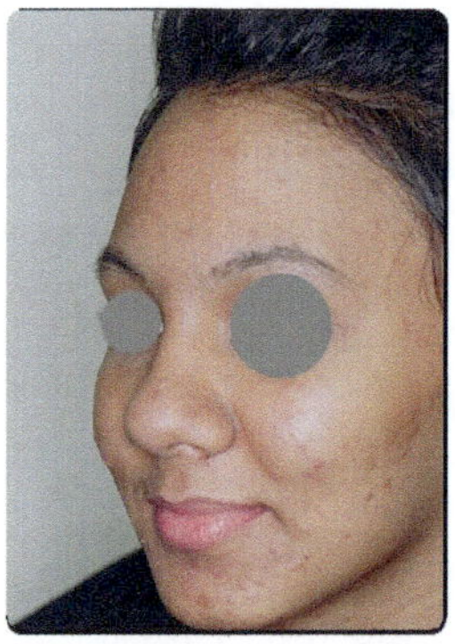
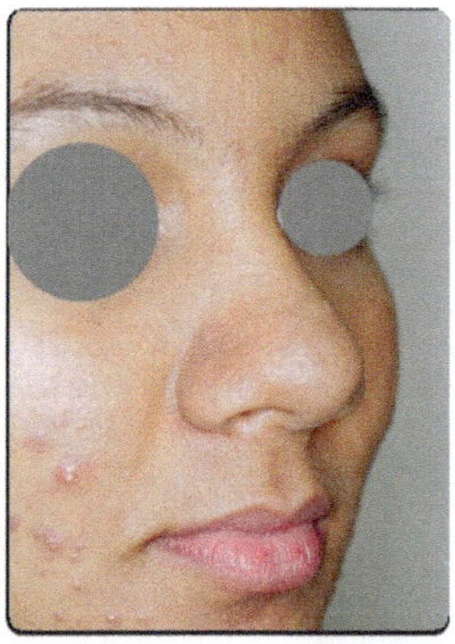
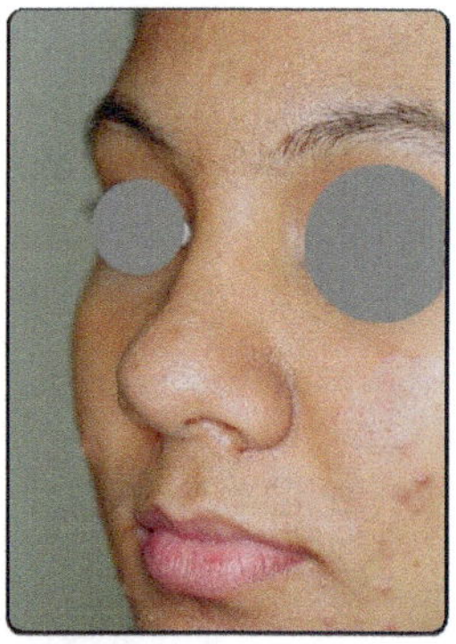

Postoperative

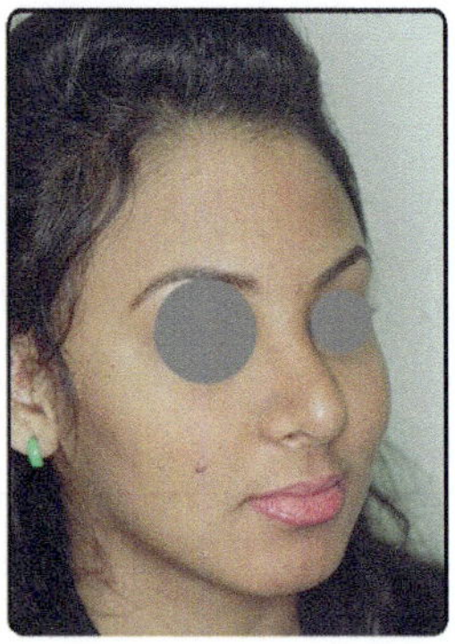
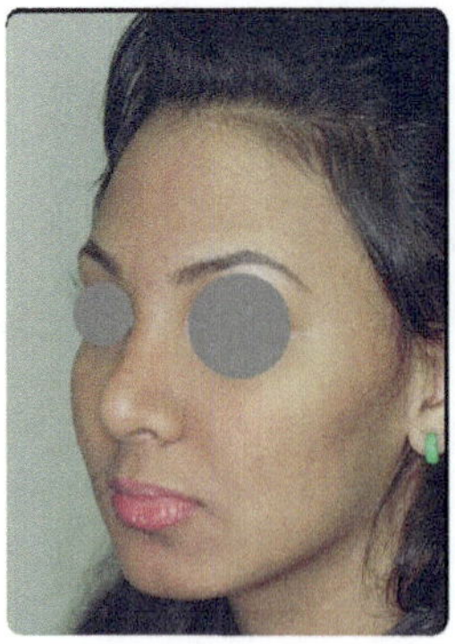
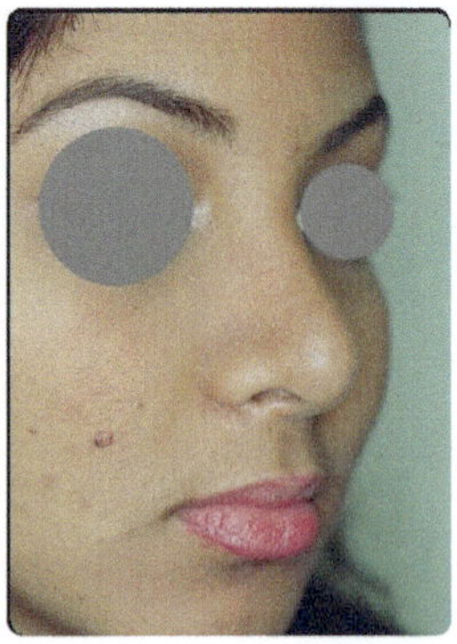
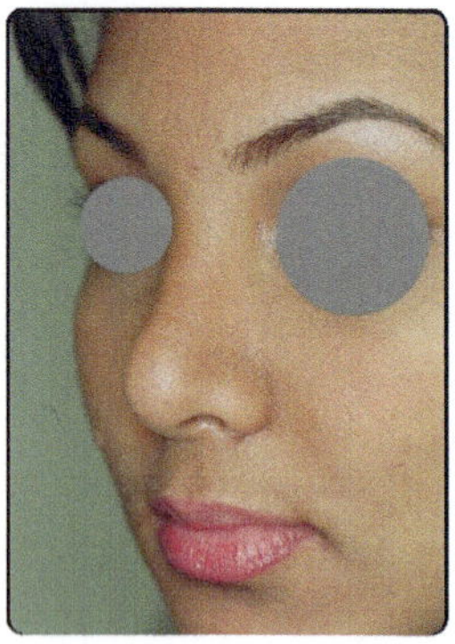

Right Oblique Cheek Margin Full Face | Left Oblique Cheek Margin Full Face | Right Oblique Cheek Margin Middle Third | Left Oblique Cheek Margin Middle Third

Preoperative

Postoperative

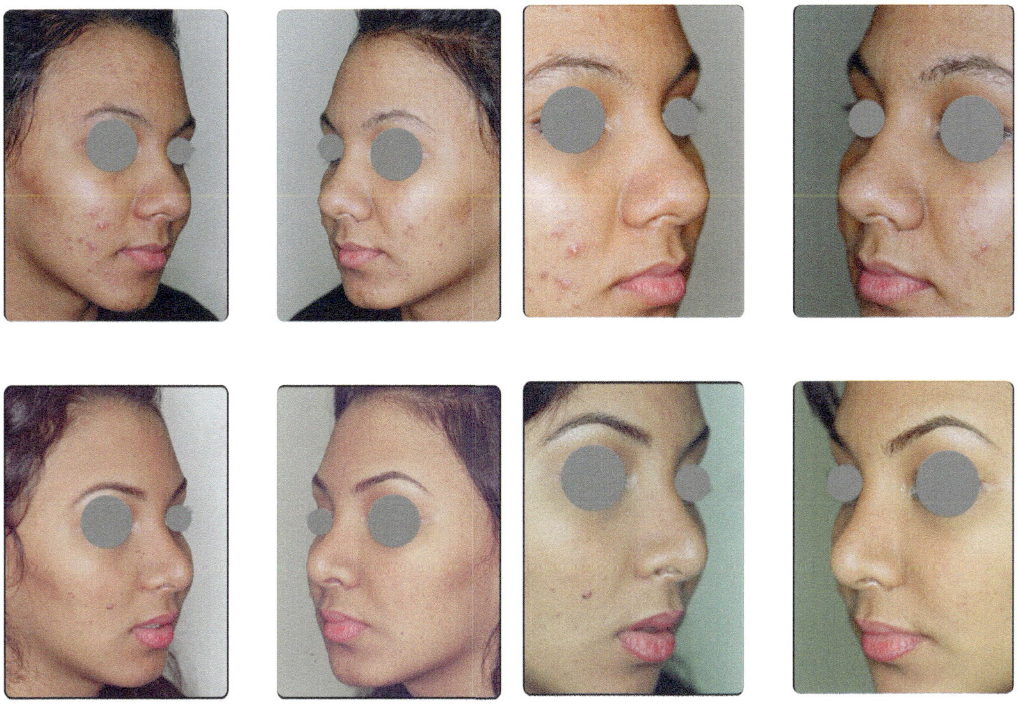

Right Lateral | Left Lateral | Right Lateral Smiling | Left Lateral Smiling

Preoperative

Postoperative

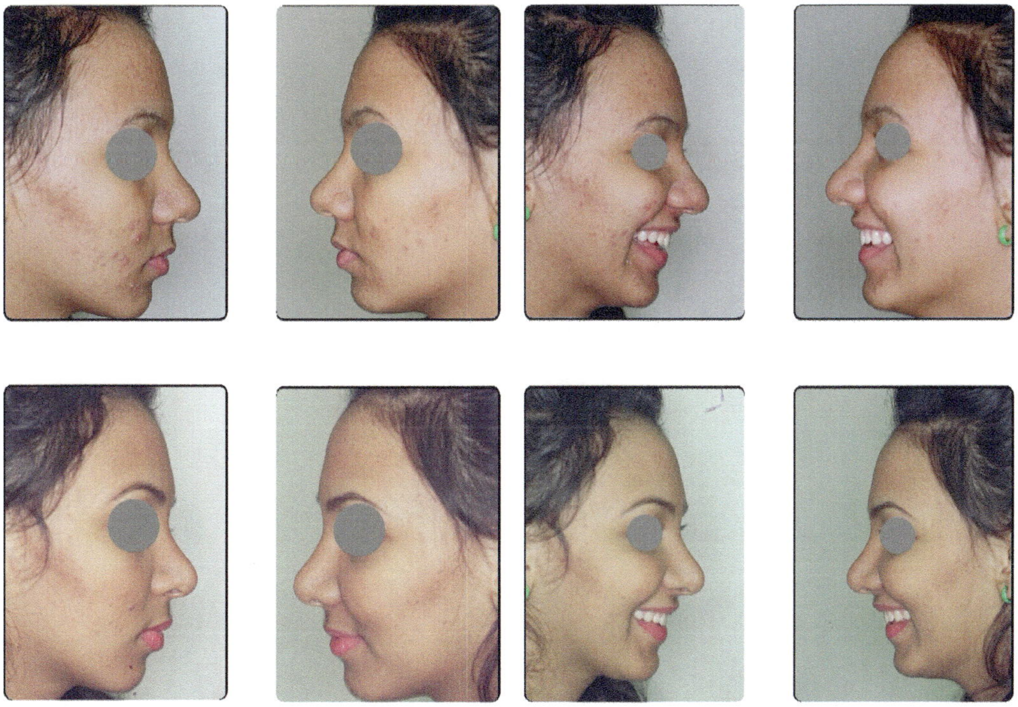

29 Part III: Clinical Case 14

Preoperative Assessment

1. **Frontolateral walls**
   a. Bulky tip as well as the lower two thirds of the nose. The alae nasi were hidden behind the bulky tip. (Frontal and Direct Dorsal Views).
   b. There is a small mole on the left ala nasi (Frontal and Direct Dorsal Views).
2. **Medial Wall**
   Nil of note.
3. **Bony pyramid**
   a. Small osteocartilaginous hump (Backward Tilting, Lateral and Oblique Views).
   b. Wide base of the bony pyramid (Direct Dorsal and Backward Tilting Views).
   c. Bulky middle third due to excess subdermal fat over the upper lateral cartilage.
4. **Alar base**
   a. Bulky alar base due to thick posterior segments of the rim sill folds. The naso-labial angles are acute producing a flat tire appearance (Backward, Tilting and Basal and Nasal Aperture Views).
   b. Wide alar base due to long inferior segments of rim-sill folds. (Backward Tilting and Basal Views).

Aims of Surgery

The overall reduction of the bulk and the size of the nose that includes the following:

1. Reduction of the bulk of the frontolateral walls and the middle third of the nose.
2. Reduction of the size of the bony pyramid.
3. Reduction of the size and bulk of the alar base.

Surgical Plan

1. **Frontolateral walls**
   a. DDD including the weak triangle to reduce the bulk of frontolateral walls and midvault.
   b. Cephalic trim of the lateral crurae to reduce the size of frontolateral wals.
   c. Removal of fat over the upper lateral cartilage to reduce the bulk of the middle third.
   d. Removal of the mole off the left ala nasi.
2. **Medial Wall**
   Nil of note.
3. **Bony pyramid**
   a. Excision of the osteocartilaginous hump.
   b. Osteotomies and medialization of the lateral bony walls.
4. **Alar base**
   Excision of the posterior and inferior segments of the rim sill folds. See illustration in the right nasal aperture view with rim sill test.

Surgical Procedure

a. As per Surgical Plan.
b. Longitudinal bilateral medial division of the attachments of the upper lateral cartilage to the nasal septum. This had an additional effect in reducing the width of the middle third of the nose. In these condition the distal triangular 2 mm of the upper lateral cartilage is trimmed in order to widen the internal valve angle (see Anatomy and Physiology of the Nasal Valve).

M. H. A. Shafy, *Atlas of Clinical Cases in Rhinoplasty*,
https://doi.org/10.1007/978-3-031-07504-9_29

Post-Operative Analysis

1. **Frontolateral Wall**
   a. Tip definition improved i.e. the tip is slimmer and prominently well identified. The alae nasi come into view to share in nasal aesthetics (Frontal, Direct Dorsal, Overhead, Backward Tilting and Basal Views).
   b. Tip projection: The nasal tip at the same level of the nasal dorsum with good aesthetic angle. This is coupled with good aesthetic nasolabial angle (lateral and oblique views).
   c. Tip light reflex is seen as one spot off the nasal tip. (Frontal and Backward Tilting Views).
2. **Medial Wall**
   Nil of Note.
3. **Bony Pyramid**
   a. Bony pyramid aesthetics: the nasal dorsum is straight and the sidewalls are smooth and narrow (all views except the Basal Views).
   b. Dorsal light reflex is seen as a regular one line off the nasal dorsum (Direct Dorsal Views).
4. **Alar Base**
   a. The superior alar grooves now clear off fat, become deeper, longer and visible (Direct Dorsal, Oblique and Lateral Views).
   b. Posterior alar groove aesthetics improved by excising the posterior segment of the rim-sill folds. Flat tire appearance is no longer present. (Backward Tilting, Basal and Nasal Aperture Views).
   c. Alae nasi aesthetics improved. They are pulled medially, better seen and are elegantly smaller. (Nasal Aperture, Oblique and Lateral Views).
   d. Nasal aperture aesthetics:
      i. Aperture size: Excision of the inferior segments of the rim sill folds have reduced the size of the nasal openings. The scars are seen as longitudinal lines at the lateral end of the nasal sill bands. The latter disappear in few weeks.
      ii. Aperture bulk: Excising the posterior segment of the rim sill fold greatly reduced the bulk of the alar base. The posterior and inferior segments are clearly seen as a pale area in the right rim sill test photograph. Postoperatively the scars are hardly seen and well camouflaged as they are hidden in the posterior alar grooves.
      iii. Aperture shape: the nasal apertures have thin walls and look aesthetically smaller and better.
   e. Marginal light reflexes are clearly seen at:
      i. Inferior alar margins (Nasal Aperture Views).
      ii. Nasal sill bands (Oblique Views).
      iii. Lateral crural prominences (Lateral Views).

Commentary

a. Postoperative photographs are taken 10 days after surgery.
b. Defatting not only had the aesthetic advantage of reducing the bulk of the middle and lower thirds of the nose, but it also clearly changed the nature of the skin to become thinner with a smooth attractive surface. Her face looked younger.
c. The Psychological impact was quite noticeable in this lady. She felt proud and confident of her normal young age as she would have always wished for.

Frontal

Preoperative

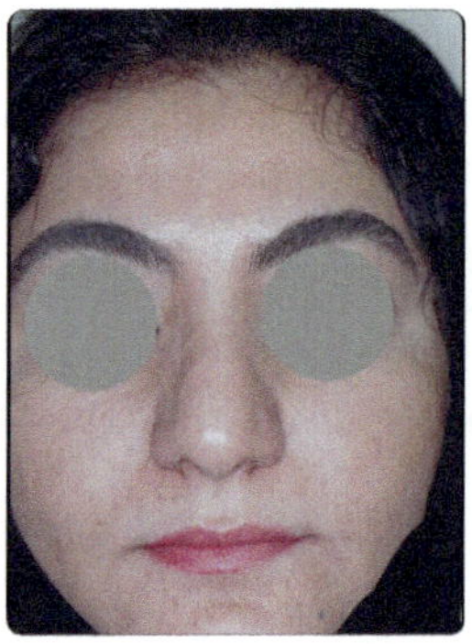

Postoperative

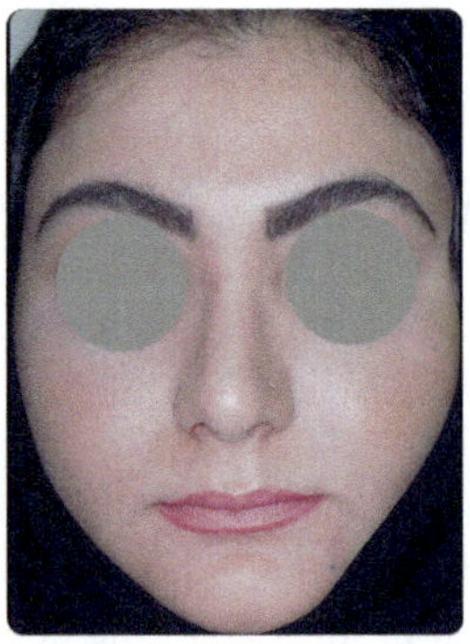

Direct Dorsal

Preoperative

Postoperative

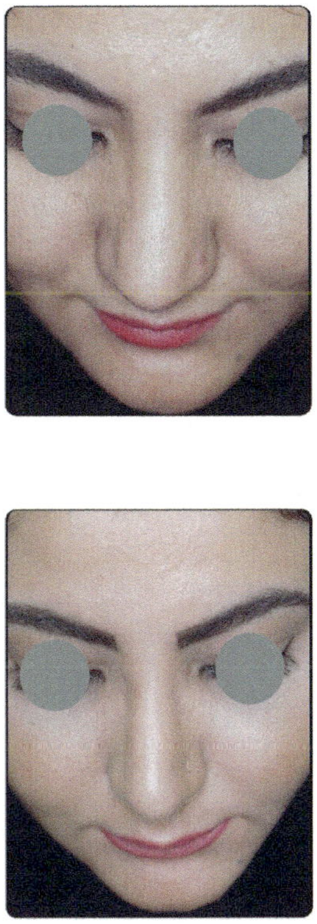

Steeper Backward Tilting

Basal

Preoperative

Postoperative

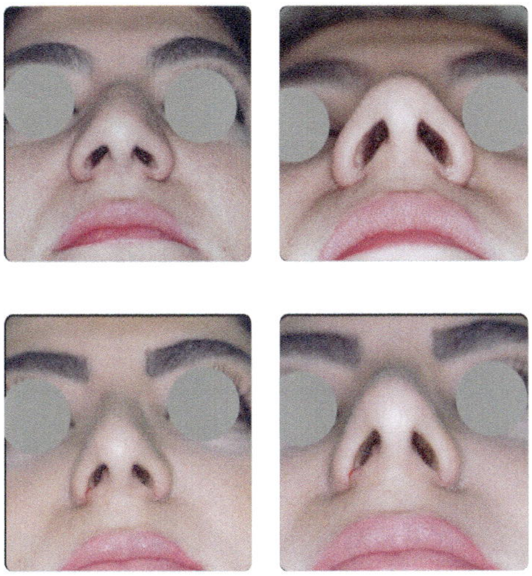

Right Nasal Aperture

Right Nasal Aperture Rim Sill Test

Left Nasal Aperture Rim Sill Test

Left Nasal Aperture

Preoperative

Postoperative

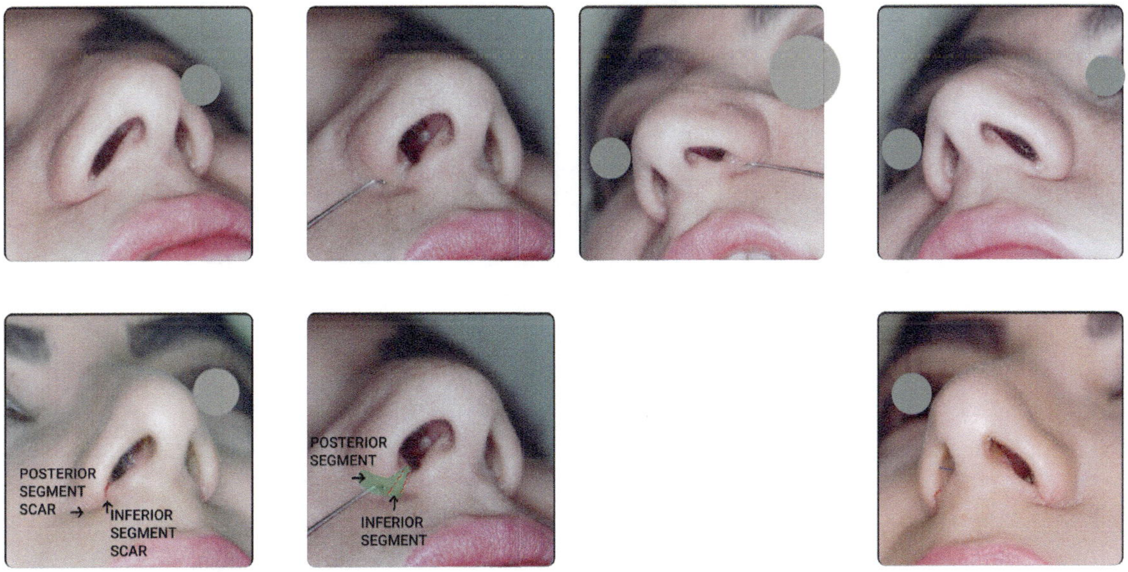

	Right Oblique Mid Cheek Middle Third	Left Oblique Mid Cheek Middle Third	Right Oblique Cheek Margin Full Face	Left Oblique Cheek Margin Full Face
Preoperative	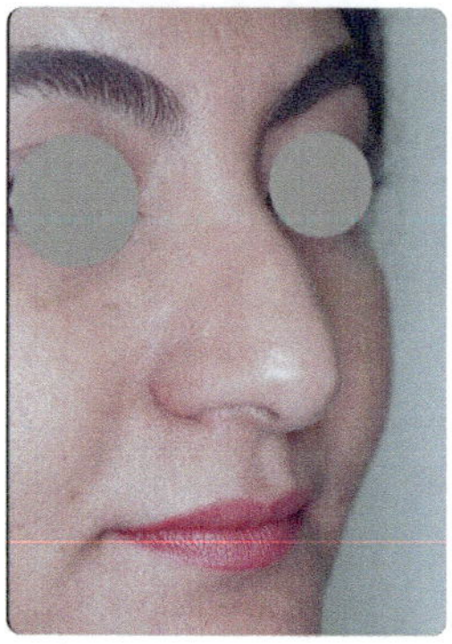	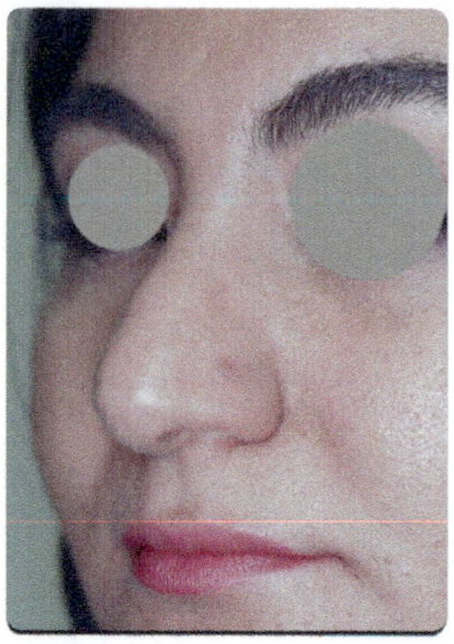	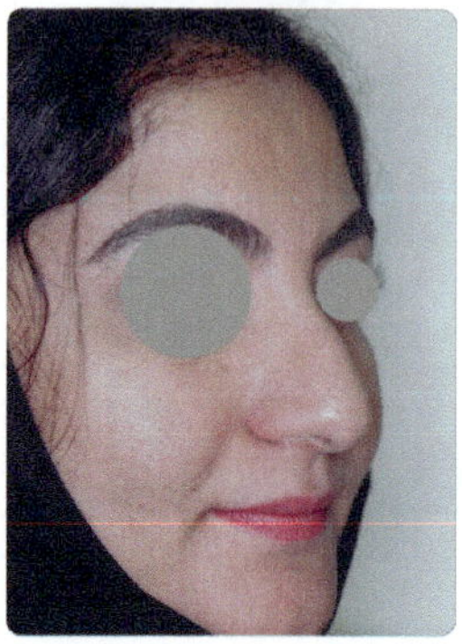	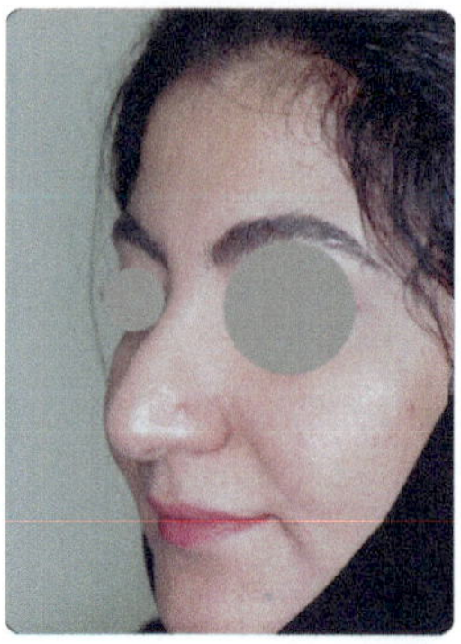
Postoperative	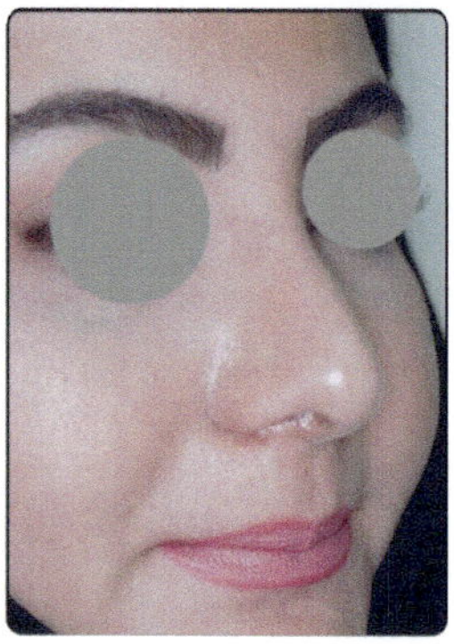	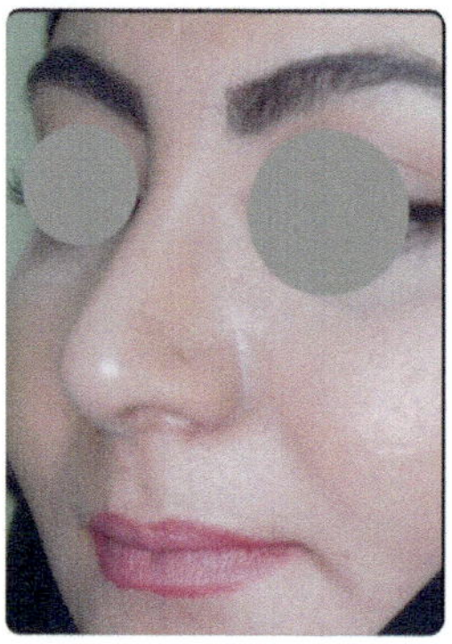	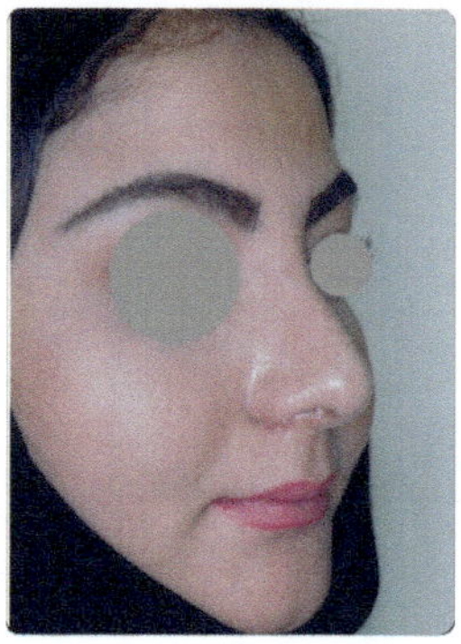	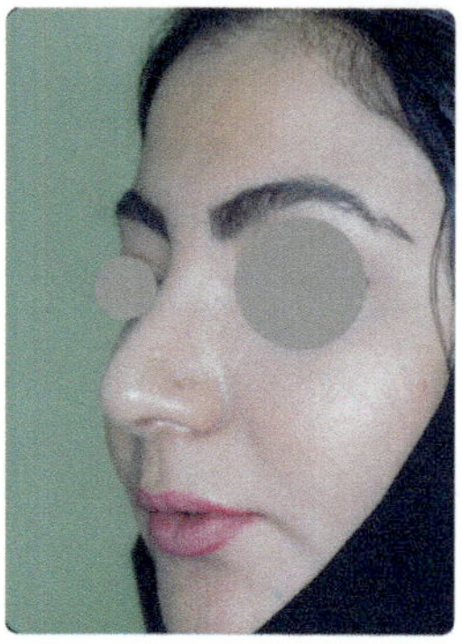

	Right Lateral	Left Lateral
Preoperative	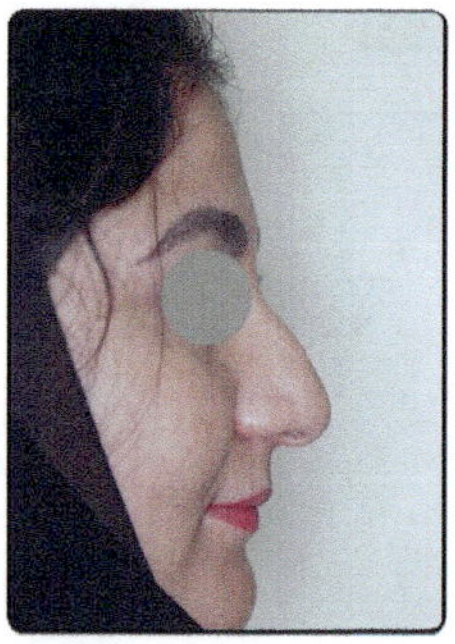	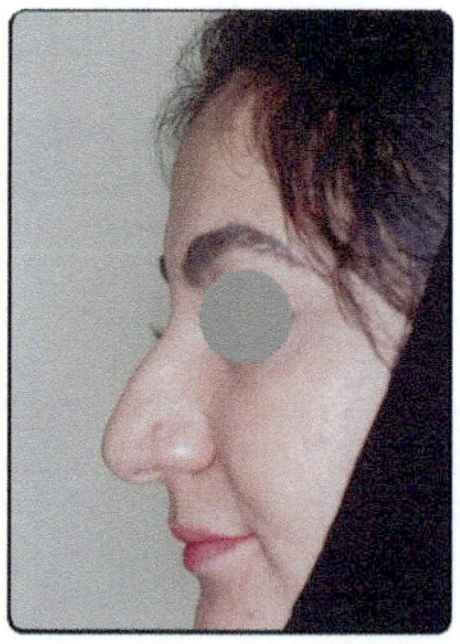
Postoperative	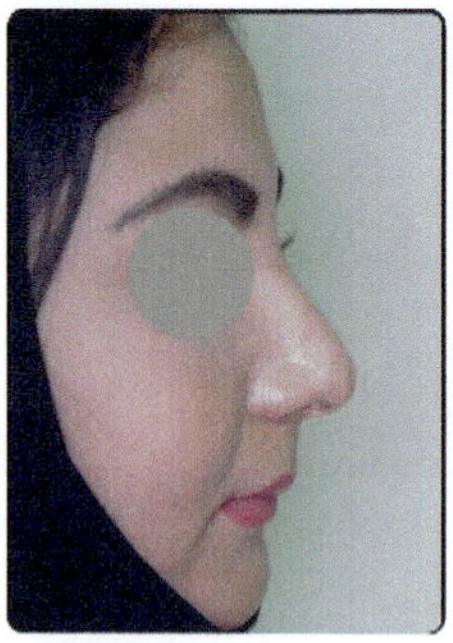	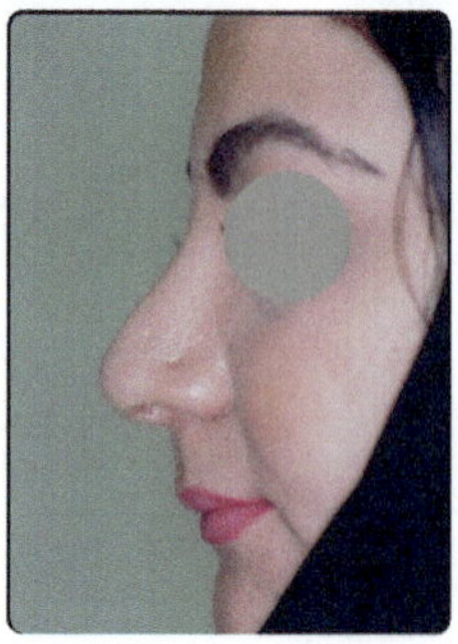

Part III: Clinical Case 15

30

Preoperative Assessment

1. **Frontolateral walls**
   Excessively bulky tip overshadowing the alae nasi (Frontal, Direct Dorsal and Overhead Views).
2. **Medial Wall**
   Nil of note.
3. **Boney pyramid**
   a. Wide base of the bony pyramid (Direct Dorsal and Backward Tilting Views).
   b. Bulky middle third due to excess subdermal fat over the upper lateral cartilage and supra tip area of the weak triangle.
   c. The dorsal. Light reflex is diffuse, (Direct Dorsal Views).
4. **Alar base**
   Wide, thick alar base due to long inferior segments and thick posterior segments of the rim sill folds successively. The posterior segments have acute angles with the upper lip, i.e. a flat car tire appearance.

Aims of Surgery

The overall reduction of the bulk and the size of the nose that includes the following:

1. Reduction of the bulk of the frontolateral walls and the middle third of the nose.
2. Reduction of the size of the bony pyramid.
3. Reduction of the size and bulk of the alar base.

Surgical Plan

1. **Frontolateral walls**
   a. DDD including the weak triangle to reduce the bulk of the nasal tip and midvault.
   b. Cephalic trim of the lateral crurae to reduce the size.
2. **Medial Wall**
   Nil of Note.
3. **Boney pyramid**
   a. Osteotomies and medialization of the lateral bony walls.
   b. Defatting the upper lateral cartilage.
4. **Alar base**
   Excision of the posterior and inferior segments of the rim sill folds.

Surgical Procedure

a. As per Surgical Plan.
b. After defatening it was found that the left side of the nasal tip (the left dome) is at a lower level than the right side (right dome). Tip augmentation with small pieces of crushed septal cartilages was used over the left dome to balance the levels between the two sides.

Post-Operative Analysis

1. **Frontolateral Walls**
   a. Tip definition improved i.e. slimmer and prominently well identified with thinner overlying skin. The alae nasi come into view to share in nasal aesthetics (Frontal, Direct Dorsal, Overhead, Backward Tilting and Basal Views).
   b. Tip projection: The nasal tip is at the same level of the nasal dorsum with good aesthetic angle. This is coupled with good aesthetic nasolabial angle (lateral and oblique views).
   c. Tip light reflex of the nasal tip is seen as one spot off the nasal tip. (Frontal, Backward Tilting and Basal Views).
2. **Medial Wall**
   Nil of Note.
3. **Bony Pyramid**
   a. Bony pyramid aesthetics improved: the nasal dorsum is straight and the sidewalls are smooth and narrow (all views except the Basal Views).

M. H. A. Shafy, *Atlas of Clinical Cases in Rhinoplasty*,
https://doi.org/10.1007/978-3-031-07504-9_30

b. Dorsal light reflex is seen as a regular one line off the nasal dorsum (Direct Dorsal Views).

4. **Alar Base**
   a. The superior alar grooves now clear off fat, become deeper, longer and visible (Direct Dorsal, Oblique and Lateral Views).
   b. Posterior alar groove aesthetics improved by excising the rim-sill folds. Flat tire appearance is no longer present. (Backward Tilting, Basal and Nasal Aperture Views).
   c. Alae nasi aesthetics improved. They are pulled medially, better seen and are elegantly smaller.
   d. Nasal aperture aesthetics improved by defatting and excising the rim-sill folds:
      i. The size of the nasal openings is smaller. (Backward Tilting, Basal and Nasal Aperture views).
      ii. The shape of nasal openings transformed from thick walled wide and rounded openings with transverse long axes to thin walled small oval openings with anterior long axes. (Backward Tilting, Basal and Nasal Aperture views).
   e. Marginal light reflexes are clearly seen at:
      i. Inferior alar margins (Nasal Aperture Views).
      ii. Nasal sill bands (Oblique Views).

Commentary

a. The amount subdermal and the capsular fatty layers of middle and lateral crurae were extensive. Nevertheless there was no redundant skin as anticipated.
b. The patient was happy that her characteristic personal image of nose and face was not changed, despite the dramatic reduction in the size of the nose.
c. There might be a temptation to carry out extra work defining the tip, e.g. a tip graft. This would have produced an unnatural surgical looking nose which would not suit the patient's, rounded face. Besides she would have lost her original nasal print.

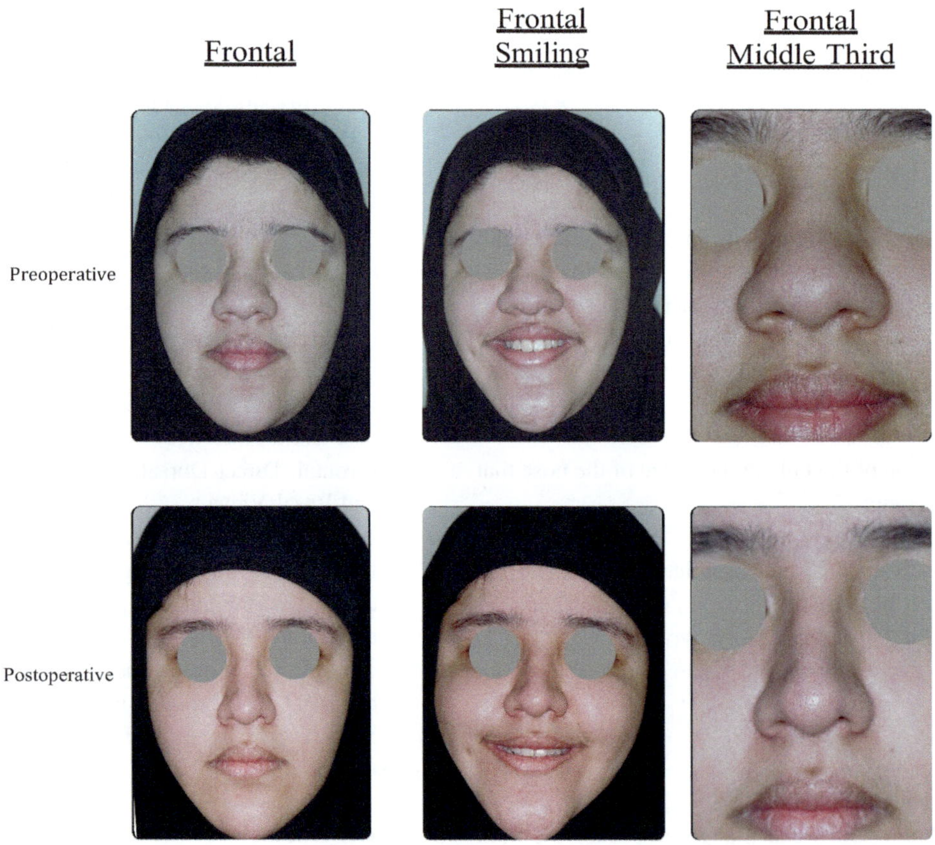

Direct Dorsal | Direct Dorsal Smiling | Overhead

Preoperative

Postoperative

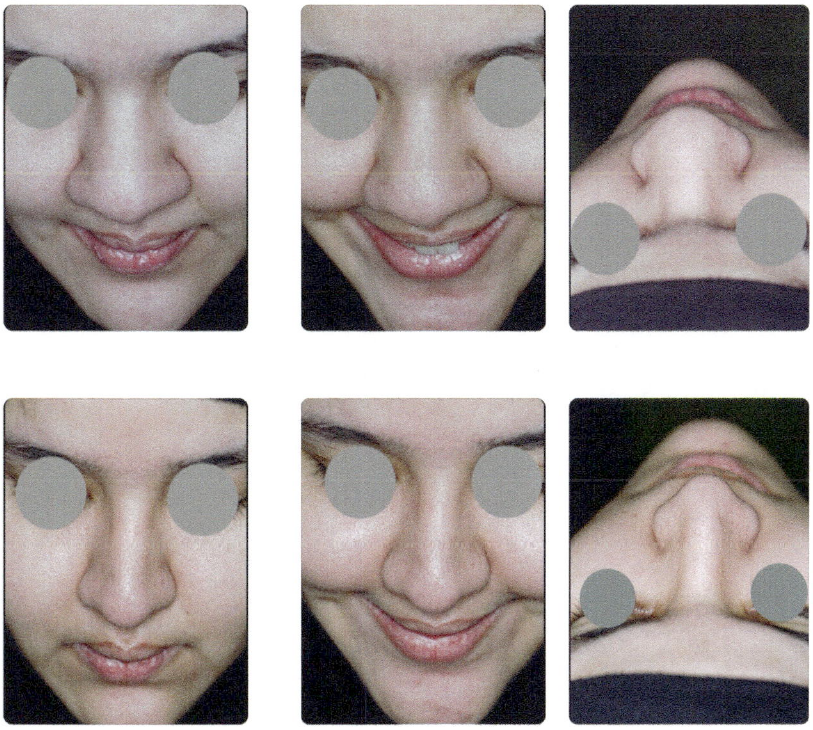

Backward Tilting | Steeper Backward Tilting | Basal | Basal Smiling

Preoperative

Postoperative

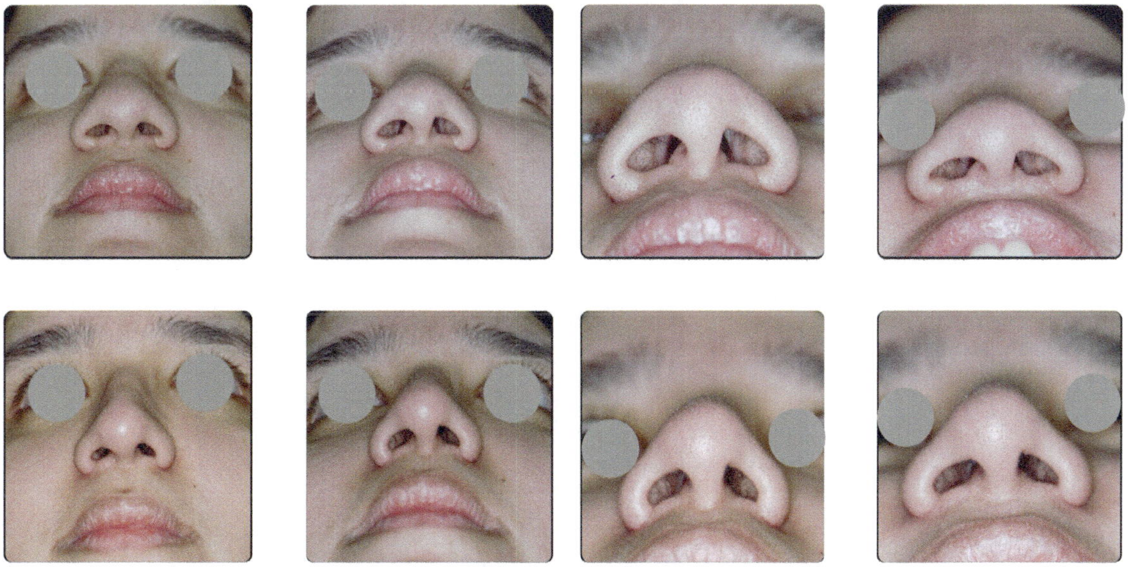

Right Nasal Aperture | Right Nasal Aperture Rim Sill Test | Left Nasal Aperture Rim Sill Test | Left Nasal Aperture

Preoperative

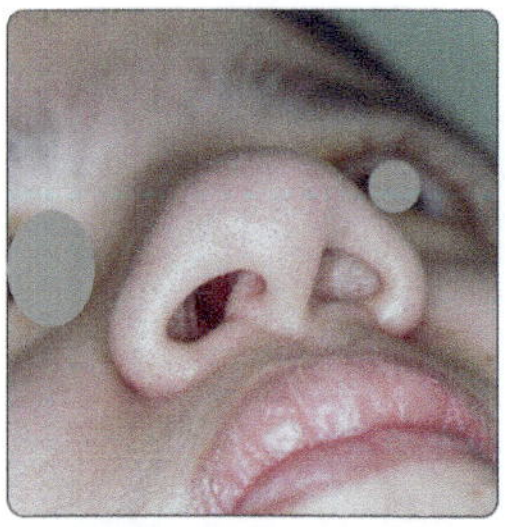

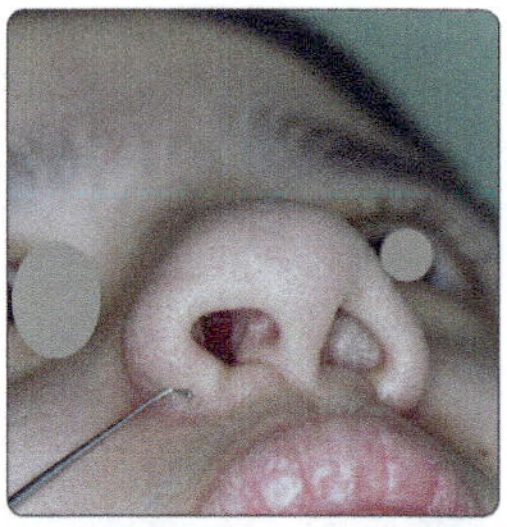

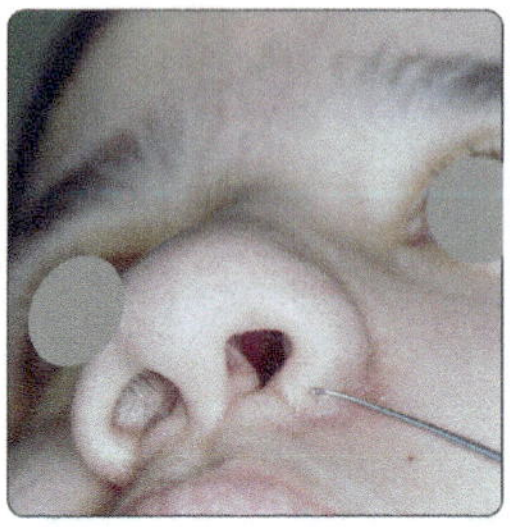

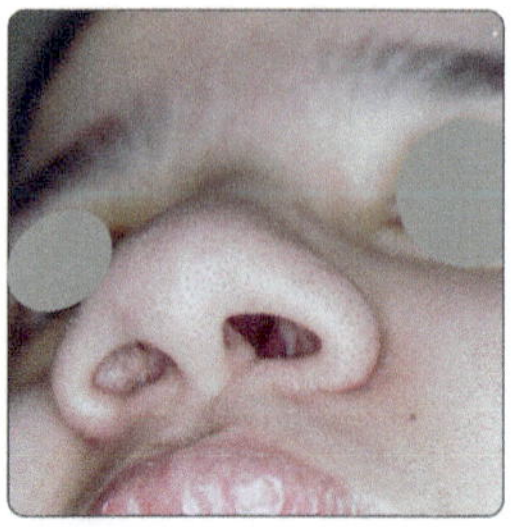

Postoperative

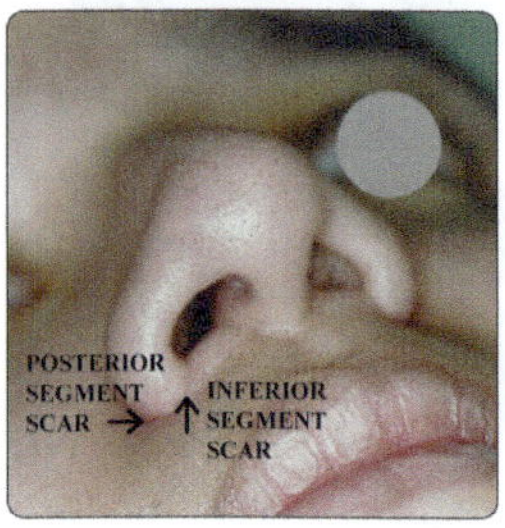

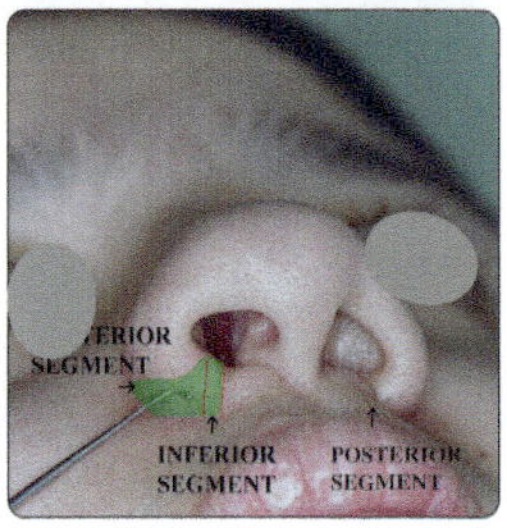

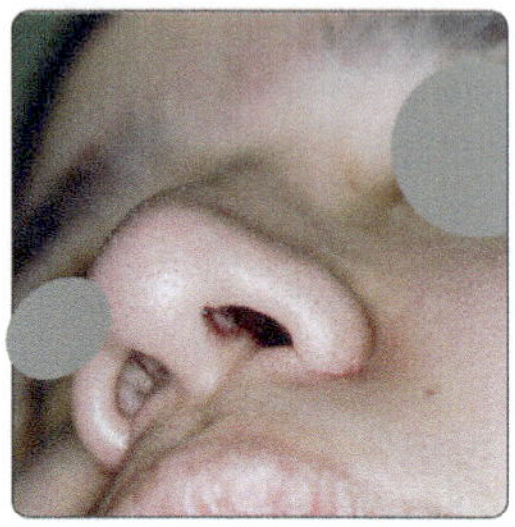

Right Oblique Mid Cheek Full Face | Left Oblique Mid Cheek Full Face

Preoperative

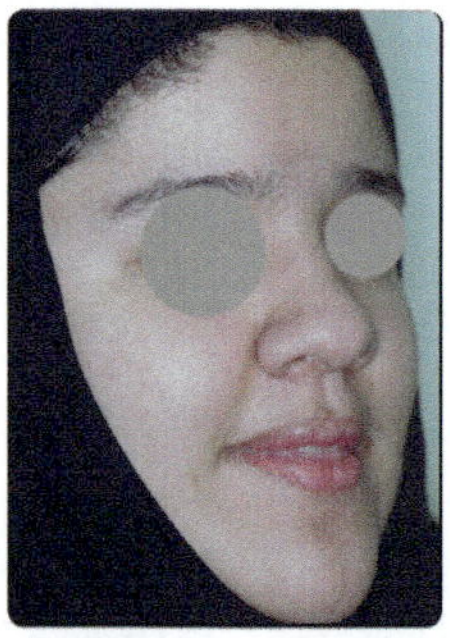

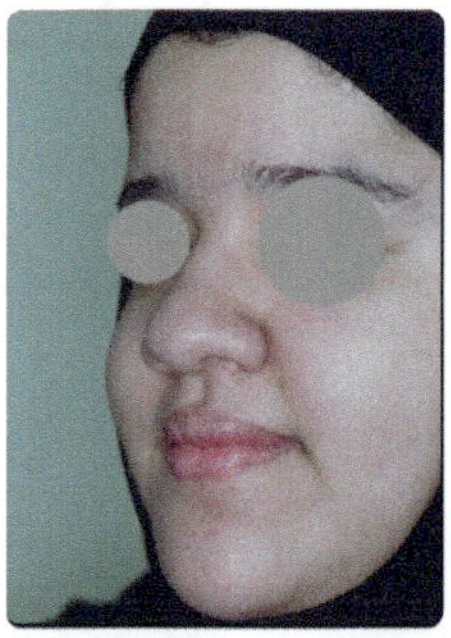

Postoperative

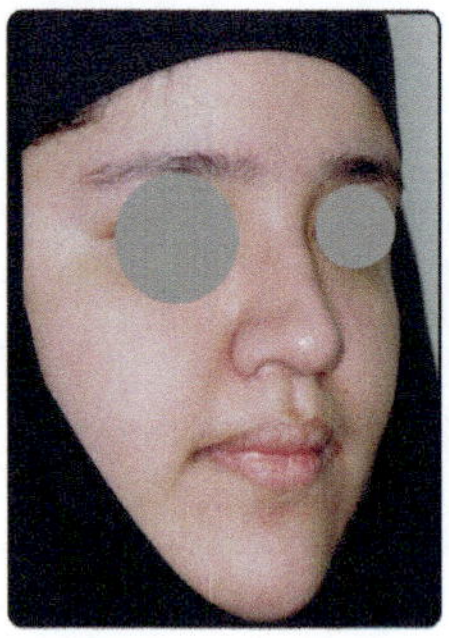

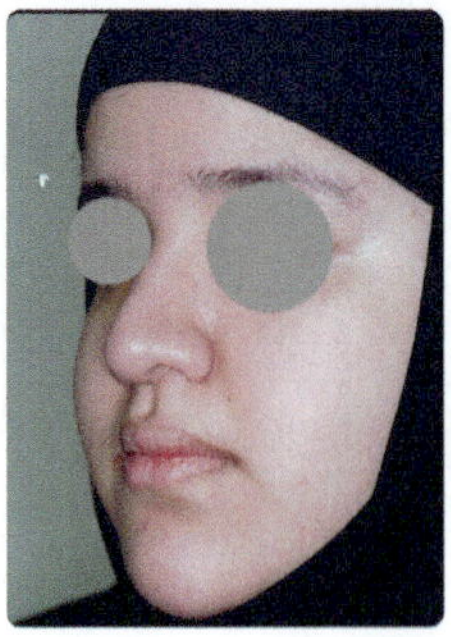

Right Oblique Cheek Margin Full Face	Left Oblique Cheek Margin Full Face	Right Oblique Cheek Margin Middle Third	Left Oblique Cheek Margin Middle Third

Preoperative

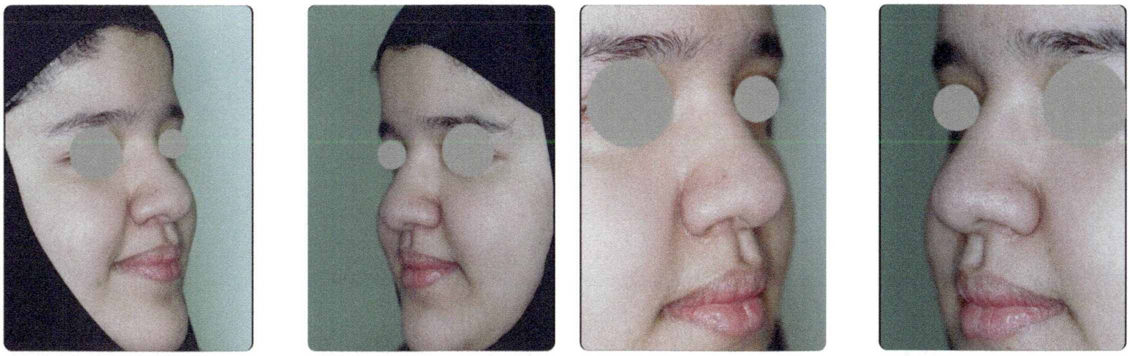

Postoperative

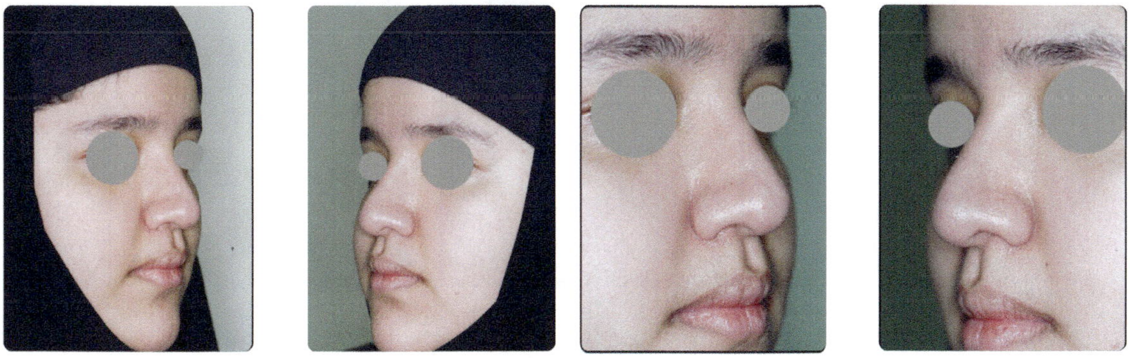

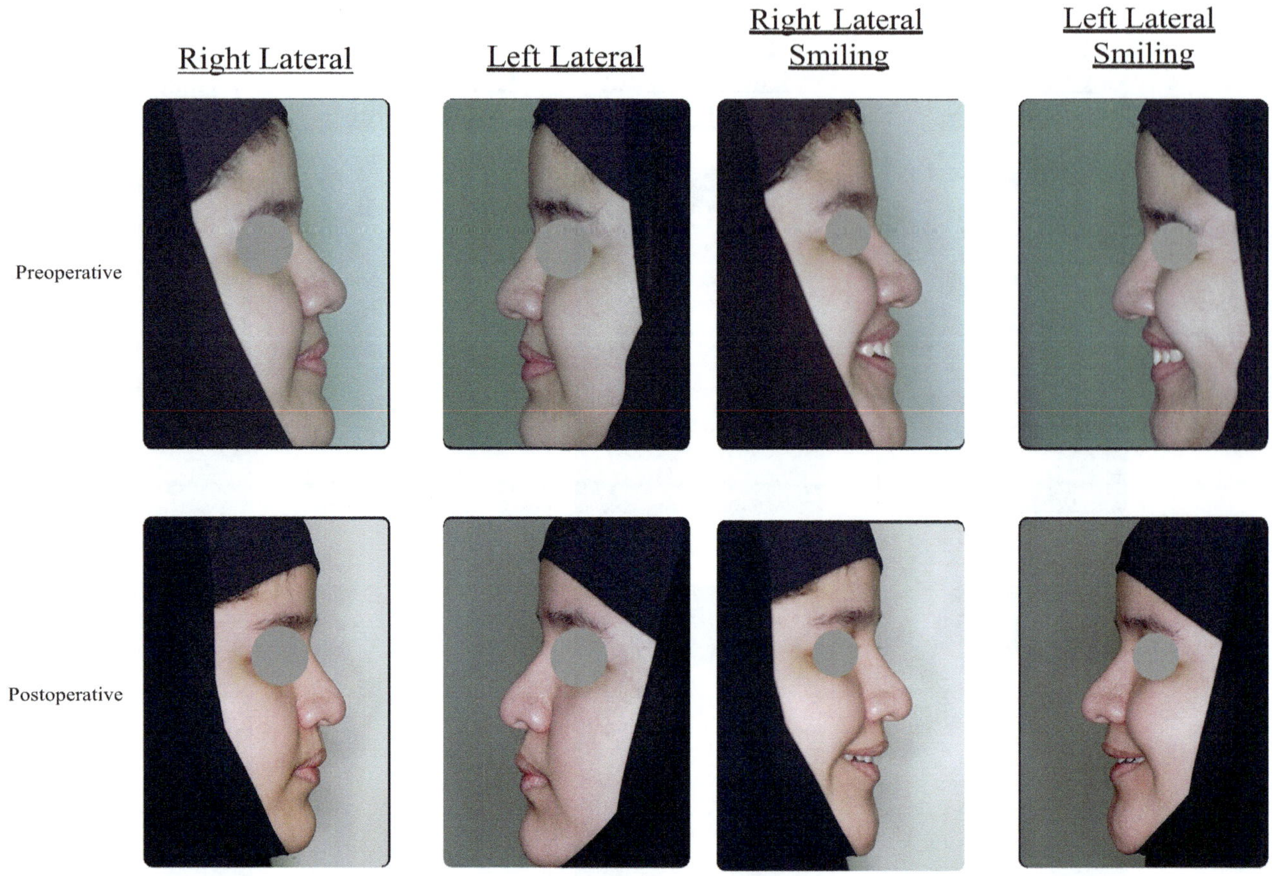
Right Lateral
Left Lateral
Right Lateral Smiling
Left Lateral Smiling
Preoperative
Postoperative

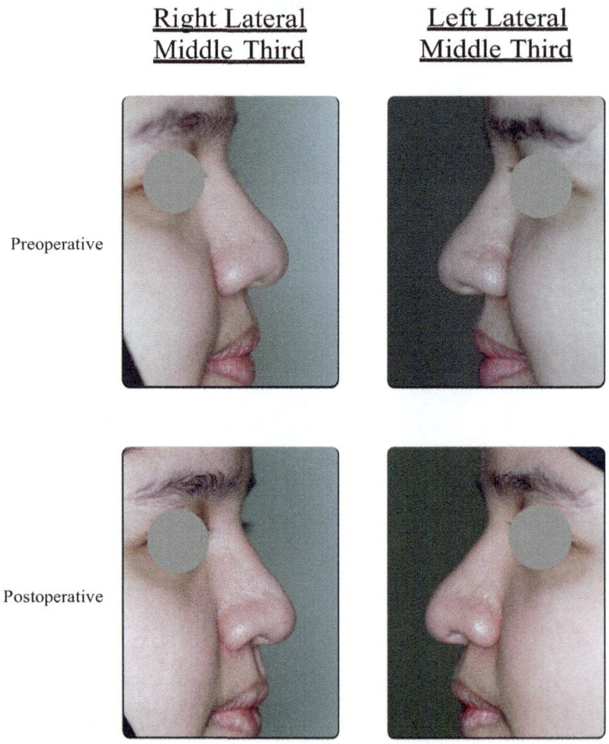
Right Lateral Middle Third
Left Lateral Middle Third
Preoperative
Postoperative

Part IV

Crooked Nose Rhinoplasty

31 Part IV: Clinical Case 1

Preoperative Assessment

1. **Frontolateral walls**
   a. Large boxy square and bulky tip leading to large and wide flat (soft) triangles. (Frontal, Backward Tilting and Nasal Aperture Views). The nasal tip is counter deviated to the left while the bony pyramid is deviated to the right (Frontal Views).
   b. The size and bulk of the tip is overshadowing the alae nasi (Frontal and Direct Dorsal Views).
2. **Medial Wall**
   a. Left caudal cartilaginous deviation and dislocation of the septum (Basal and left Nasal Aperture Views).
   b. C-shaped septal deviation to the right (Right Nasal Aperture View).
   c. Mobile nasal tip (Lateral Smiling Views).
3. **Bony pyramid**
   a. Wide base of the bony pyramid (Direct Dorsal and Backward Tilting Views).
   b. Osteocartilaginous hump. Bilateral maxillary asymmetry, leading to oblique and deviation of the bony pyramid to the right (Frontal and Backward Tilting Views). The left cheek is wide and low while the right cheek is narrow and high.
4. **Alar base**
   a. The nasal openings are thick walled rounded in shape.
   b. The flat triangles (soft triangles) were large with prominent margins, giving the nasal tip its square boxy appearance (Frontal, Backward Tilting and Nasal Aperture Views). Note the light reflex of the margins of the flat triangles (Nasal Aperture Views).

Aims of Surgery

1. Reduction of the size and bulk of the nasal tip.
2. Correction of the caudal septal deviation.
3. Correction of the crooked nose.

Surgical Plan

1. **Frontolateral walls**
   a. DDD including the weak triangle to reduce the size and bulk of the tip and supratip area.
   b. Cephalic trim of the lateral crurae to reduce the size of the tip.
2. **Medial Wall**
   a. Septoplasty.
   b. Division of the Depressor Septi muscles.
3. **Bony pyramid**
   a. Excision of the osteocartilaginous hump.
   b. Osteotomies and Kasanjian maneuver to the left i.e. cross fracture of the bony pyramid after osteotomies (Refer to Surgery of the Bony Pyramid).
4. **Alar base**
   Nil of note.

Surgical Procedure

a. As per Surgical Plan.
b. Supra tip depression was noticed during surgery. Corrected with crushed cartilage graft from the septum.
c. Intercrural stitch to thin the columella.

Post-Operative Analysis

1. **Frontolateral Wall**
   a. Tip definition: the nasal tip is slimmer, more prominent and well identified from the alae nasi on both sides. The alae nasi become clearly visible and share in nasal aesthetics (Frontal, Direct Dorsal, Overhead, Backward Tilting and Basal Views).
   b. Tip projection: The nasal tip is at the same level of the nasal dorsum with good aesthetic angle. This is coupled with good aesthetic nasolabial angle (lateral and oblique views).

M. H. A. Shafy, *Atlas of Clinical Cases in Rhinoplasty*,
https://doi.org/10.1007/978-3-031-07504-9_31

c. Tip light reflex is seen as one spot off the nasal tip (Frontal and Backward Tilting Views).

2. **Medial Wall**

The deviated septum was corrected with better looking basal and nasal aperture views.

3. **Bony Pyramid**
   a. Bony pyramid aesthetics: the nasal dorsum is straight and the sidewalls are smooth and narrow (all views except the Basal Views).
   b. Dorsal light reflex is seen as an uninterrupted line off the nasal dorsum (Direct Dorsal Views).
4. **Alar Base**
   a. Superior alar groove aesthetics improved by defatting. The grooves become longer and deeper (Frontal, Direct Dorsal, Oblique and Lateral Views).
   b. Posterior alar groove aesthetics improved by defatting alone. The alae nasi are pulled medially producing wider angles with the upper lip (Basal and Nasal Aperture Views).
   c. Alae nasi aesthetics improved as they are pulled medially and become more elegantly visible (Frontal, Nasal Aperture, Oblique and Lateral Views).
   d. Nasal aperture aesthetics: The shape of nasal openings improved by defatting alone. They become thin walled and more elegantly oval in shape (Nasal Aperture, Backward Tilting and Basal Views).
   e. Marginal light reflexes are clearly seen at:
      i. Inferior alar margins (Nasal Aperture Views).
      ii. Nasal sill bands (Oblique Views).
      iii. Lateral crural prominences (Lateral Views).

Commentary

a. Crookedness of this lady's nose is developmental due to bilateral maxillary asymmetry that led to the right deviation of the bony pyramid and counter deviation of the nasal tip to the left. No history of trauma.

b. The boxy shaped nasal tip with the noticable wide flat triangles both disappeared after the two step defatting process of the middle and lateral crurae. This resulted in reduction of the bulk and size of the middle and lateral crurae.

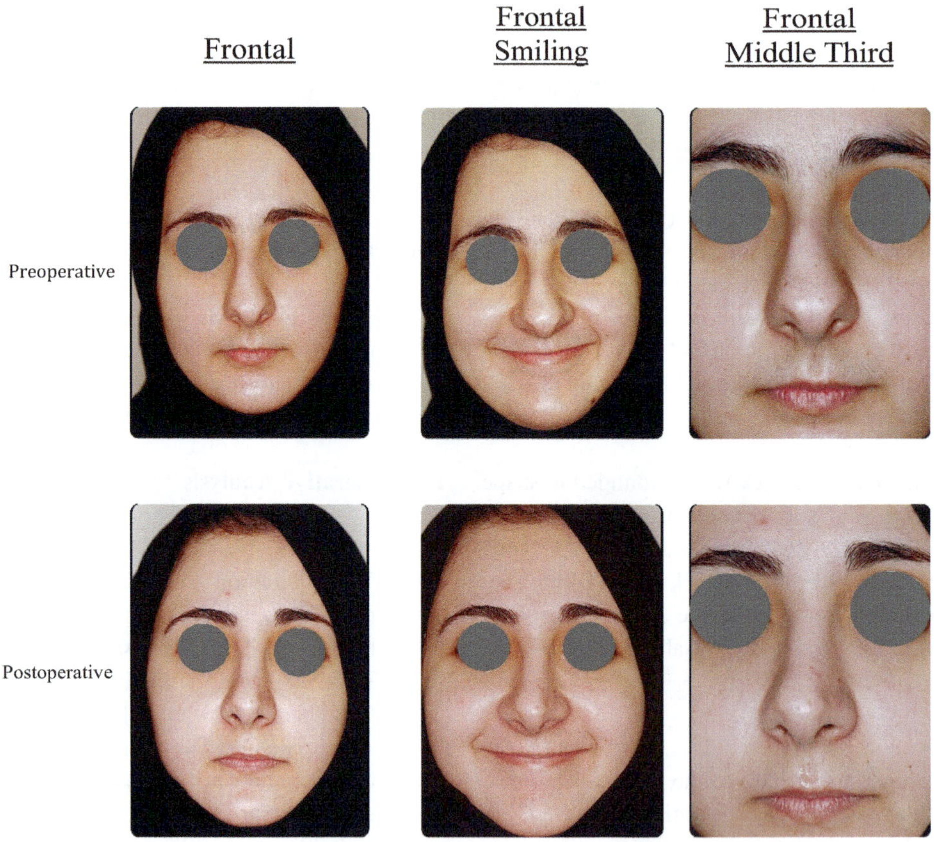

Direct Dorsal | Direct Dorsal Smiling | Overhead | Overhead Smiling

Preoperative

Postoperative

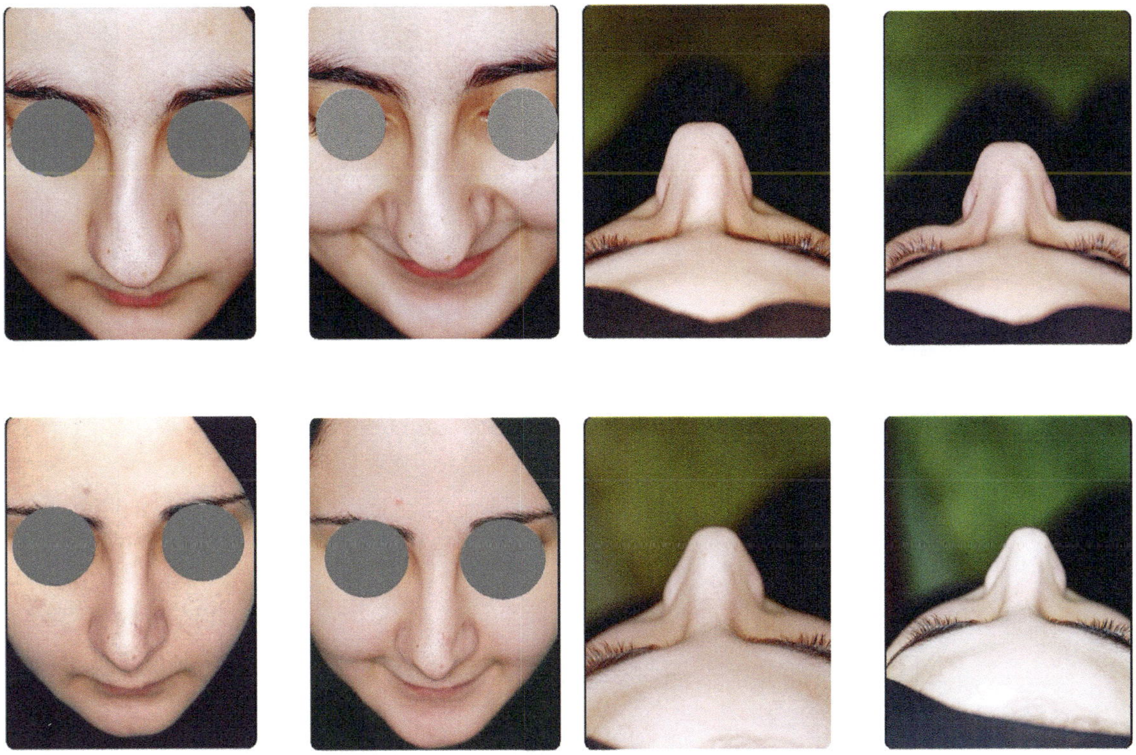

Backward Tilting | Steeper Backward Tilting | Basal

Preoperative

Postoperative

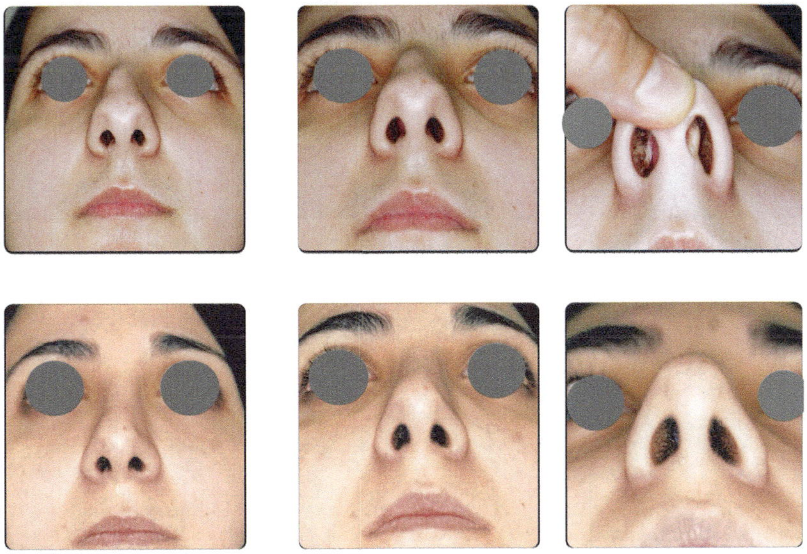

Right Nasal Aperture | Right Nasal Aperture Rim Sill Test | Left Nasal Aperture Rim Sill Test | Left Nasal Aperture

Preoperative

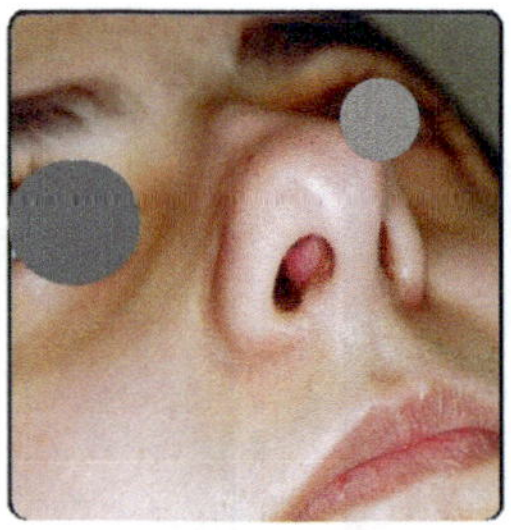
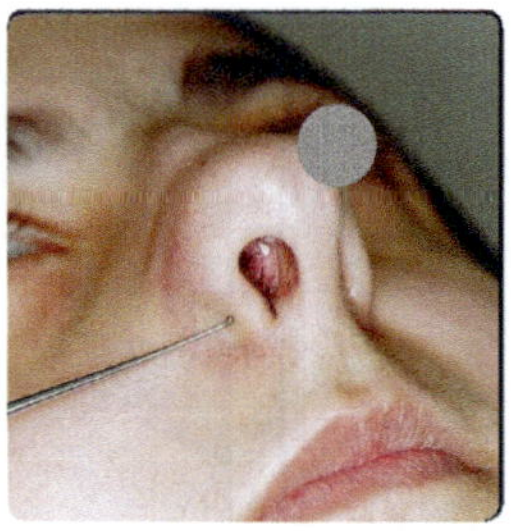
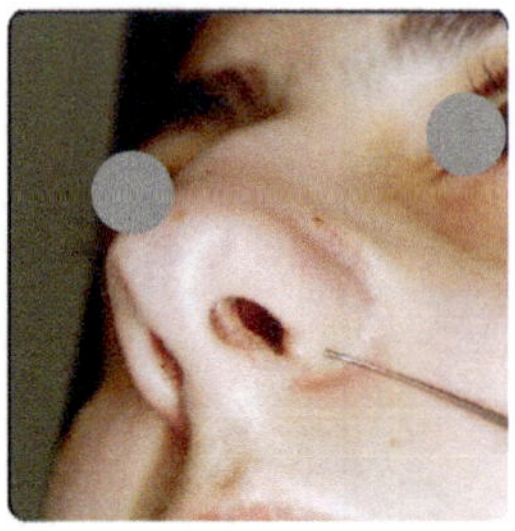
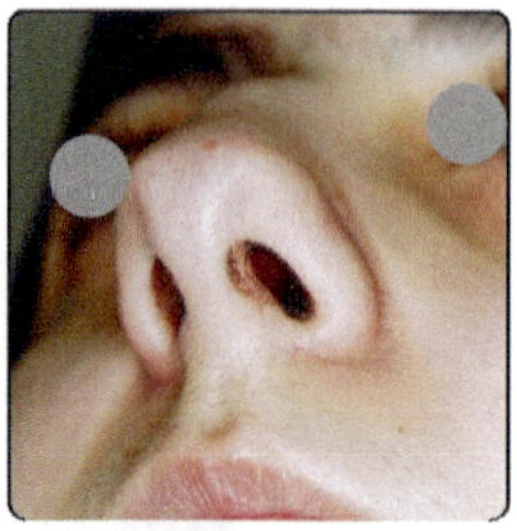

Postoperative

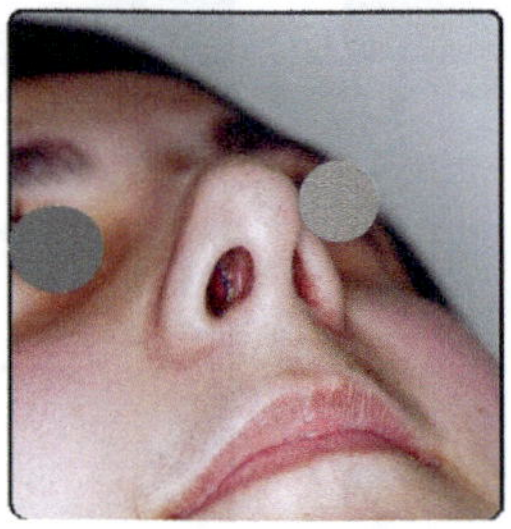
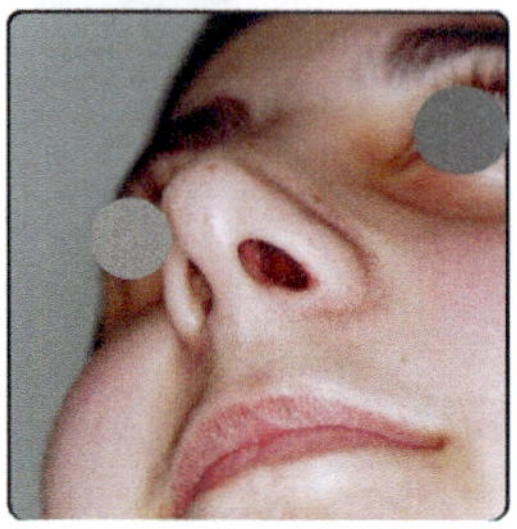

Right Oblique Mid Cheek Full Face | Left Oblique Mid Cheek Full Face | Right Oblique Mid Cheek Middle Third | Left Oblique Mid Cheek Middle Third

Preoperative

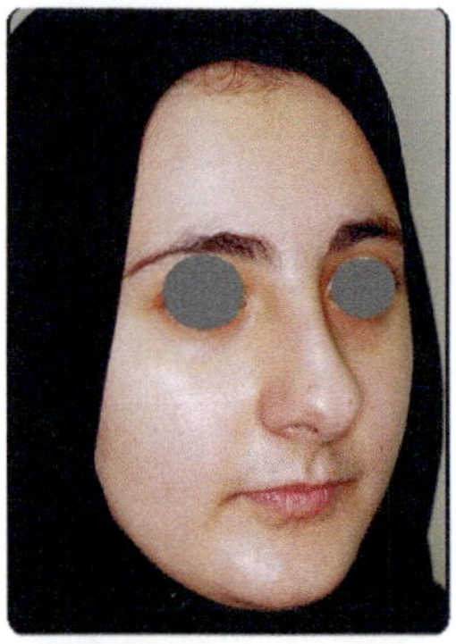
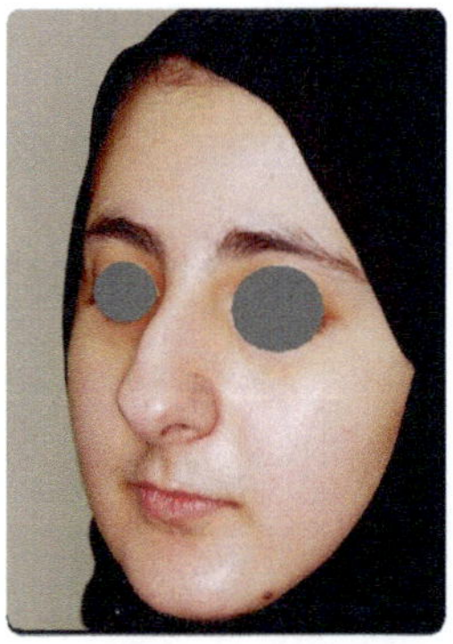
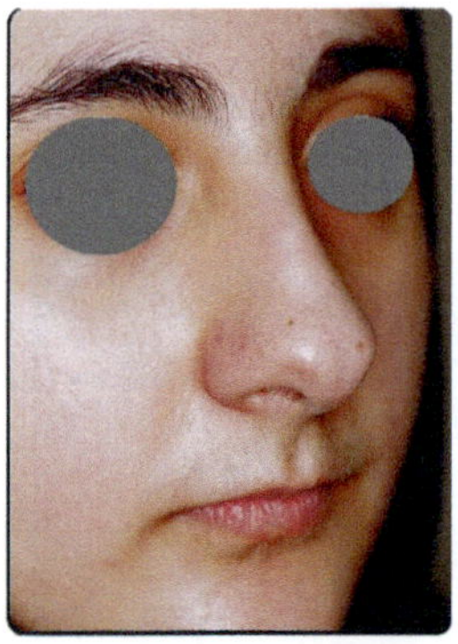
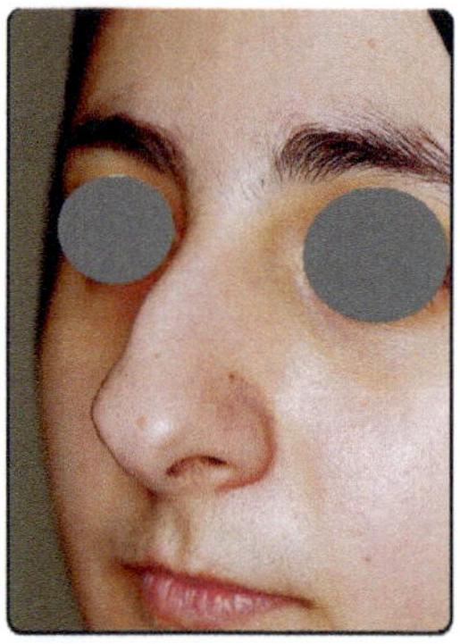

Postoperative

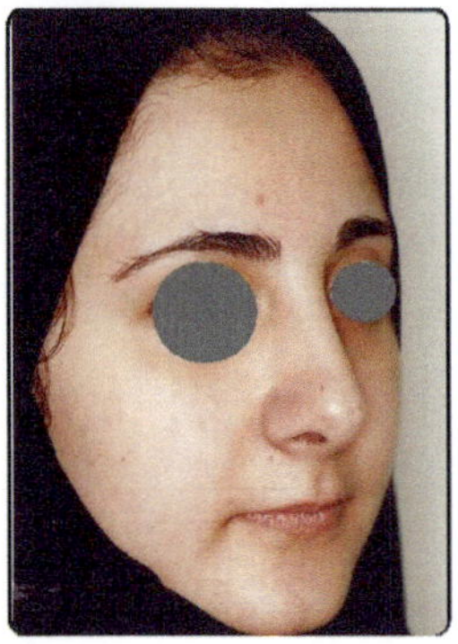
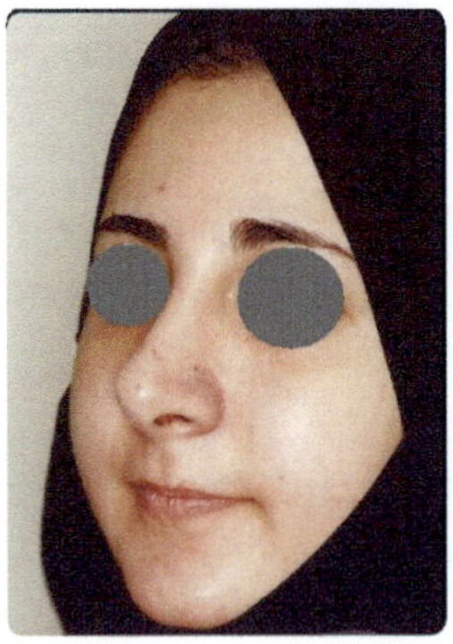
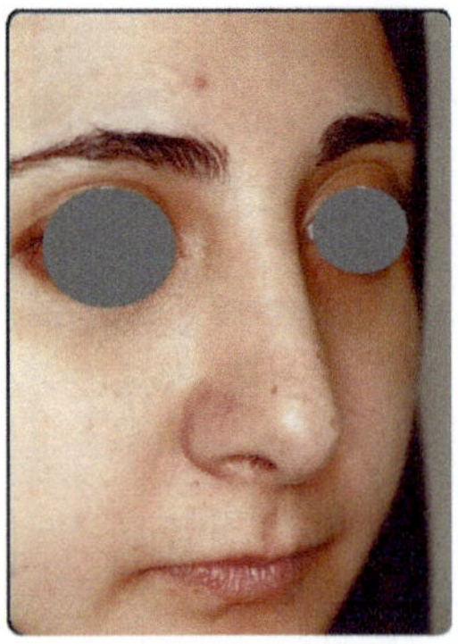
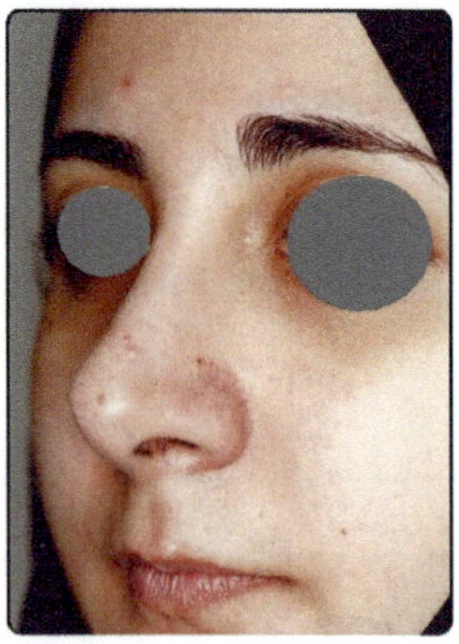

Right Oblique Cheek Margin Full Face	Left Oblique Cheek Margin Full Face	Right Oblique Cheek Margin Middle Third	Left Oblique Cheek Margin Middle Third

Preoperative

Postoperative

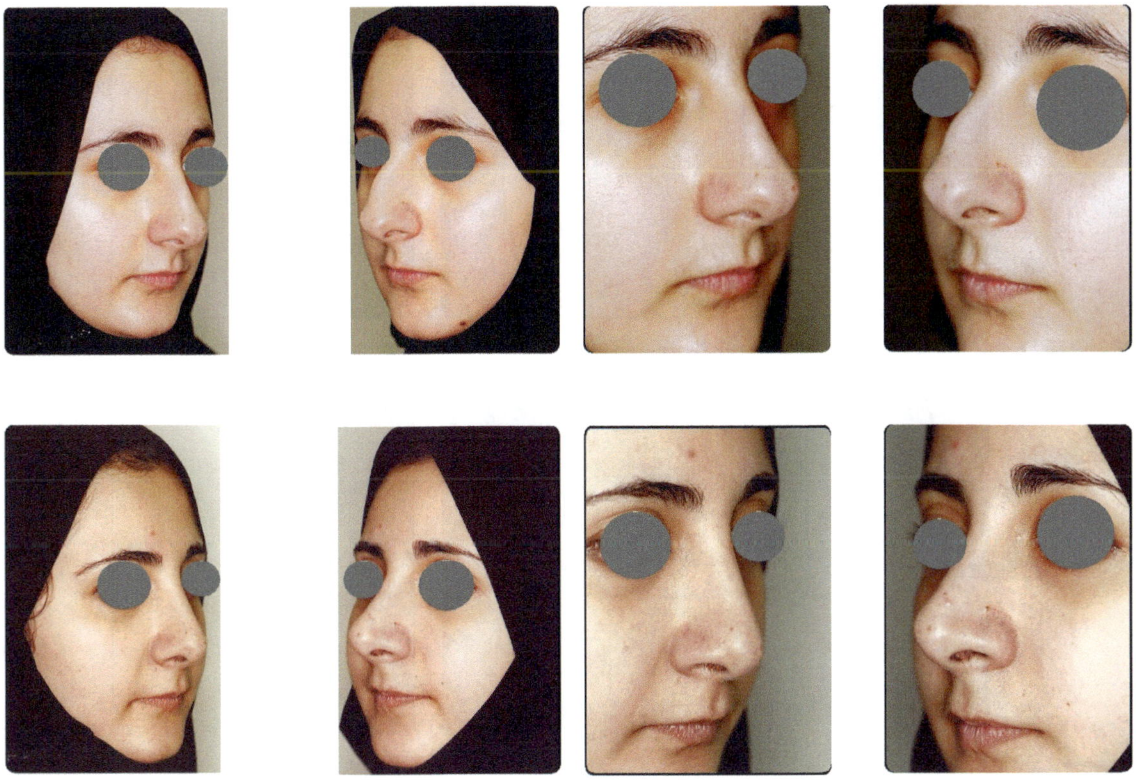

Right Lateral | Left Lateral | Right Lateral **Smiling** | Left Lateral **Smiling**

Preoperative

Postoperative

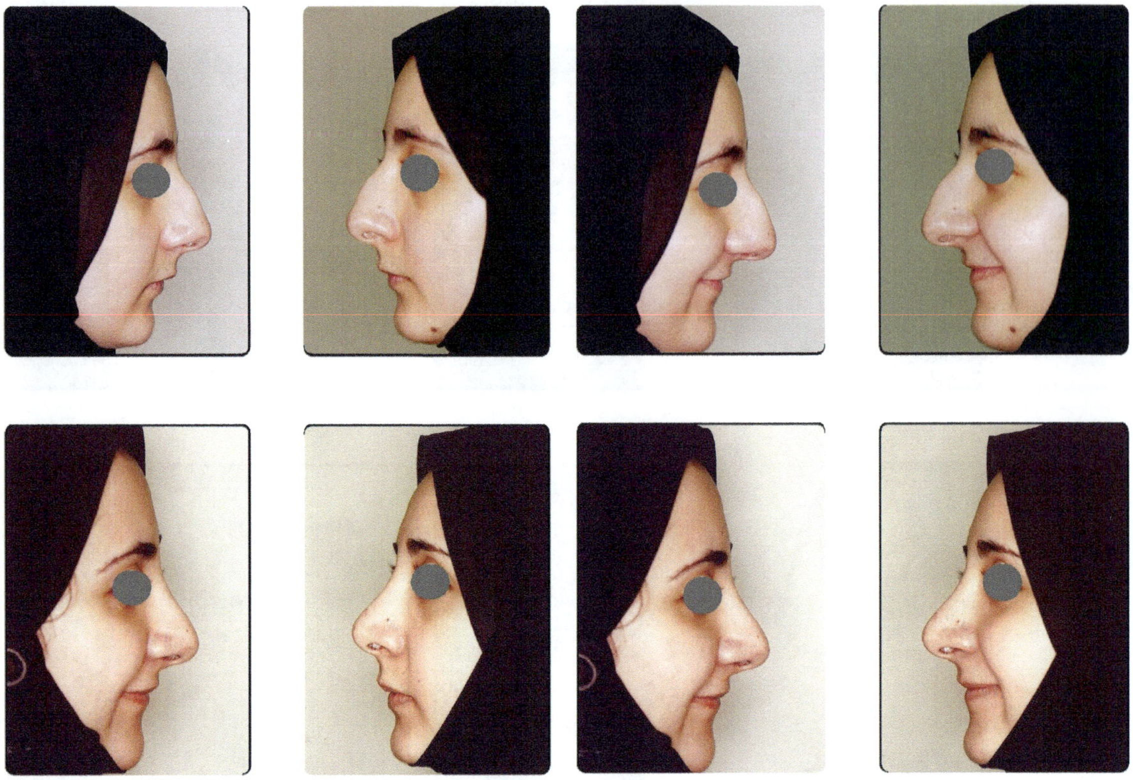

Right Lateral Middle Third | Left Lateral Middle Third

Preoperative

Postoperative

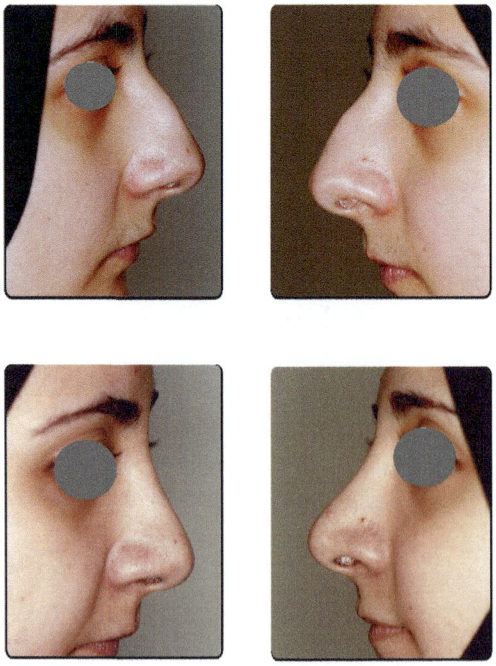

32 Part IV: Clinical Case 2

Preoperative Assessment

1. **Frontolateral walls**
   Large and bulky frontolateral walls overshadowing the alae nasi (Frontal, Direct Dorsal and Overhead Views). The nasal tip is counter deviated to the right side as compared with the left deviation of the bony pyramid.
2. **Medial Wall**
   a. Left caudal dislocation of the septum enchroaching upon and distorting the shape of the left nasal aperture (Basal and Left Nasal Aperture Views).
   b. Mobile tip (Smiling Lateral Views).
3. **Bony pyramid**
   a. Oblique and deviated boney pyramid to the left due to bilateral maxilary asymmetry. The right cheek is wide and low while the left cheek is narrow and high. (Frontal, Direct Dorsal Overhead and Backward Tilting Views).
   b. Osteocartilaginous hump predominantly oblique and deviated to the left side (Backward Tilting, Oblique and Lateral Views).
   c. Observation and palpation of the side walls of the boney pyramid, they are smooth and regular, unlike post traumatic cases where the walls may look and feel irregular and ragged.
4. **Alar base**
   a. The right ala nasi is naturally larger than the left.
   b. The caudal cartilagenous septum was protruding through the left nasal opening, distorting its appearance.

Aims of Surgery

1. Reduce the overall size of the nose including the size and bulk of the nasal tip.
2. Excision of the osteocartilaginous hump and correction of the deviation of the boney pyramid.

Surgical Plan

1. **Frontolateral walls**
   a. D.D.D. including weak triangle to reduce the bulk of the nasal tip and Supra tip area.
   b. Bilateral cephalic trim of the lateral crurae to reduce the tip size.
2. **Medial Wall**
   a. Septoplasty.
   b. Division of the Depressor Septi Muscles.
3. **Bony pyramid**
   a. Excision of the osteocartilaginous hump.
   b. Osteotomies. Kassanjian maneuver to the right side i.e. cross fracture of the bony pyramid after osteotomies (refer to Surgery of the Bony Pyramid).
4. **Alar base**
   Nil of note.

Surgical Procedure

As per Surgical Plan.

Post-Operative Analysis

1. **Frontolateral Wall**
   a. Tip definition: the nasal tip is smaller with thinner and smoother overlying skin. It is more prominent and well identified from the alae nasi on both sides. The alae nasi come into view to become clearly visible and share in nasal aesthetics (Frontal, Direct Dorsal, Overhead, Backward Tilting and Basal Views).
   b. Tip projection: The nasal tip at the same level of the nasal dorsum with good aesthetic angle. This is coupled with good aesthetic nasolabial angle (lateral and oblique views).

M. H. A. Shafy, *Atlas of Clinical Cases in Rhinoplasty*,
https://doi.org/10.1007/978-3-031-07504-9_32

c. Tip light reflex is seen as one spot off the nasal tip (Frontal and Backward Tilting Views).

2. **Medial Wall**

Nasal apertures are clear off the protruding caudal septum after septoplasty. Mobility of the nasal tip is abolished.

3. **Bony Pyramid**

a. Bony pyramid aesthetics: the nasal dorsum is straight and the sidewalls are smooth and narrow (all views except the Basal Views).

b. Dorsal light reflex is seen as an uninterrupted line off the nasal dorsum (Direct Dorsal Views).

4. **Alar Base**

a. Superior alar groove aesthetics improved by defatting. The grooves become longer and deeper (Oblique, Lateral and Direct Dorsal Views).

b. Aesthetics of the alae nasi and posterior alar grooves improved after defatting. The alae nasi pulled medially widening the posterior groove angles. The alae are better seen and aesthetically more elegant.

c. Nasal apertures became closer to each other in size and shape after correction of the caudal septal deviation. Their aesthetics further improved after defatting.

d. Marginal light reflexes are clearly seen at:

i. Inferior alar margins (Nasal Aperture Views).

ii. Nasal sill bands (Oblique Views).

iii. Lateral crural prominences (Lateral Views).

Commentary

a. Postoperative photographs are taken only one month after surgery. The nasafrontal area, midvault and nasal tip will continue to pleasantly reduced in size on the long term.

b. The continuing difference in size between the two alae nasi had no negative aesthetic effects post-operatively.

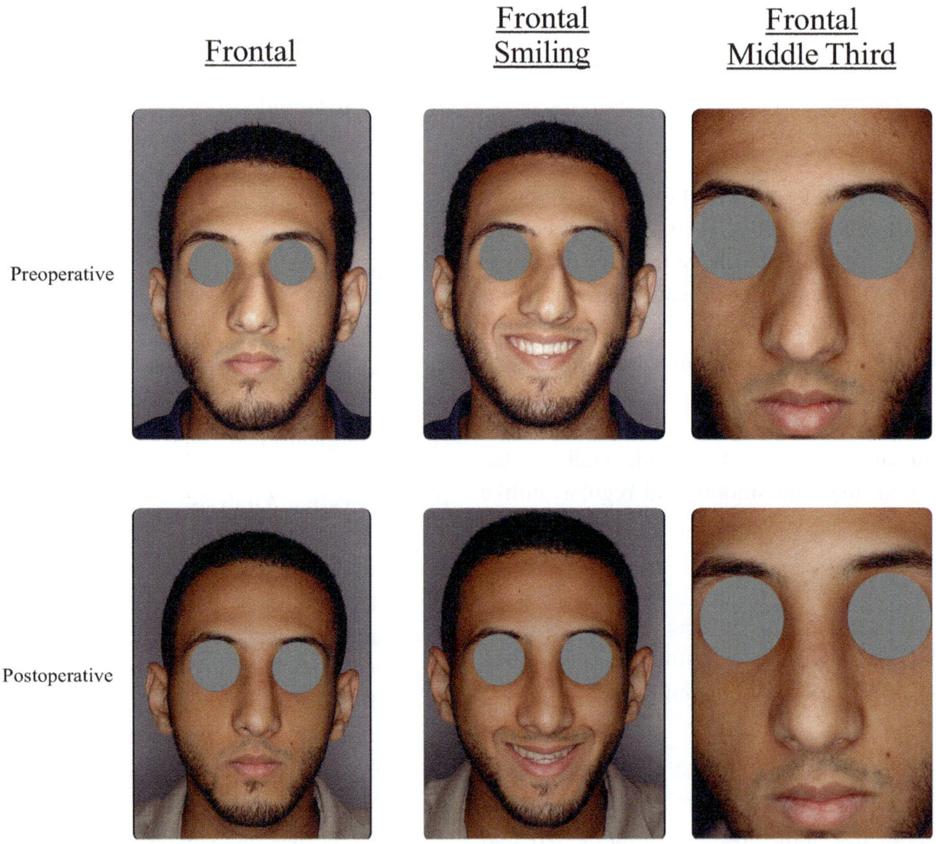

Direct Dorsal | Direct Dorsal Smiling | Overhead | Overhead Smiling

Preoperative

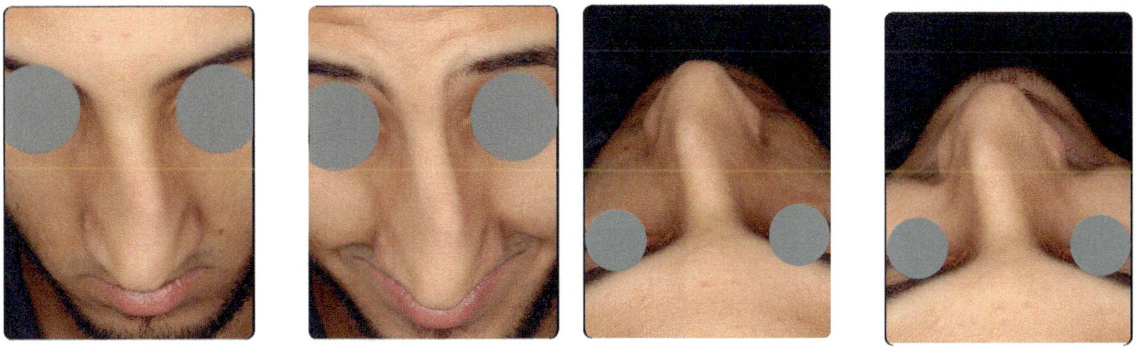

Postoperative

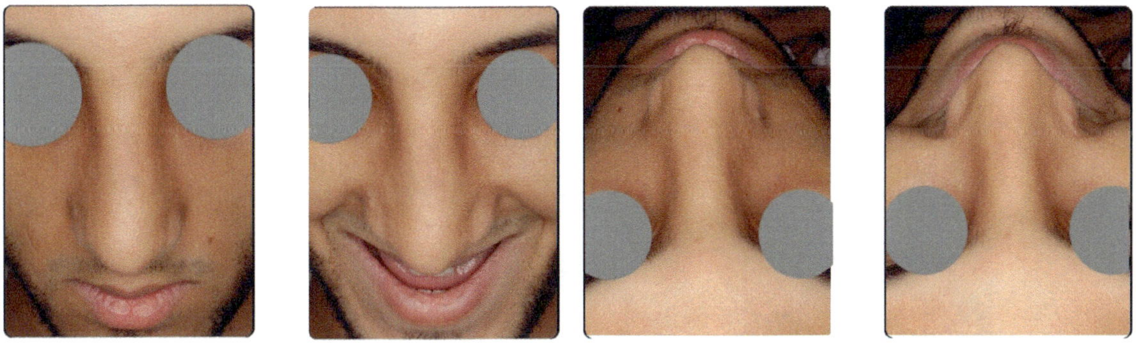

Backward Tilting | Steeper Backward Tilting | Basal | Basal Smiling

Preoperative

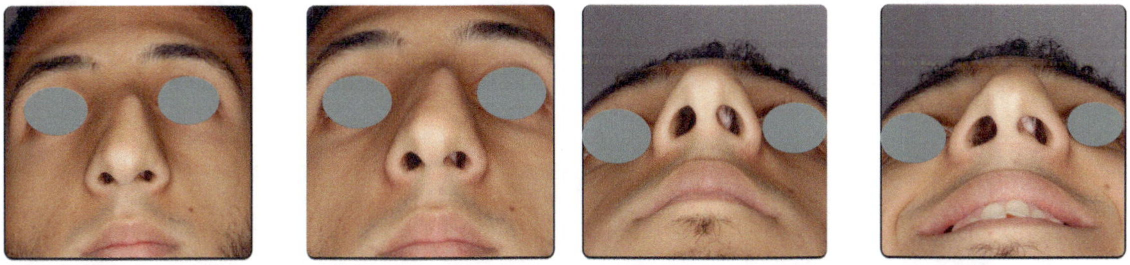

Postoperative

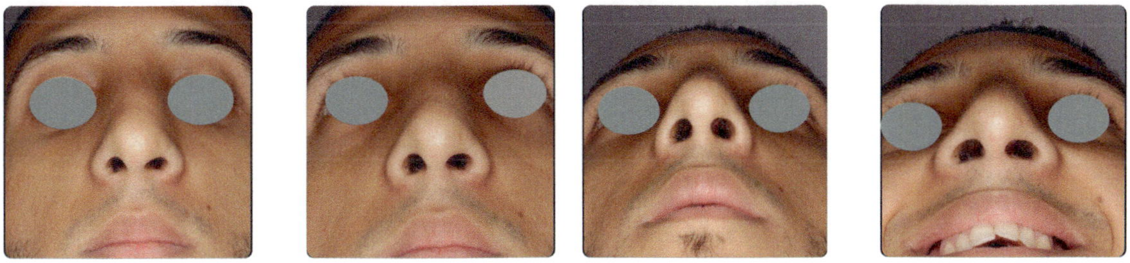

Right Nasal Aperture | Left Nasal Aperture

Preoperative

Postoperative

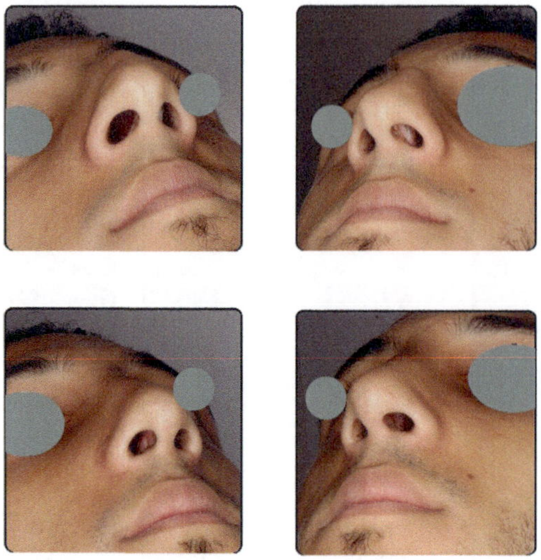

Right Oblique Mid Cheek Full Face | Left Oblique Mid Cheek Full Face | Right Oblique Mid Cheek Middle Third | Left Oblique Mid Cheek Middle Third

Preoperative

Postoperative

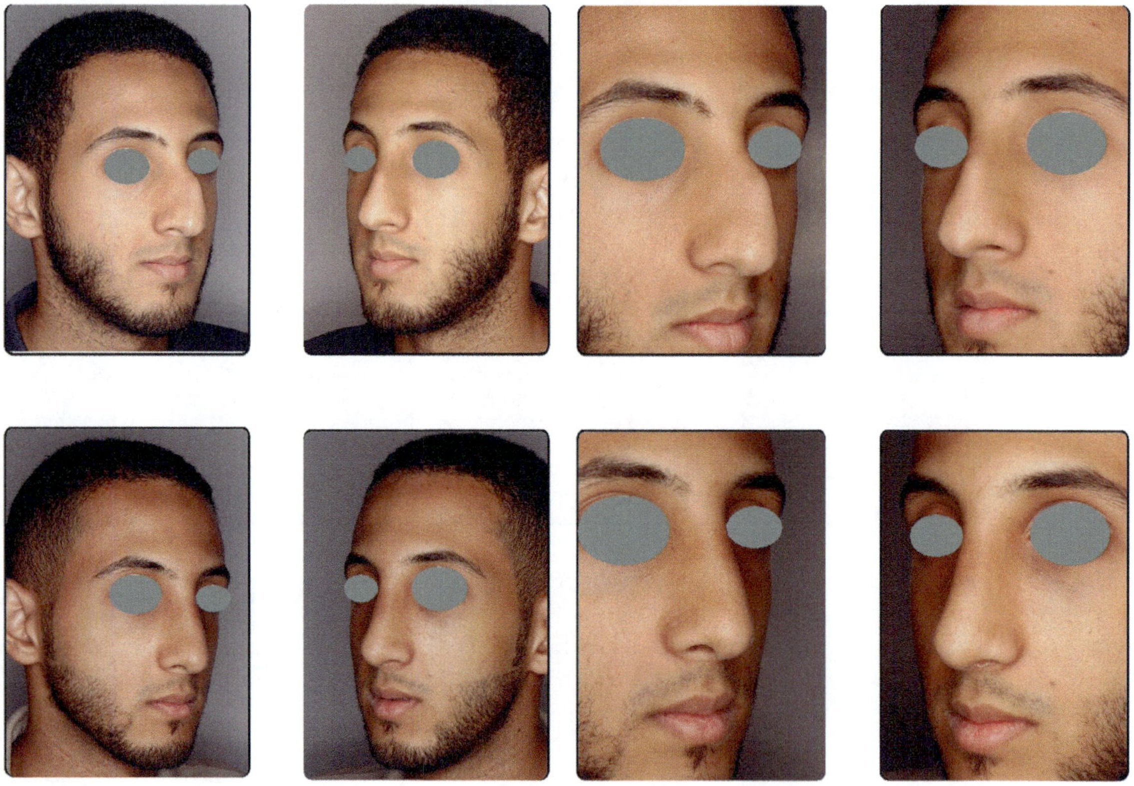

	Right Oblique Cheek Margin Full Face	Left Oblique Cheek Margin Full Face	Right Oblique Cheek Margin Middle Third	Left Oblique Cheek Margin Middle Third

Preoperative

Postoperative

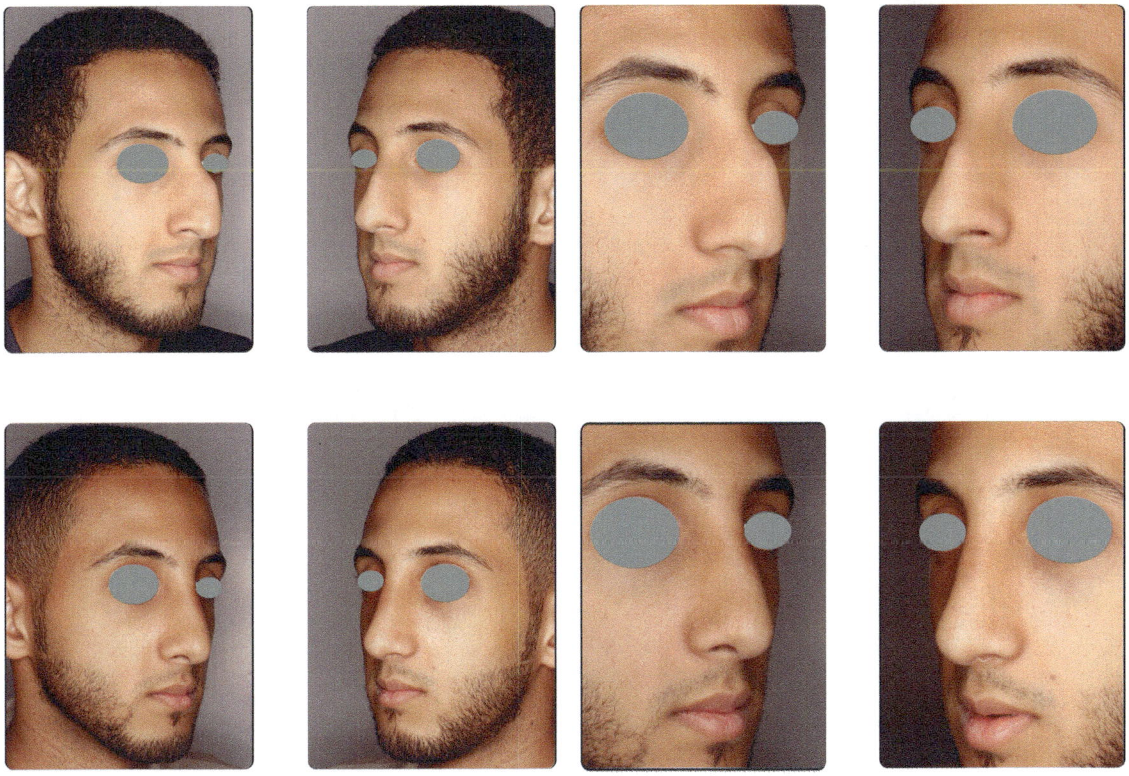

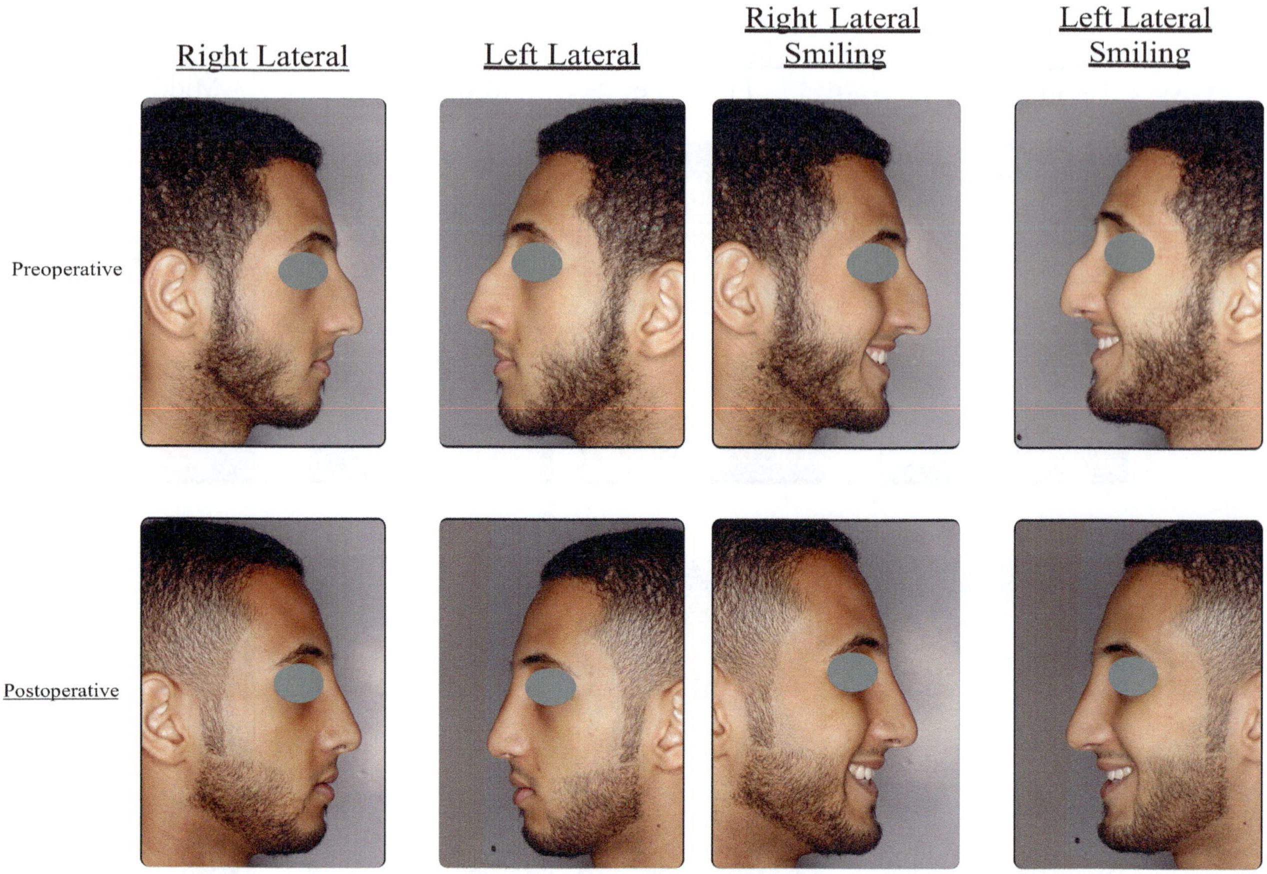
Right Lateral
Left Lateral
Right Lateral Smiling
Left Lateral Smiling
Preoperative
Postoperative

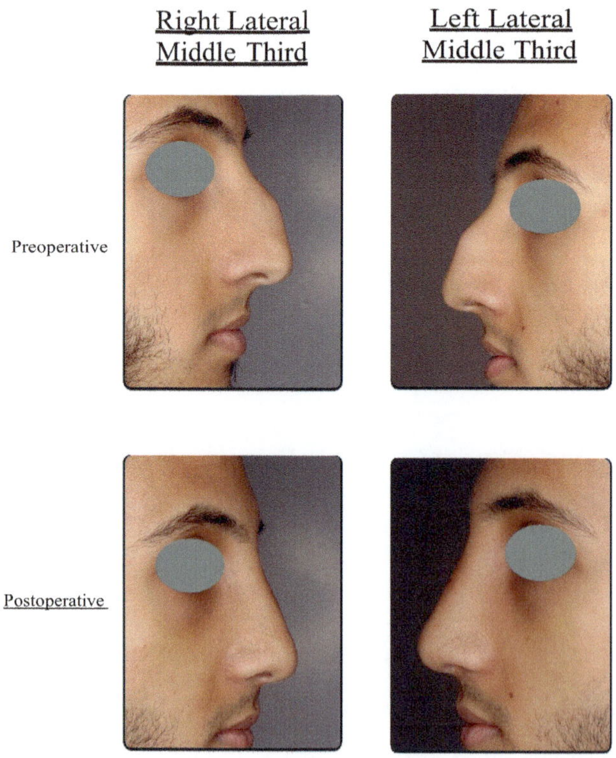
Right Lateral Middle Third
Left Lateral Middle Third
Preoperative
Postoperative

Part IV: Clinical Case 3

33

Preoperative Assessment

1. **Frontolateral walls**
   a. Bulbous tip which was counter deviated to the right side while the bony pyramid is diverted to the left side (Frontal, Direct Dorsal, Overhead and Backward Tilting views). A crooked nose by definition is the nose that has a bend, or a twist in its structural body.
   b. The alae nasi could not be seen behind the bulky tip. (Frontal, Direct Dorsal and Overhead Views).
2. **Medial Wall**
   a. C-shaped deviated nasal septum. There is left caudal dislocation that pushed the medial crus laterally into the left nasal aperture. The medial crus appears as a bulge that distorts the shape of the left nasal opening (Basal and Left Nasal Aperture Views).
   b. Protruding columella (Lateral Views).
   c. Mobile tip (Lateral Smiling Views).
3. **Bony pyramid**
   a. Wide base of the boney pyramid (Direct Dorsal and Backward Tilting Views).
   b. Osteocartilaginous hump, which is oblique (Backward Tilting Views) and deviated (Frontal, Direct Dorsal and Overhead Views) to the left side due bilateral maxillary. The right maxilla is wide and low, while the left maxilla is narrow and high i.e. the right cheek is larger than the left cheek.
4. **Alar base**
   a. Laterally angulated left alar margin, due to an oblique inferior segment of the rim sill fold. This aperture is, therefore, rectangular in shape, i.e. it has four walls. This is best seen in the Basal, Basal Smiling and Left Nasal Aperture Views.
   b. The alar base is not bulky but slightly wide due to long inferior segments of the rim sill folds (Basal Views).
   c. Note the light reflex off the inferior alar margins, margins of the flat triangles and the nasal sill bands. (Pre-operative Nasal Aperture Views). No light is reflected from the rim-sill folds.

Aims of Surgery

1. Reduce bulk of the nasal tip.
2. Abolish the mobile tip.
3. Reduce the protruding columella.
4. Correction of upper and lower nasal deformities by the following procedures:
   a. Excision of the nasal hump.
   b. Correction of the oblique and deviated bony pyramid as well as the counter deviated lower third.
5. To enhance the aesthetics of the alar base.

Surgical Plan

1. **Frontolateral walls**
   a. DDD including the weak triangle to reduce the size and bulk of the nasal tip and supra tip area.
   b. Bilateral cephalic trim of lateral crura to reduce the size.
2. **Medial Wall**
   a. Septoplasty.
   b. Minimal trim of the membranous septum including part of the caudal cartilage.
   c. Division of the Depressor Septi muscles.
3. **Bony pyramid**
   a. Excision of the osteocartilaginous hump.
   b. Osteotomies and Kasanjian maneuver to the patient's right i.e. cross fracture of the bony pyramid after osteotomies (See Surgery of the Bony Pyramid in the Text).
4. **Alar base**
   Excision of the inferior segments of the rim sill folds on both sides to reduce the size of the nasal apertures.

M. H. A. Shafy, *Atlas of Clinical Cases in Rhinoplasty*,
https://doi.org/10.1007/978-3-031-07504-9_33

Surgical Procedure

a. As per Surgical Plan.
b. Supra tip depression was noticed in the course of surgery. A graft using cephalic trimmings of the lateral crural cartilages.

Post-Operative Analysis

1. **Frontolateral Wall**
   a. Tip definition: the nasal tip is smaller with thinner and smoother overlying skin. It is more prominent and well identified from the alae nasi on both sides. The alae nasi come into view to become clearly visible and share in nasal aesthetics (Frontal, Direct Dorsal, Overhead, Backward Tilting and Basal Views).
   b. Tip projection: The nasal tip at the same level of the nasal dorsum with good aesthetic angle. This is coupled with good aesthetic nasolabial angle (Lateral and Oblique Views).
   c. Tip light reflex is seen as one spot off the nasal tip (Frontal and Backward Tilting Views).
2. **Medial Wall**
   a. Protruding columella disappeared.
   b. Mobile tip is abolished.
3. **Bony Pyramid**
   a. Bony pyramid aesthetics improved: the nasal dorsum is straight and the sidewalls are smooth and narrow (all views except the Basal Views).
   b. Dorsal light reflex is seen as an uninterrupted line off the nasal dorsum (Direct Dorsal Views).
4. **Alar Base**
   a. Superior alar groove aesthetics improved by defatting. The grooves become longer and deeper (Oblique, Lateral and Direct Dorsal Views).
   b. Posterior alar groove aesthetics improved by defatting and excision of the inferior segments of the rim-sill folds. The alae nasi medialized with better alar lip angles. (Basal and Nasal Aperture Views).
   c. Alae nasi aesthetics improved. They are pulled medially, become more visible and smaller in size.
   d. Nasal aperture aesthetics improved after septoplasty and by defatting and excision of the inferior segments of the rim-sill folds:
      i. The size of the nasal openings: they appear smaller and equal.
      ii. The shapes became thin walled and elegantly oval. The left opening is no more rectangular in shape.
   e. Marginal light reflexes are clearly seen at:
      i. Inferior alar margins (Nasal Aperture Views).
      ii. Nasal sill bands (Oblique Views).
      iii. Lateral crural prominences (Lateral Views).

Commentary

a. Although the two nasal openings were equal in size, they had different shapes. Excision of the inferior segment of the left rim sill fold has transformed the rectangular shape of the nasal aperture to a triangular one.
b. Resection of the inferior segment on the right side had to be done to equalize the sizes of both nasal openings.

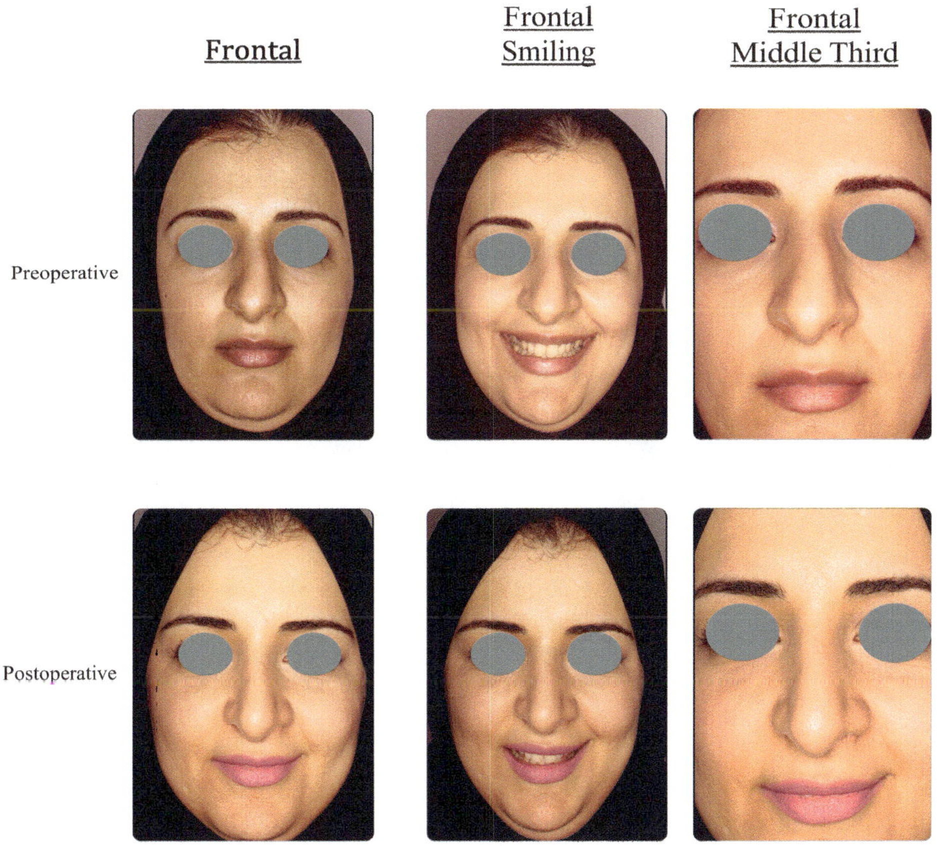
Frontal
Frontal Smiling
Frontal Middle Third
Preoperative
Postoperative

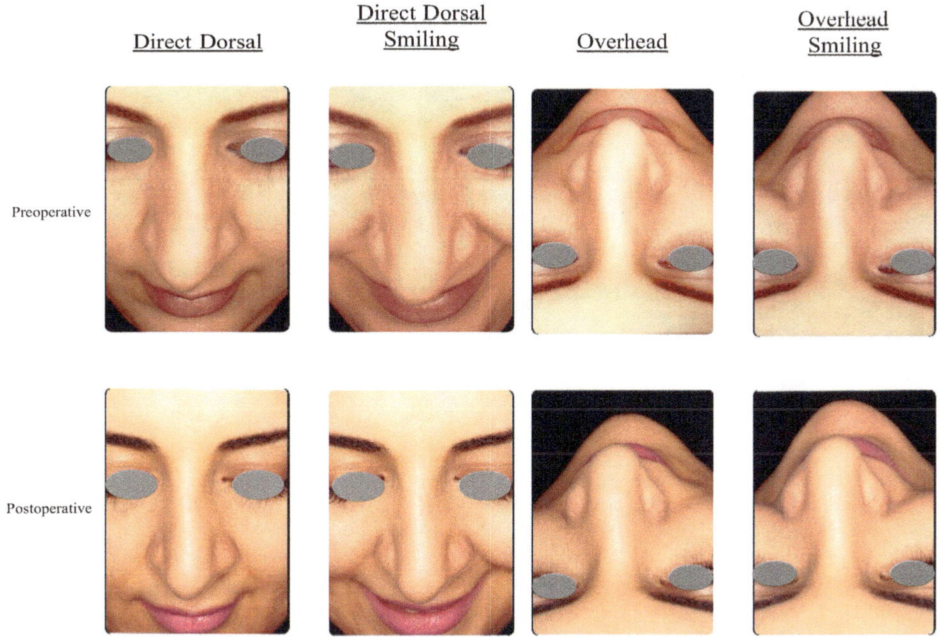
Direct Dorsal
Direct Dorsal Smiling
Overhead
Overhead Smiling
Preoperative
Postoperative

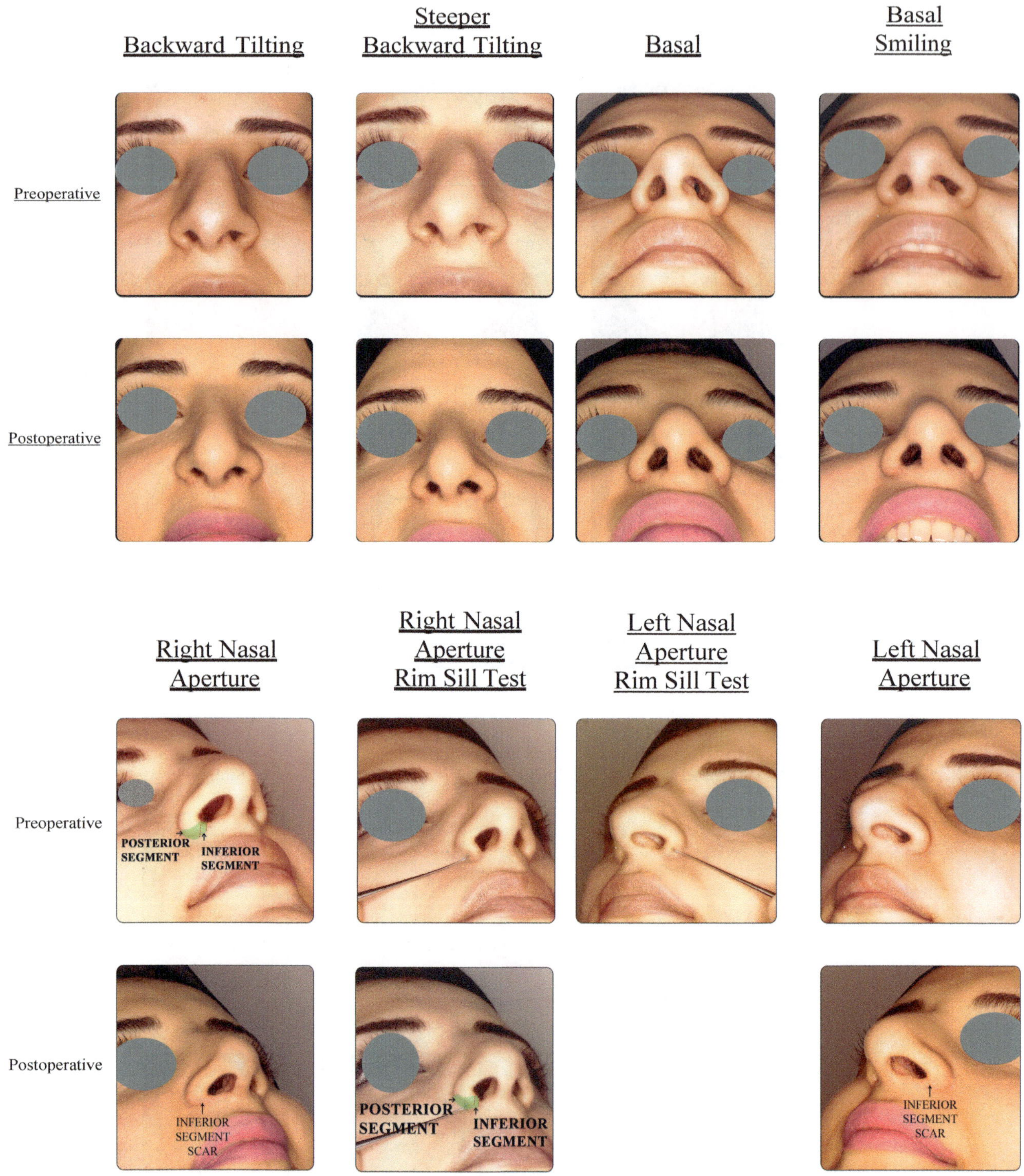
Backward Tilting
Steeper Backward Tilting
Basal
Basal Smiling
Preoperative
Postoperative
Right Nasal Aperture
Right Nasal Aperture Rim Sill Test
Left Nasal Aperture Rim Sill Test
Left Nasal Aperture
Preoperative
POSTERIOR SEGMENT
INFERIOR SEGMENT
Postoperative
INFERIOR SEGMENT SCAR
POSTERIOR SEGMENT
INFERIOR SEGMENT
INFERIOR SEGMENT SCAR

Right Oblique Mid Cheek Full Face	Left Oblique Mid Cheek Full Face	Right Oblique Mid Cheek Middle Third	Left Oblique Mid Cheek Middle Third

Preoperative

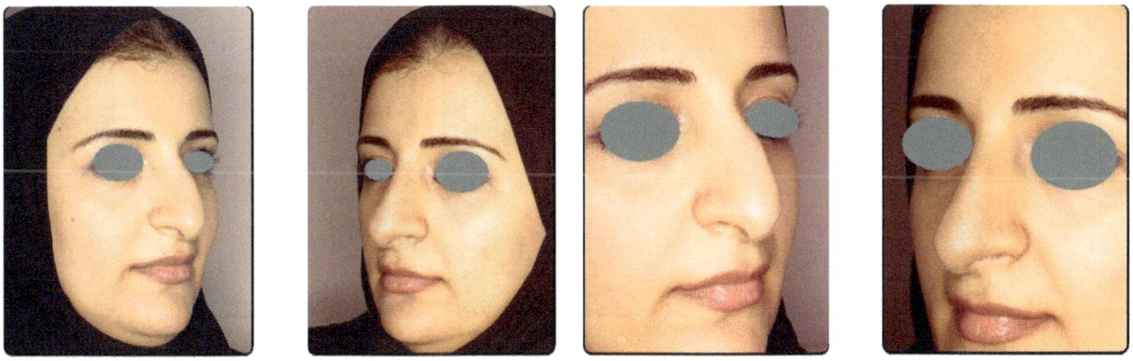

Postoperative

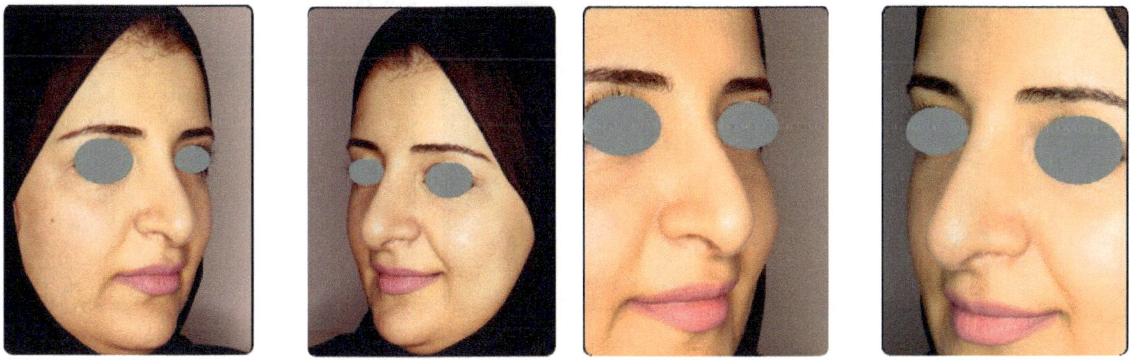

Right Oblique Cheek Margin Full Face	Left Oblique Cheek Margin Full Face	Right Oblique Cheek Margin Middle Third	Left Oblique Cheek Margin Middle Third

Preoperative

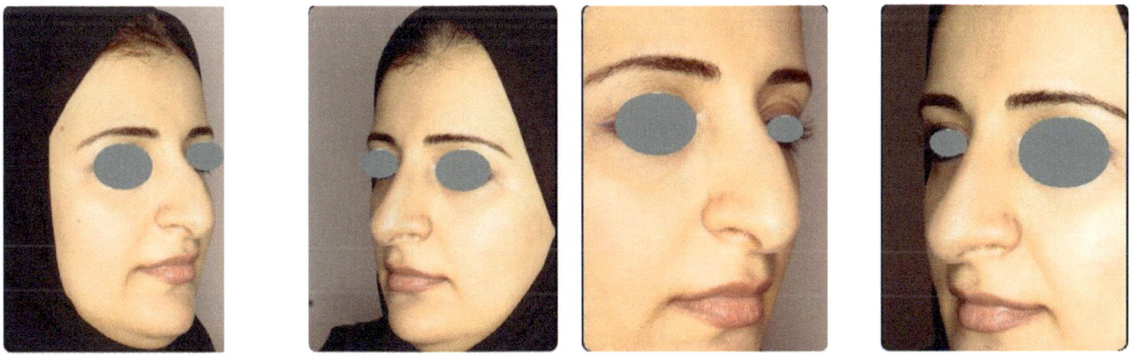

Postoperative

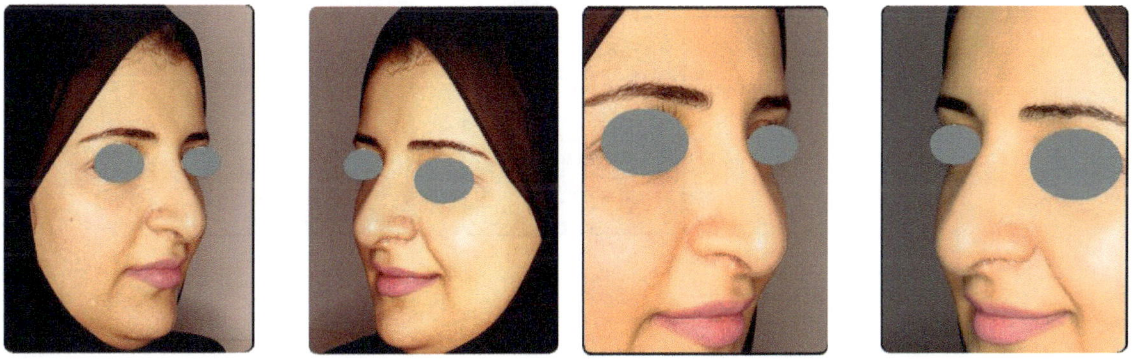

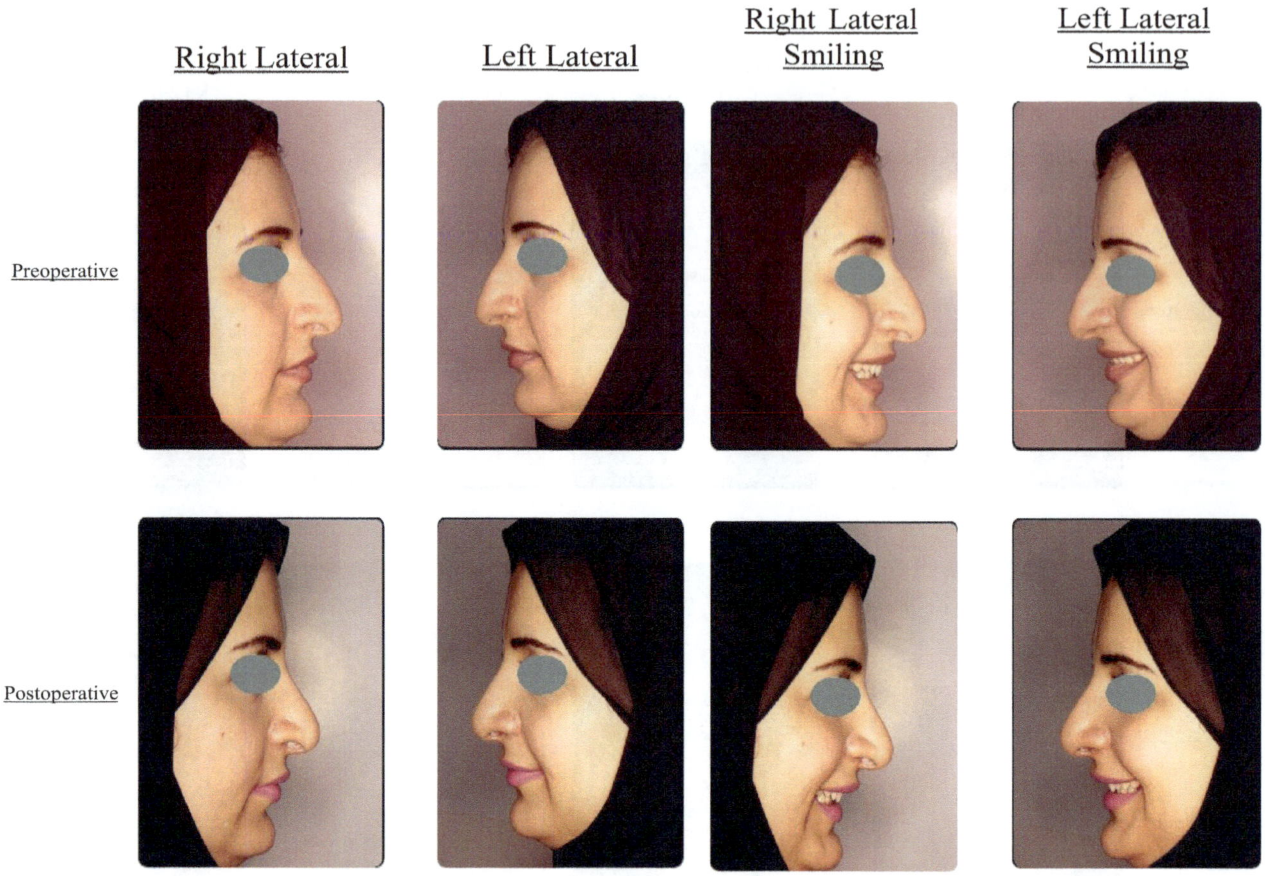
Right Lateral
Left Lateral
Right Lateral Smiling
Left Lateral Smiling
Preoperative
Postoperative

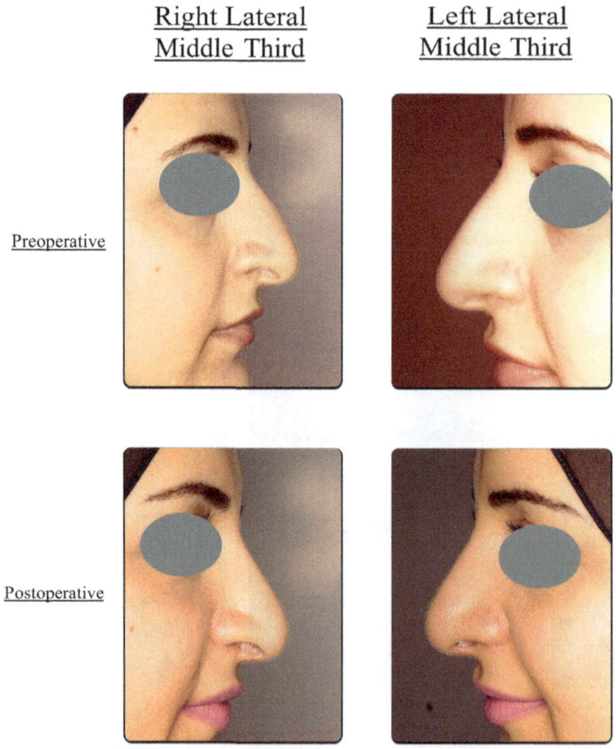
Right Lateral Middle Third
Left Lateral Middle Third
Preoperative
Postoperative

34 Part IV: Clinical Case 4

Preoperative Assessment

1. **Frontolateral walls**
   a. Bulbous bulky tip overshadowing the alae nasi on both sides (Frontal and Direct Dorsal Views).
   b. Tip counter-deviated to the left side while he bony pyramid is deviated right side (Frontal, Direct Dorsal and Backward Tilting Views).
2. **Medial Wall**
   a. Right caudal dislocation of the septum (Backward Tilting, Basal and Right Nasal Aperture Views).
   b. C-Shaped deviated septum with its convexity to the left side.
3. **Bony pyramid**
   a. Wide base of thc boncy pyramid (Direct Dorsal and Backward Tilting Views).
   b. Osteocartilaginous hump which is oblique to the right side.
   c. There is bilateral maxillary asymmetry. The left cheek is narrow and more forward than the right cheek which is wider and more backward. The boney pyramid is oblique and deviated to the right side i.e. the opposite direction of the nasal tip. (Frontal and Backward Tilting Views).
4. **Alar base**
   a. Apparent unequal sizes and shapes of the nasal openings due to right caudal septal deviation (Backward Tilting and Basal Views).
   b. Nasal openings are thick walled and rounded (preoperative, Basal Views).

Aims of Surgery

1. Reduce the size and bulk of the nasal tip.
2. Excise the osteocartilaginous hump.
3. To correct the nasal crookedness.

Surgical Plan

1. **Frontolateral walls**
   a. DDD including the weak triangle to reduce the size bulk of the nasal tip.
   b. Cephalic trim of the lateral crurae to reduce the size of nasal tip.
2. **Medial Wall**
   Septoplasty and correction of caudal deviation.
3. **Bony pyramid**
   a. Excision of the osteocartilaginous hump.
   b. Osteotomies to centralize the bony pyramid.
   c. Kasanjian maneuver to the left i.e. cross fracture of the bony pyramid after osteotomies (see Surgery of the bony pyramid in the text).
4. **Alar base**
   Nil of note.

Surgical Procedure

a. As per Surgical Plan.
b. Depressed area appeared at the left side of the upper lateral cartilage. Crushed cartilaginous graft was used to fill in the defect.

Post-Operative Analysis

1. **Frontolateral Wall**
   a. Tip definition: nasal tip is smaller with thinner and smoother thinner overlying skin. It is more prominent and well identified from the alae nasi on both sides. The alae nasi come into view to become clearly visible and share in nasal aesthetics (Frontal, Direct Dorsal, Overhead, Backward Tilting and Basal Views).

M. H. A. Shafy, *Atlas of Clinical Cases in Rhinoplasty*,
https://doi.org/10.1007/978-3-031-07504-9_34

   b. Tip projection: The nasal tip is at the same level of the nasal dorsum with good aesthetic angle. This is coupled with good aesthetic nasolabial angle (lateral and oblique views).
   c. Tip light reflex is seen as one spot off the nasal tip (Frontal and Backward Tilting. Views).
2. **Medial Wall**
   The caudal deviation of septum is corrected.
3. **Bony Pyramid**
   a. Bony pyramid aesthetics improved: the nasal dorsum is straight and the sidewalls are smooth and narrow (all views except the Basal Views).
   b. Dorsal light reflex is seen a straight line off the nasal dorsum post-operatively as compared to the distorted reflex pre-operatively (Direct Dorsal Views).
4. **Alar Base**
   a. Superior alar groove aesthetics improved by defatting. The grooves become longer and deeper (Oblique, Lateral and Direct Dorsal grooves).
   b. Posterior alar groove aesthetic improved by defatting only. The alae nasi are pulled medially and the angles of posterior alar grooves become wider (Basal, Backward Tilting and Nasal Aperture Views).
   c. Alae nasi aesthetics improved after defatting. They are pulled medially widening the posterior alar grooves, become better seen and look smaller.
   d. Nasal aperture aesthetics improved after defatting and correction of the caudal septal deviation:
      i. The size of nasal apertures became equal (basal and Backward Tilting Views).
      ii. The shapes of the nasal apertures became symmetrical with thin elegantly oval walls (Basal and Backward Tilting Views).
   e. Marginal light reflexes are clearly seen at:
      i. Inferior alar margins (Nasal Aperture Views).
      ii. Nasal sill bands (Oblique Views).
      iii. Lateral crural prominences (Lateral Views).

Commentary

a. After her pre-operative trivial nasal injury, looking at the mirror became more frequent, she became more critical and obsessed by the deformity in her nose, which was originally developmental, and had no relation to the injury.
b. Deviation of the bony pyramid was to the right side, while counter deviation of the nasal tip was to the left. (Frontal and Direct Dorsal Views).
c. The bony pyramid was more oblique than deviated to the left side (Backward Tilting Views).

Frontal | Frontal Smiling | Frontal Middle Third

Preoperative

Postoperative

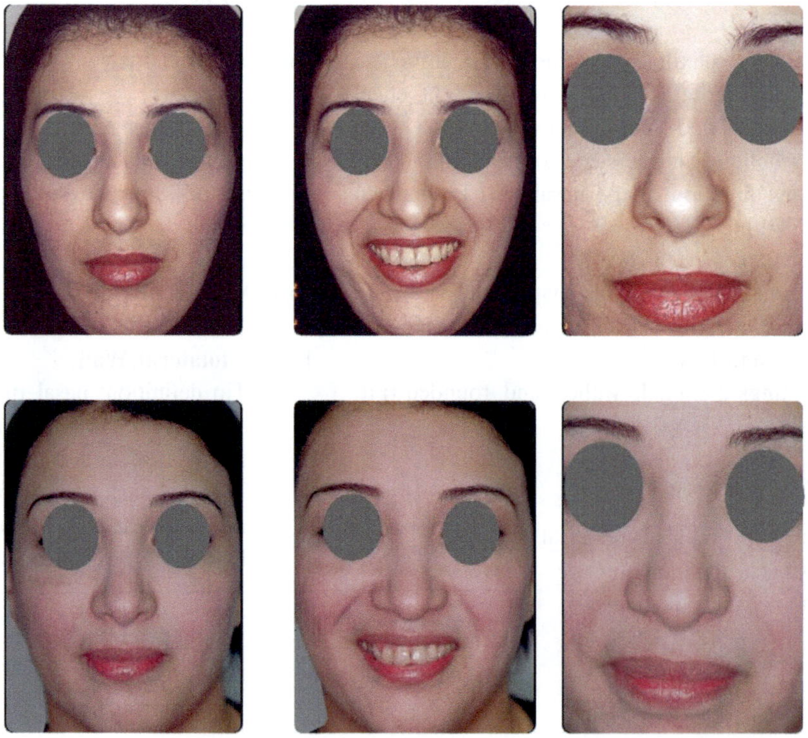

Direct Dorsal | Direct Dorsal Smiling

Preoperative

Postoperative

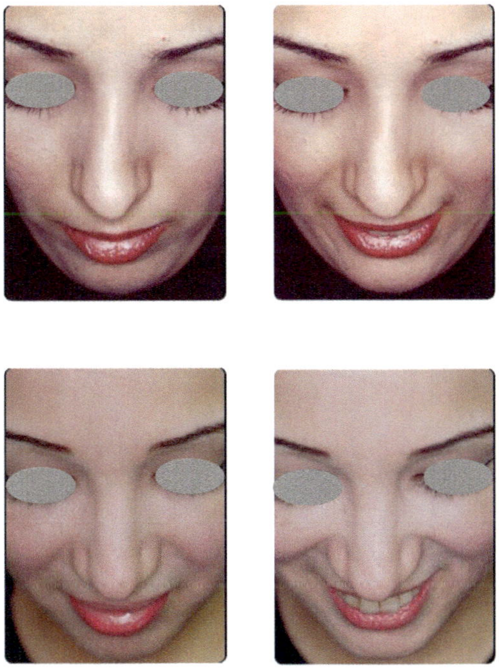

Backward Tilting | Steeper Backward Tilting | Basal | Basal Smiling

Preoperative

Postoperative

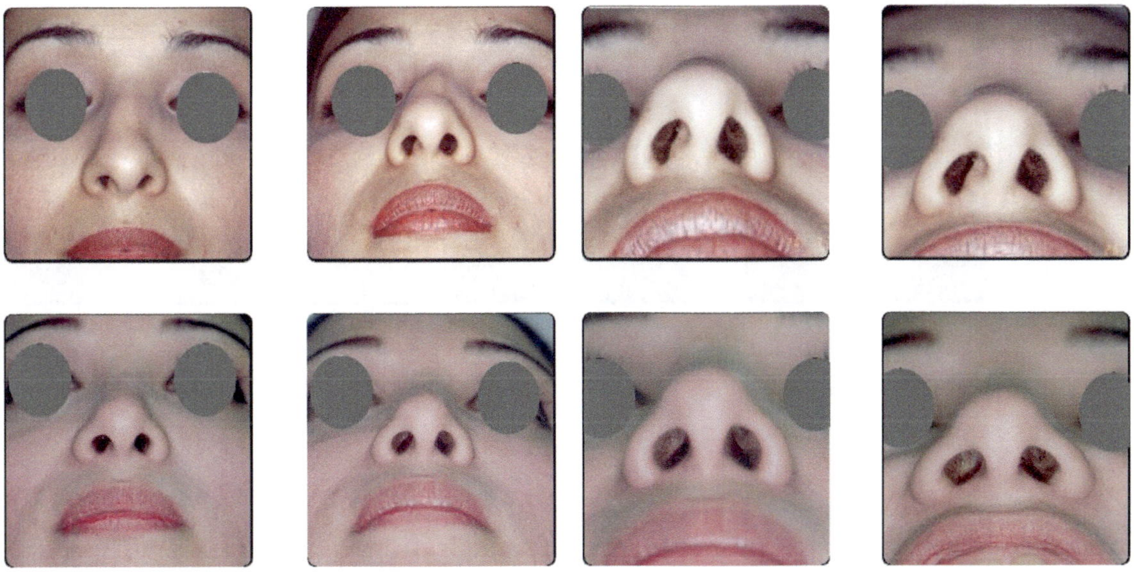

Right Nasal Aperture | Right Nasal Aperture Rim Sill Test | Left Nasal Aperture Rim Sill Test | Left Nasal Aperture

Preoperative

Postoperative

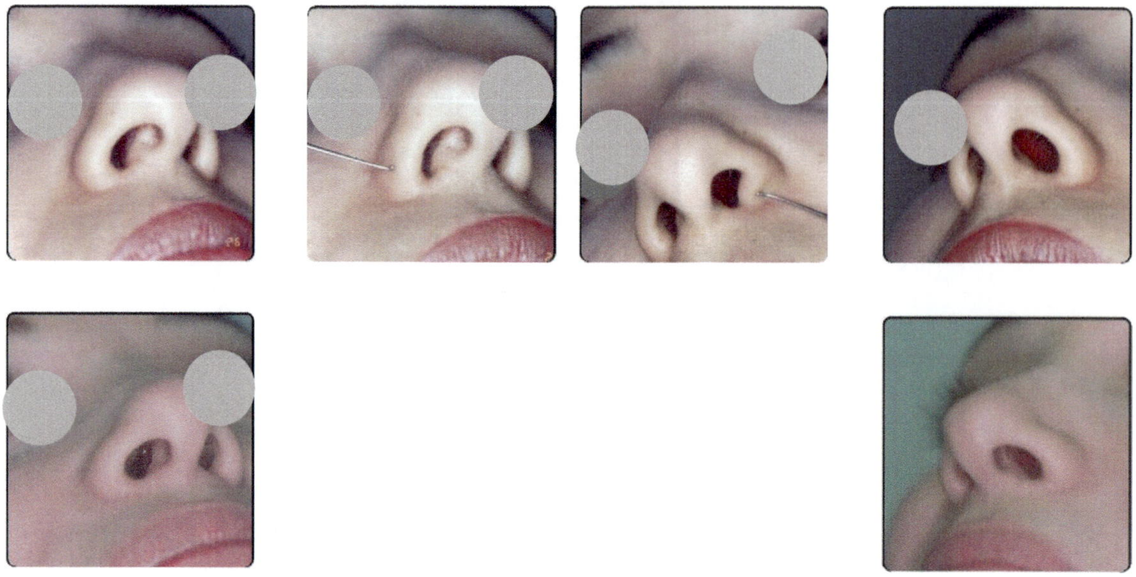

Right Oblique Mid Cheek Full Face | Left Oblique Mid Cheek Full Face | Right Oblique Mid Cheek Middle Third | Left Oblique Mid Cheek Middle Third

Preoperative

Postoperative

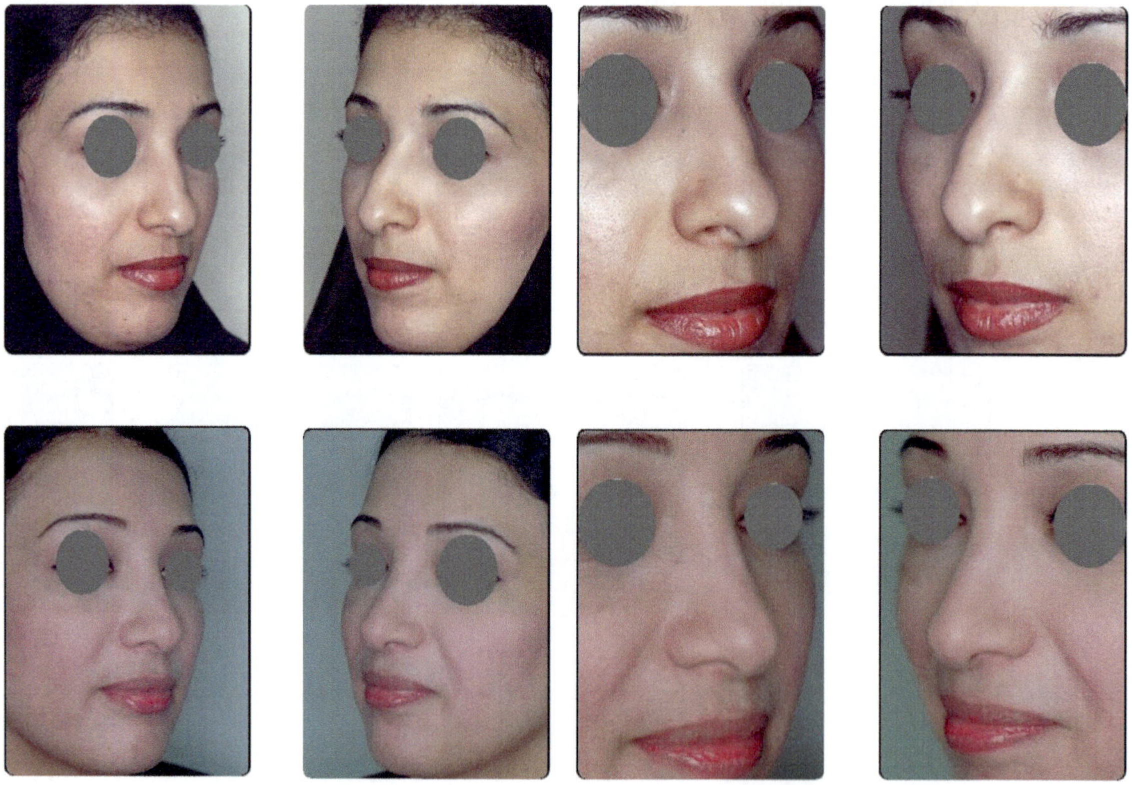

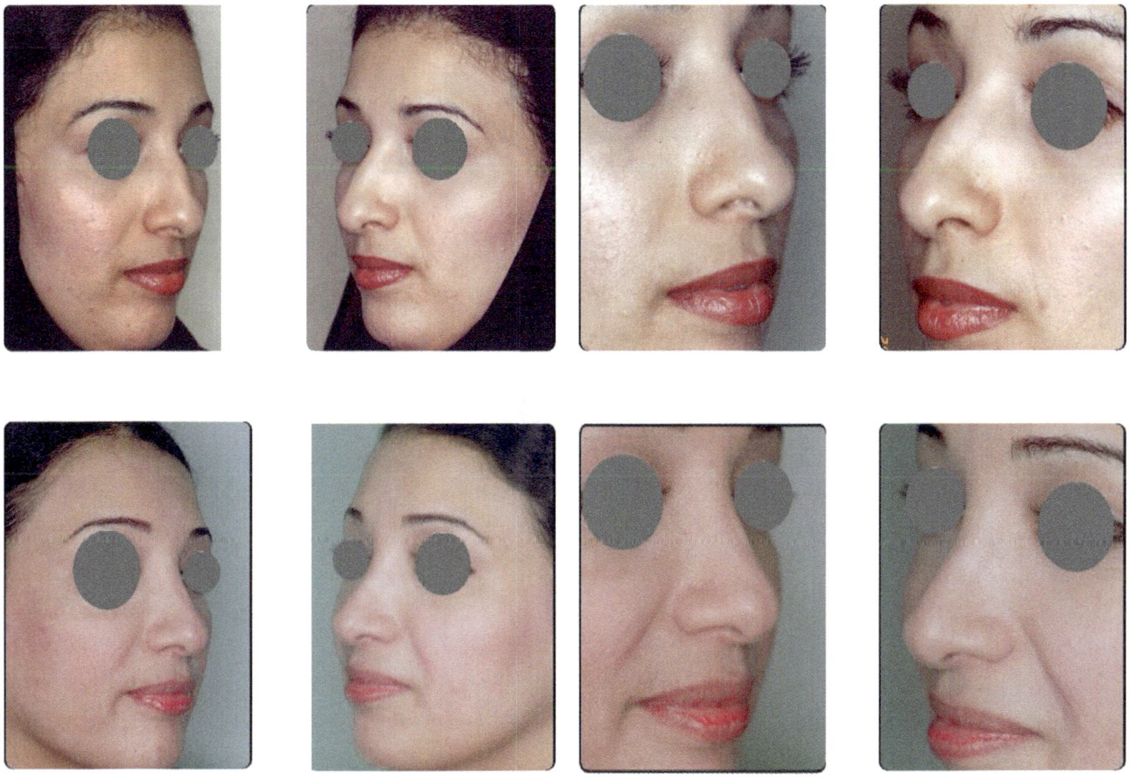
Right Oblique
Cheek Margin
Full Face
Left Oblique
Cheek Margin
Full Face
Right Oblique
Cheek Margin
Middle Third
Left Oblique
Cheek Margin
Middle Third
Preoperative
Postoperative

Right Lateral | Left Lateral | Right Lateral Smiling | Left Lateral Smiling

Preoperative

Postoperative

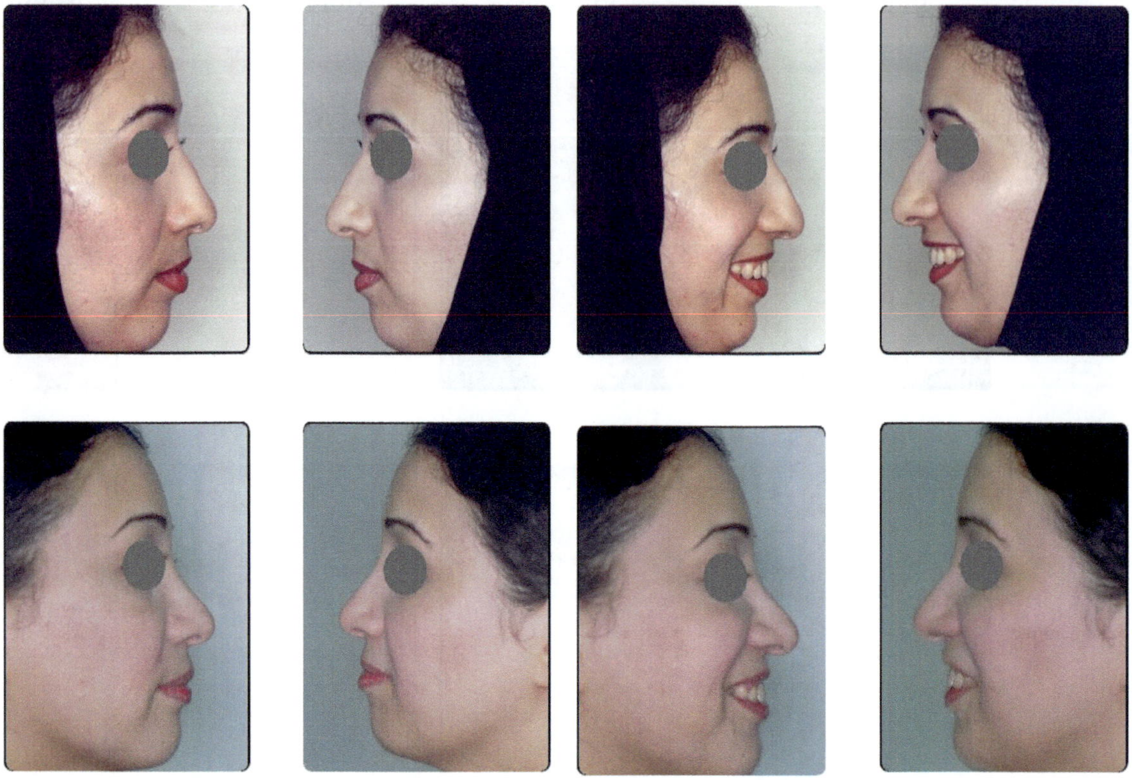

Right Lateral Middle Third | Left Lateral Middle Third

Preoperative

Postoperative

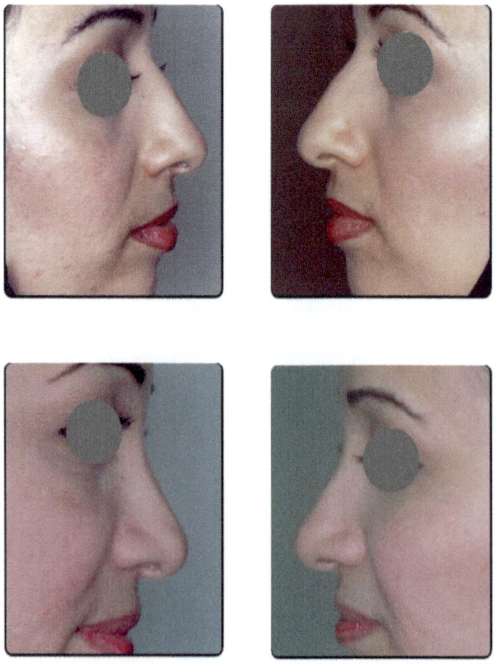

35 Part IV: Clinical Case 5

Preoperative Assessment

1. **Frontolateral walls**
   a. Bulky lower third: due to the bulky scroll areas (overlap of the lateral crurae over the upper lateral cartilage). The alae nasi are overshadowed behind the bulky tip (Frontal and Dorsal Dorsal Views).
   b. The nasal tip is counterdeviated to the right in opposite direction to the left deviation of the bony pyramid (Frontal, Direct Dorsal and Backward Tilting Views).
2. **Medial Wall**
   a. Severe left nasal septal deviation with left caudal dislocation. This has two effects:
      i. As the nasal tips is counter deviated to the right the dorsum had an inverted C-shaped appearance (preoperative Direct Dorsal View).
      ii. The left nasal sill band is pushed inferiorly (Frontal and Backward Tilting Views) and the left medial crus is pushed laterally (Backward Tilting and Basal Views). The left nasal aperture is distorted and became apparently different in size and shape from the right aperture (Preoperative, Backward Tilting and Basal Views).
3. **Bony pyramid**
   a. Wide base of the bony pyramid (Direct Dorsal and Backward Tilting Views).
   b. Bilateral maxillary asymmetry with oblique and deviation of the bony pyramid to the left side. The right cheek is wide and low and the left cheek is high and narrow. (Backward Tilting Views).
4. **Alar base**
   a. Apparently different nasal apertures in shape and size due to caudal septal deviation. (Backward Tilting and Basal Views).
   b. Nasal apertures are stretched and elongated forward by the long caudal septum.

Aims of Surgery

1. Correction of the crooked nose, i.e. the deviated bony pyramid, nasal septum including the caudal margin and consequently, the nasal tip.
2. Reduction of the size and bulk of the lower third of the nose including the scroll areas.

Surgical Plan

1. **Frontolateral walls**
   a. DDD not including the weak triangle to reduce the bulk and size of the nasal tip and midvault.
   b. Trim of the scroll areas on both sides to reduce their bulk.
2. **Medial Wall**
   Septoplasty and correction of caudal deviation.
3. **Bony pyramid**
   a. Osteotomies and medialization of the lateral bony walls to reduce the width and size of the bony pyramid.
   b. Kasanjian maneuver to the right i.e. cross fracture of the bony pyramid after osteotomies (see Surgery of the Bony Pyramid in Text).
4. **Alar base**
   Nil of note.

Surgical Procedure

a. As per Surgical Plan.
b. A crushed cartilaginous graft is needed to augment an area of depression that appeared over the right side of the upper lateral cartilage.

M. H. A. Shafy, *Atlas of Clinical Cases in Rhinoplasty*,
https://doi.org/10.1007/978-3-031-07504-9_35

Post-Operative Analysis

1. **Frontolateral Wall**
   a. Tip definition: nasal tip is smaller with thinner and smoother overlying skin. It is more prominent and well identified from the alae nasi on both sides. The alae nasi come into view to become clearly visible and share in nasal aesthetics (Frontal, Direct Dorsal, Overhead, Backward Tilting and Basal Views).
   b. Tip projection: The nasal tip at the same level of the nasal dorsum with good aesthetic angle. This is coupled with good aesthetic nasolabial angle (lateral and oblique views).
   c. Tip light reflex is seen as one spot off the nasal tip. (Frontal and Backward Tilting Views).
2. **Medial Wall**
   Caudal deviation of the septum was corrected.
3. **Bony Pyramid**
   a. Bony pyramid aesthetics improved: the nasal dorsum is straight in the midline and the sidewalls are smooth and narrow (all views except the Basal Views).
   b. Dorsal light reflex is seen as an uninterrupted line off the nasal dorsum (Direct Dorsal Views).
4. **Alar Base**
   a. Superior alar groove aesthetics improved by defatting. The grooves become longer and deeper (Oblique, Lateral and Direct Dorsal grooves).
   b. Posterior alar groove aesthetics improved by defatting. The alae nasi pulled medially widening the posterior groove angle. (Nasal Aperture and Oblique Views).
   c. Alae nasi aesthetics improved. They are pulled medially become better seen, smaller and share in nasal aesthetics. (Nasal Aperture, Oblique and Lateral Views).
   d. Nasal Aperture aesthetics:
      i. Correction of the left caudal septal deviation have reduced the protrusion of the left nasal sill band and the bulge of the left medial crus. The two nasal apertures became closer in size and in shape (Backward Tilting and Basal Views).
      ii. The nasal opening: they became elegantly oval. Their elongation by the caudal septum was corrected.
   e. Marginal light reflexes are clearly seen at:
      i. Inferior alar margins (Nasal Aperture Views).
      ii. Nasal sill bands (Oblique Views).
      iii. Lateral crural prominences (Lateral Views).

Commentary

This is a deceivingly simple and straightforward case. A mere septoplasty and osteotomies would have produced a straight but irregularly bulky nose. Debulking the scroll area, defatting of the lower third as well as centralizing the bony pyramid to the mid-line has contributed to a straight, regular, slim nose.

Frontal | Frontal Smiling | Frontal Middle Third

Preoperative

Postoperative

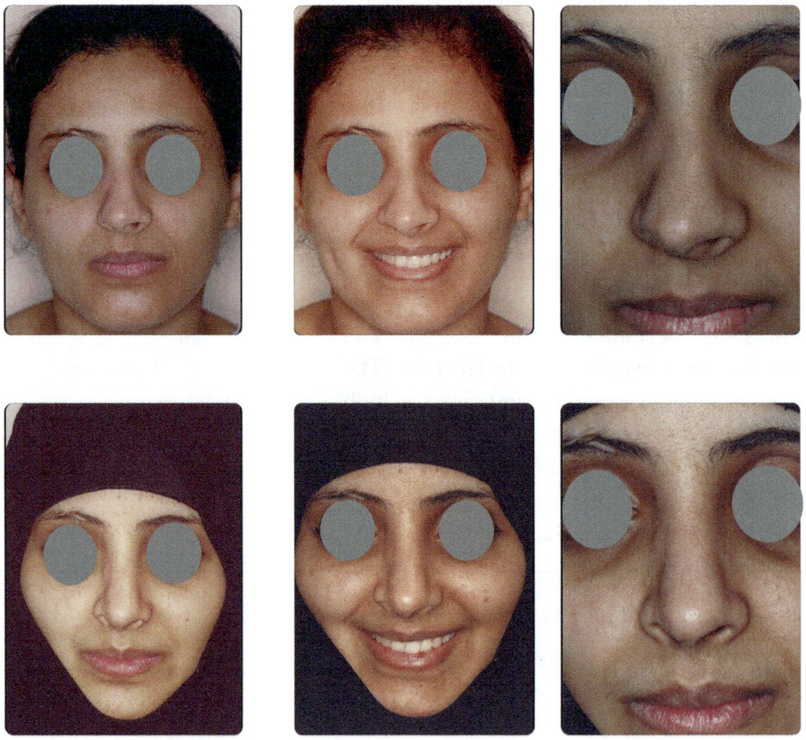

Direct Dorsal

Preoperative

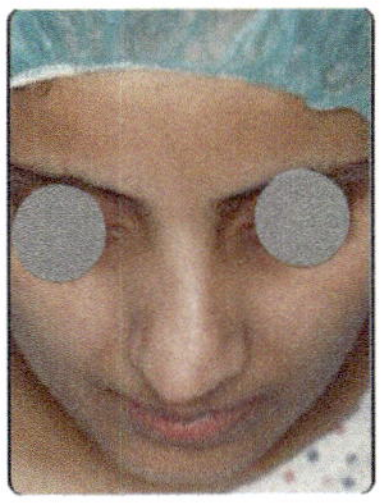

Postoperative

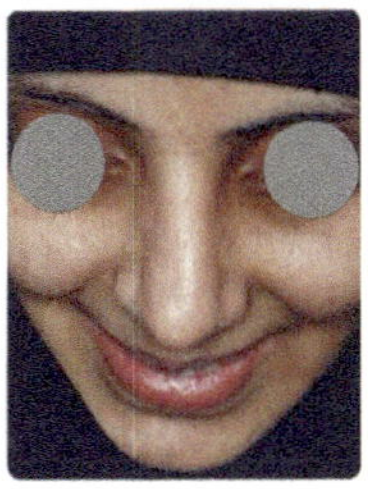

Backward Tilting	Steeper Backward Tilting	Basal	Basal Smiling

Preoperative

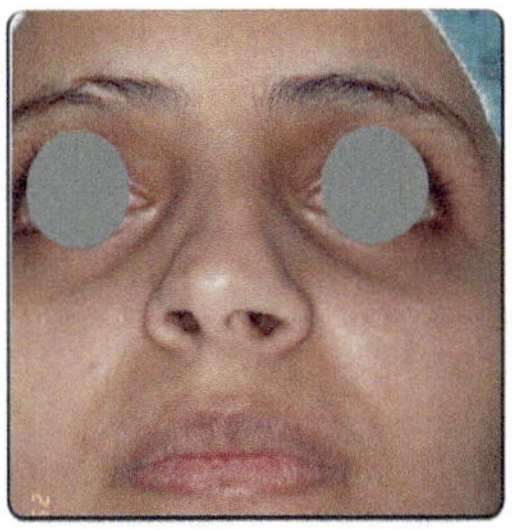
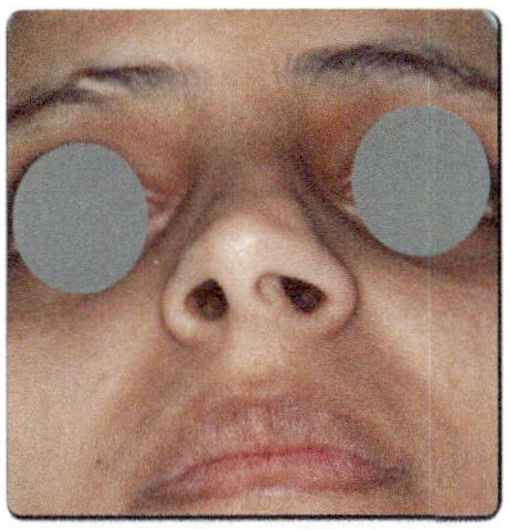
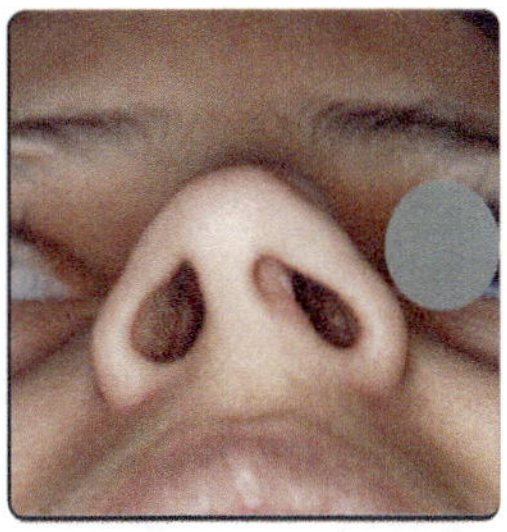
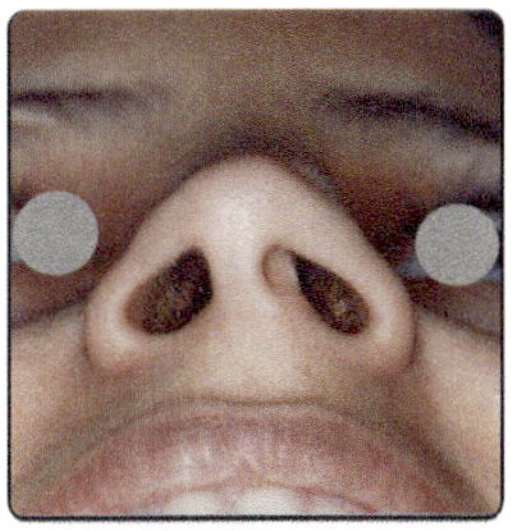

Postoperative

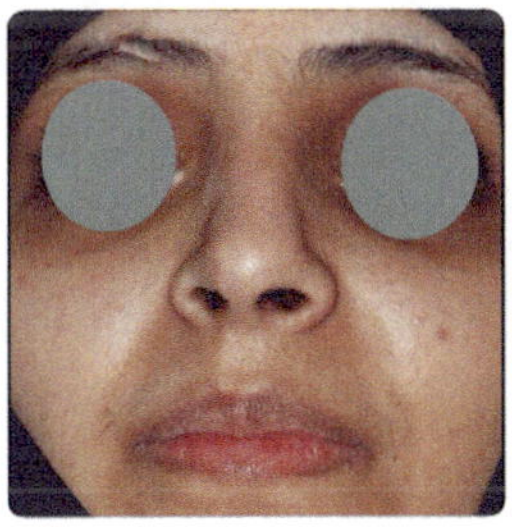
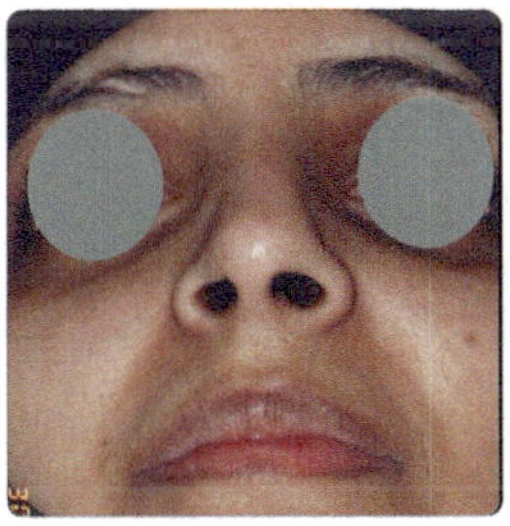
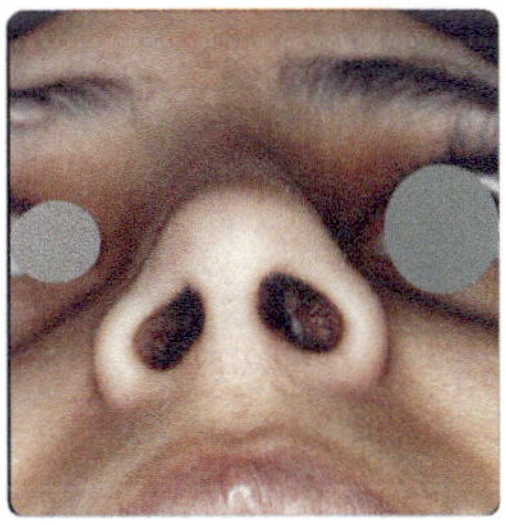
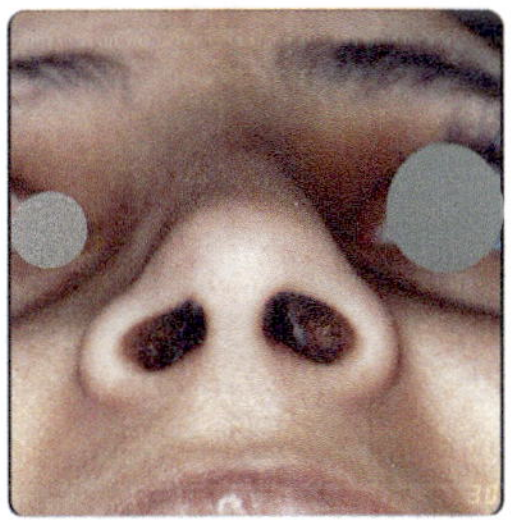

Right Nasal Aperture

Right Nasal Aperture Rim Sill Test

Left Nasal Aperture Rim Sill Test

Left Nasal Aperture

Preoperative

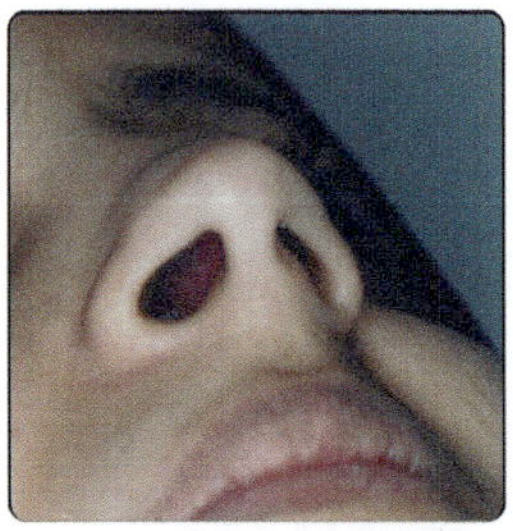
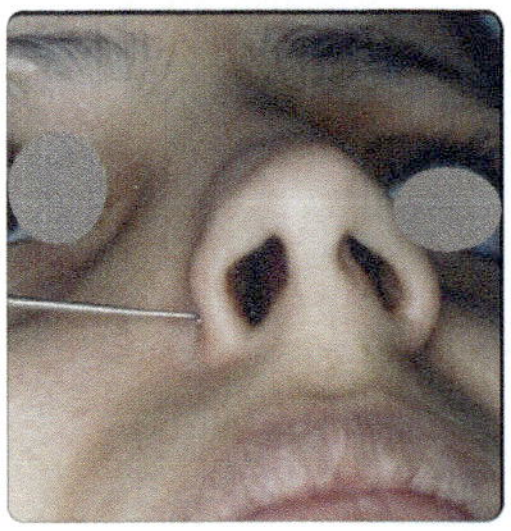
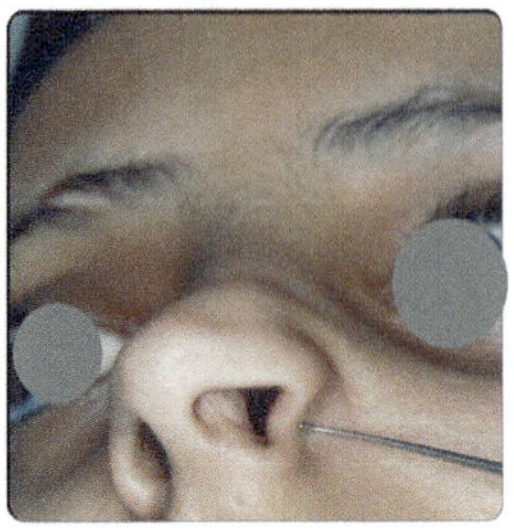
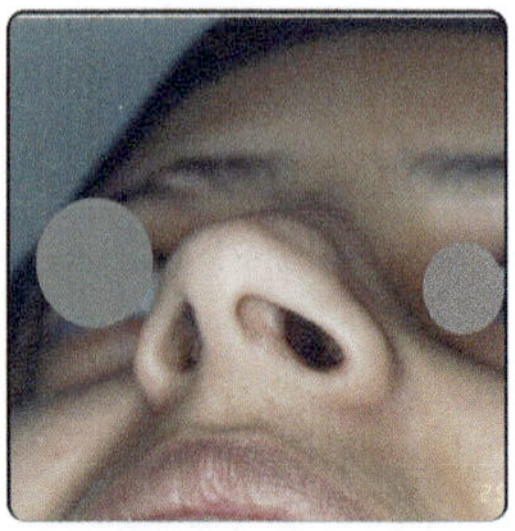

Postoperative

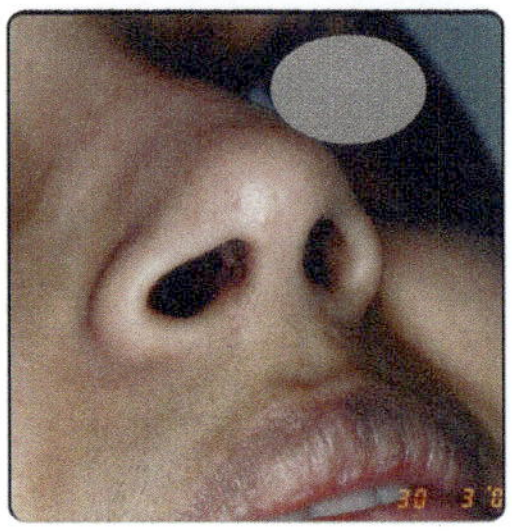
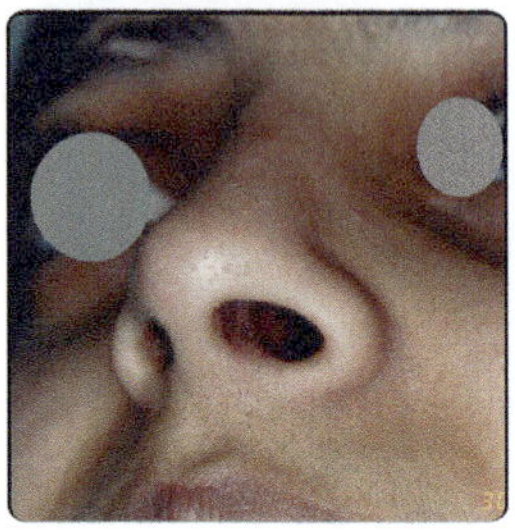

Right Oblique Mid Cheek Full Face

Left Oblique Mid Cheek Full Face

Right Oblique Mid Cheek Middle Third

Left Oblique Mid Cheek Middle Third

Preoperative

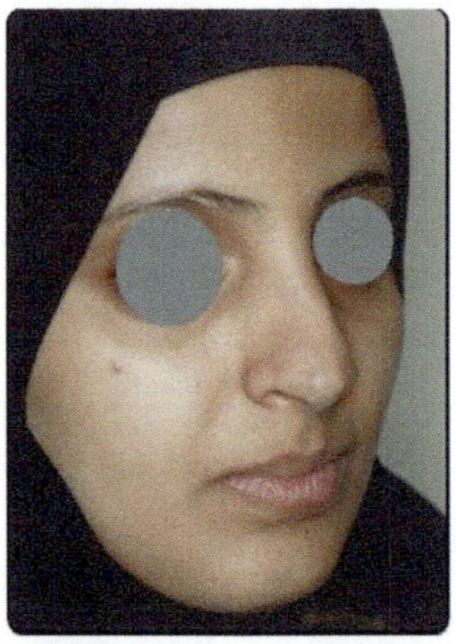
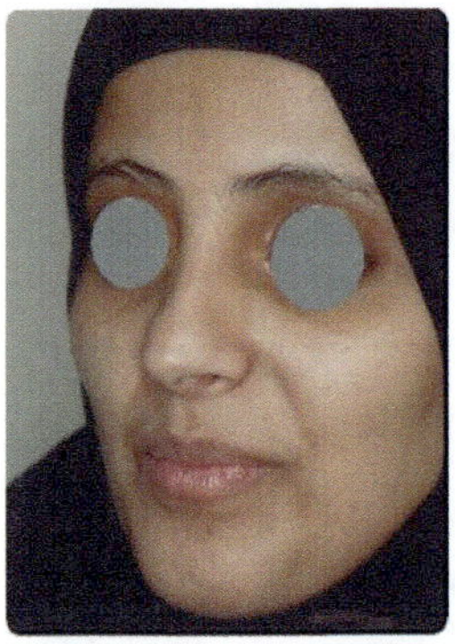
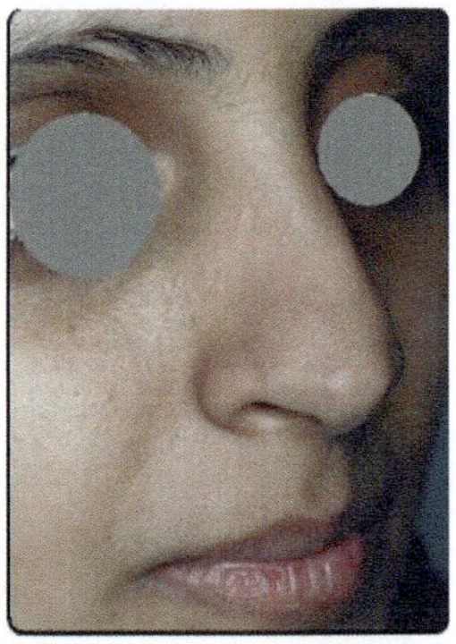
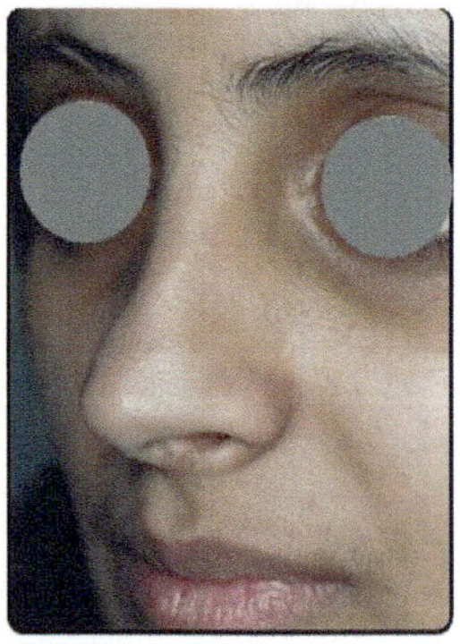

Postoperative

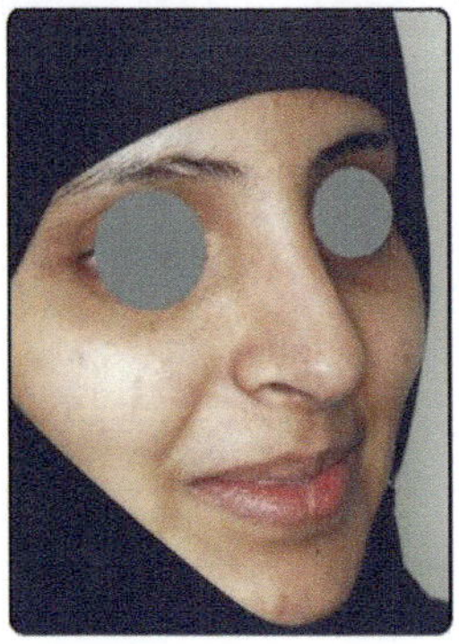
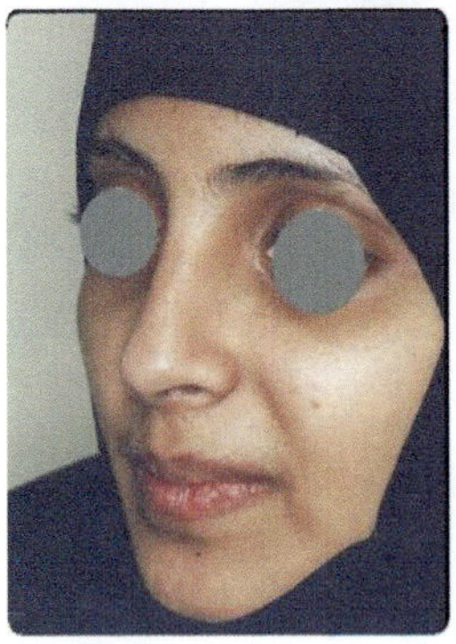
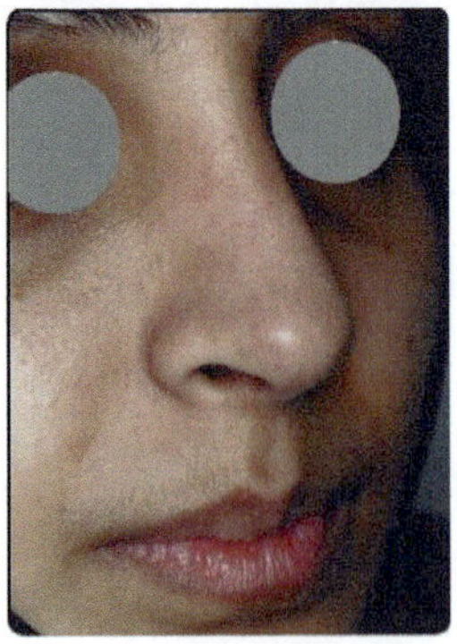

Right Oblique Cheek Margin Full Face | Left Oblique Cheek Margin Full Face | Right Oblique Cheek Margin Middle Third | Left Oblique Cheek Margin Middle Third

Preoperative

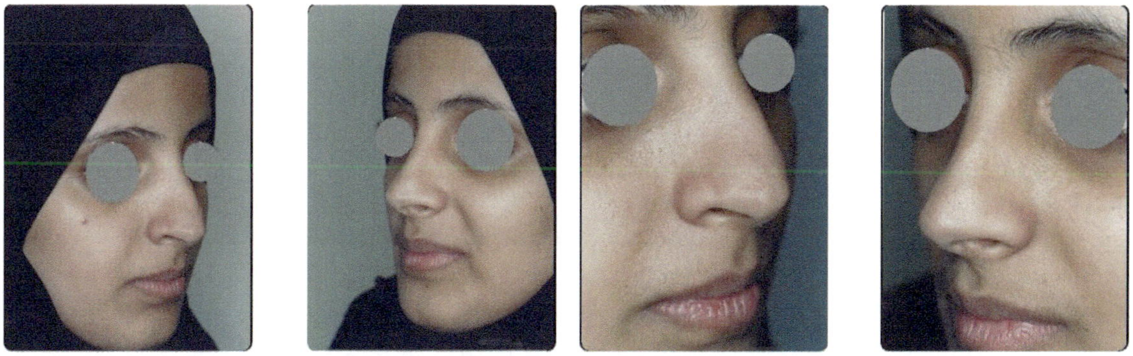

Postoperative

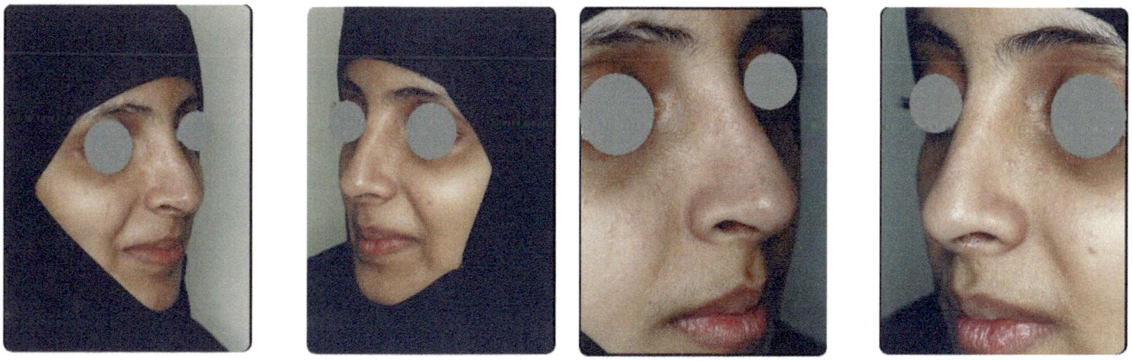

Right Lateral | Left Lateral | Right Lateral Smiling | Left Lateral Smiling

Preoperative

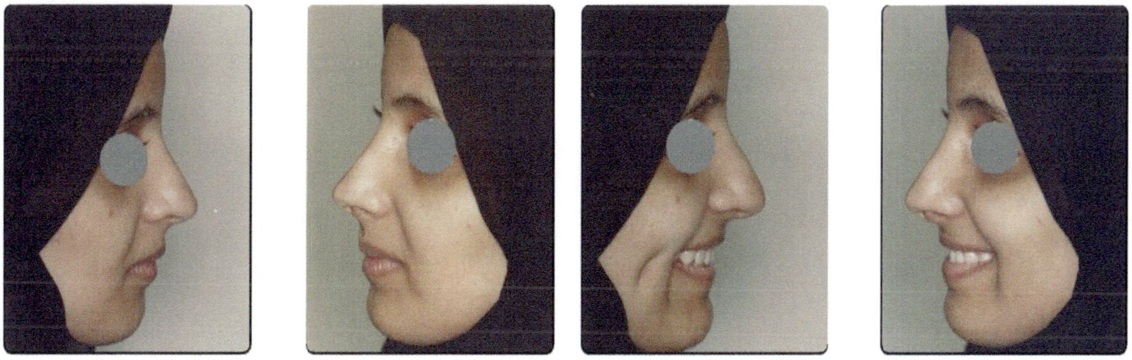

Postoperative

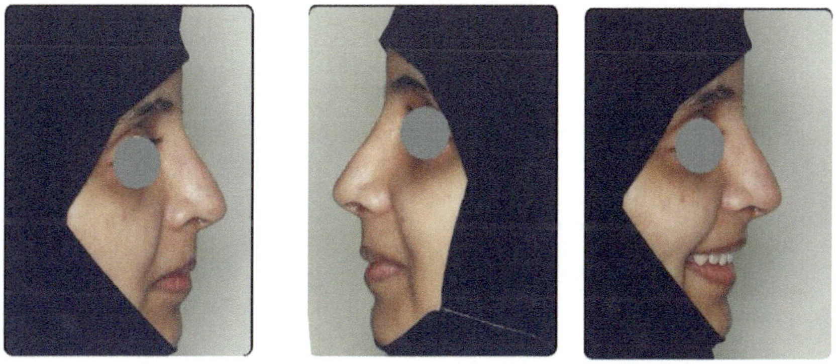

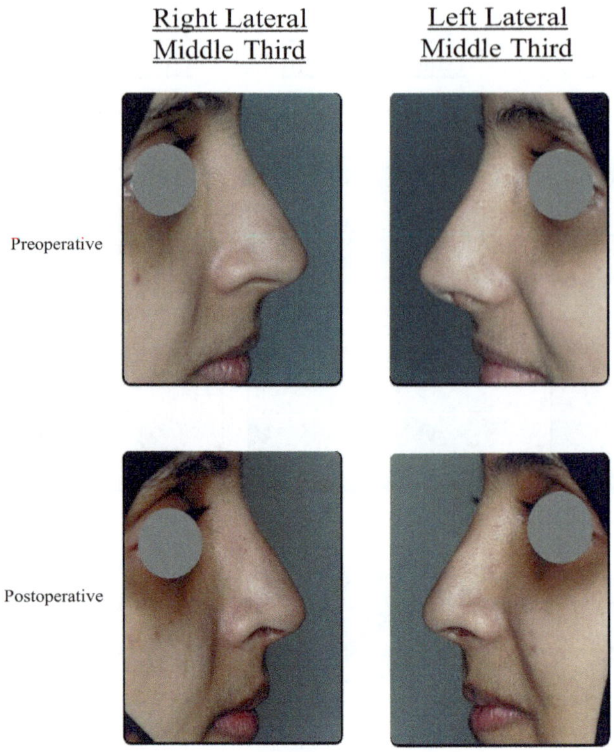
Right Lateral
Middle Third
Left Lateral
Middle Third
Preoperative
Postoperative

36 Part IV: Clinical Case 6

Preoperative Assessment

1. **Frontolateral walls**
   a. Bulky, large tip. The right side is naturally larger than the left i.e. larger right lateral crus. The nasal tip is deviated to the left especially on smiling. (Frontal and Direct Dorsal Views). The alae nasi were completely overshadowed by the large and bulky tip. (Frontal, Direct Dorsal and Overhead Views).
   b. Slight bifidity (Backward Tilting Views).
2. **Medial Wall**
   a. Mobile tip i.e. the nasal tip moves inferiorly on smiling (Lateral Smiling Views).
   b. Sliding tip i.e. the nasal tip moves posteriorly on smiling (Lateral Smiling Views).
   c. Right caudal septal deviation (Right Nasal Aperture Views).
3. **Bony pyramid**
   a. Wide base of the boney pyramid (Direct Dorsal and Backward Tilting Views).
   b. Osteocartilagenous hump which is both deviated and oblique to the right due to bilateral maxillary asymmetry. The right cheek is high and narrow while the left cheek wide and low (Backward Tilting Views).
   c. The right deviation of the bony pyramid is followed by counterdeviation of the lower 2/3rds to the left. Further deviation takes place on smiling due to movements in the lower 1/3rd of the nose. (Frontal, Direct Dorsal and Overhead Views).
4. **Alar base**
   a. The right medial crus is pushed into the nasal aperture by the caudally deviated nasal septum. The right nasal aperture was distorted and different from the left nose.
   b. The right ala nasi is larger than the left (Frontal, Backward Tilting, Direct Dorsal and Overhead Views).

Aims of Surgery

1. To reduce the size and the bulk of the nasal tip.
2. Abolish the mobile tip and the sliding tip.
3. Excision the osteocartilaginous hump.
4. Correction of the crookedness including the bony pyramid and the lower third.

Surgical Plan

1. **Frontolateral walls**
   a. DDD including the weak triangle to reduce the bulk of the nasal tip.
   b. Bilateral cephalic trim of the lateral crurae to reduce the size.
2. **Medial Wall**
   a. Septoplasty. Trim of two millimeter of the membranous septum.
   b. Division of the Depressor Septi muscles.
3. **Bony pyramid**
   a. Excision of the osteocartilaginous hump.
   b. Osteotomies with Kassanjian maneuver to the left i.e. cross fracture of the bony pyramid after osteotomies (see Surgery of the Bony Pyramid in the Text).
4. **Alar base**
   Nil of note.

Surgical Procedure

As per Surgical Plan.

Post-Operative Analysis

1. **Frontolateral Wall**
   a. Tip Definition: nasal tip is smaller with thinner and smoother overlying skin. It is more prominent and well identified from the alae nasi on both sides. The alae nasi come into view to become clearly visible

M. H. A. Shafy, *Atlas of Clinical Cases in Rhinoplasty*,
https://doi.org/10.1007/978-3-031-07504-9_36

and share in nasal aesthetics (Frontal, Direct Dorsal, Overhead, Backward Tilting and Basal Views).

b. Tip projection: The nasal tip at the same level of the nasal dorsum with good aesthetic angle. This is coupled with good aesthetic nasolabial angle (lateral and oblique views).

c. Tip light reflex is seen as one spot off the nasal tip. (Frontal and Backward Tilting Views).

2. **Medial Wall**

The caudal septal deviation is corrected.

3. **Bony Pyramid**

a. Bony pyramid aesthetics improved: the nasal dorsum is straight and the sidewalls are smooth and narrow (all views except the Basal Views).

b. Dorsal light reflex is seen as an uninterrupted line off the nasal dorsum (Direct Dorsal Views).

Caudal septal deviation is corrected.

4. **Alar Base**

a. Superior alar groove aesthetics improved by defatting. The grooves become longer and deeper (Oblique, Lateral and Direct Dorsal grooves).

b. Posterior alar groove aesthetics improved. Defatting pulled the alae nasi medially widening the posterior alar groove angles.

c. Alae nasi aesthetics improved. They are pulled medially become better seen, smaller and share in nasal aesthetics. (Nasal Aperture, Oblique and Lateral Views).

d. Nasal aperture aesthetics improved after defatting and correction of caudal septal deviation. The nasal openings became equal and they look more elegantly smaller.

e. Marginal light reflexes are clearly seen at:

i. Inferior alar margins (Nasal Aperture Views).

ii. Nasal sill bands (Oblique Views).

iii. Lateral crural prominences (Lateral Views).

Commentary

a. After DDD, the difference in size between the two sides of the frontolateral walls is greatly reduced. The larger right side was due to larger right lateral crus as well as excess of the overlying two layers of subdermal fat.

b. The post-operative photographs were taken only four months after surgery the expected final result of DDD may take up to two years.

c. Bifidity of columella is gone after defatting.

Frontal | Frontal Smiling | Frontal Middle Third

Preoperative

Postoperative

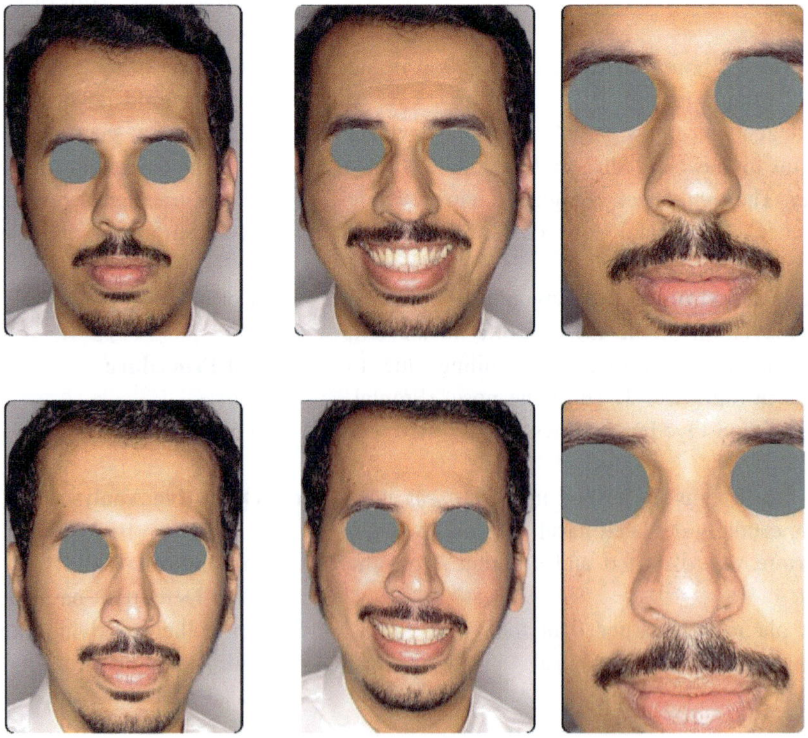

Direct Dorsal | Direct Dorsal Smiling | Overhead | Overhead Smiling

Preoperative

Postoperative

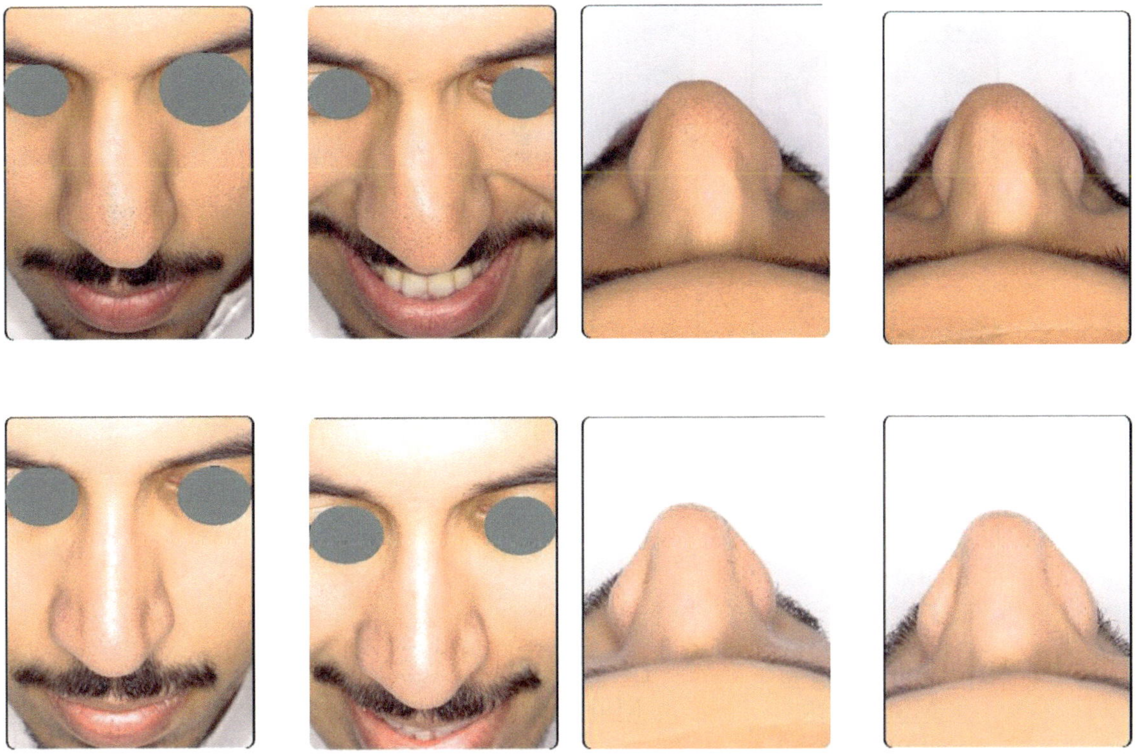

Backward Tilting | Steeper Backward Tilting | Basal | Basal Smiling

Preoperative

Postoperative

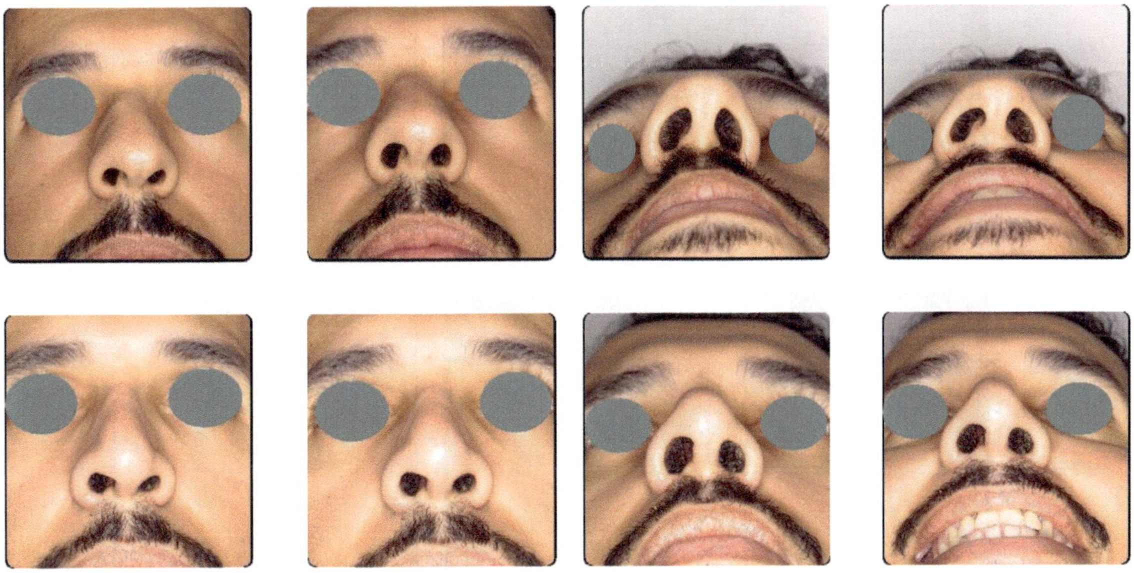

Right Nasal Aperture | Right Nasal Aperture Rim Sill Test | Left Nasal Aperture Rim Sill Test | Left Nasal Aperture

Preoperative

Postoperative

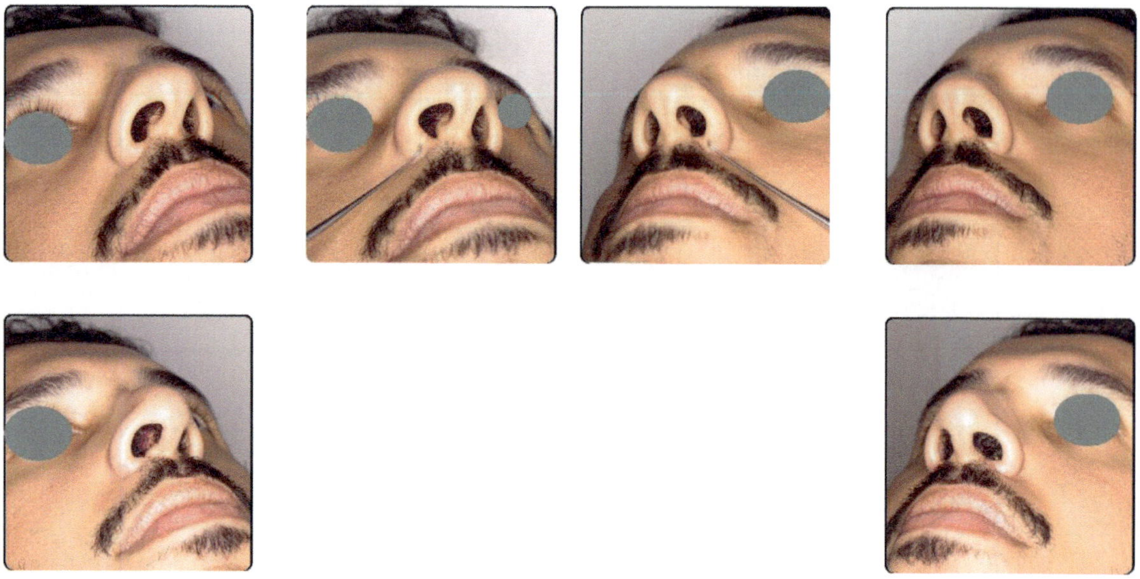

Right Oblique Mid Cheek Full Face | Left Oblique Mid Cheek Full Face | Right Oblique Mid Cheek Middle Third | Left Oblique Mid Cheek Middle Third

Preoperative

Postoperative

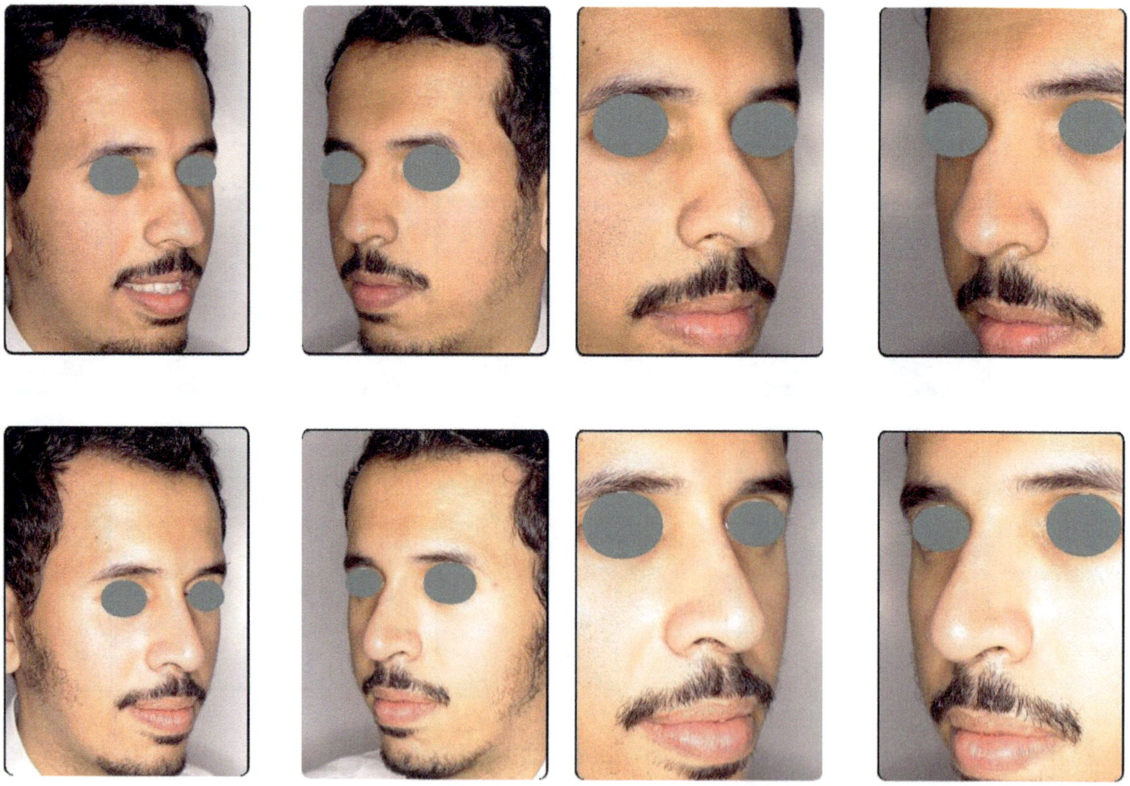

Right Oblique Cheek Margin Full Face	Left Oblique Cheek Margin Full Face	Right Oblique Cheek Margin Middle Third	Left Oblique Cheek Margin Middle Third

Preoperative

Postoperative

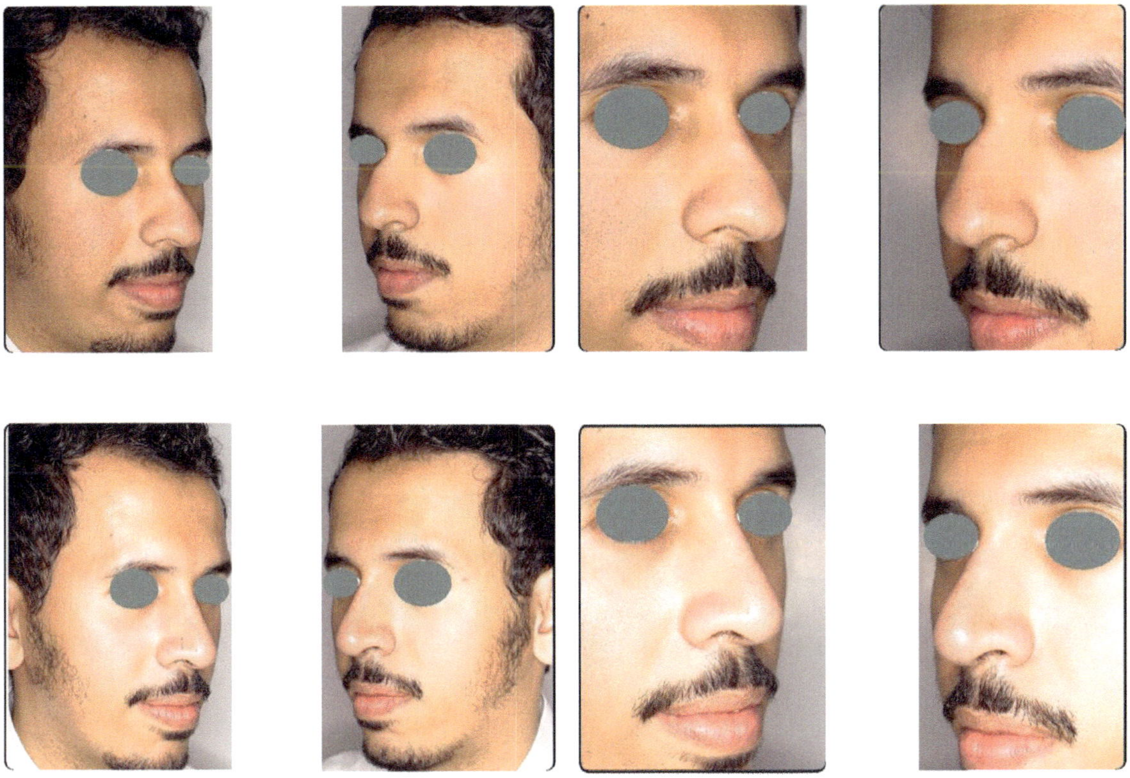

Right Lateral | **Left Lateral** | **Right Lateral Smiling** | **Left Lateral Smiling**

Preoperative

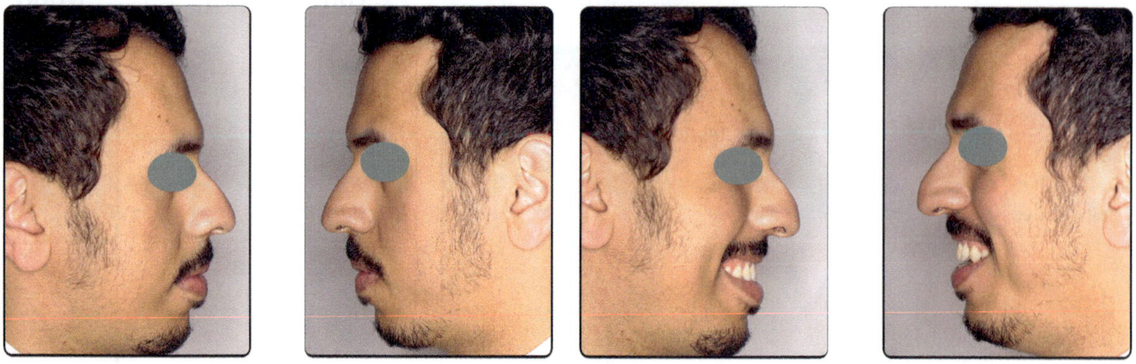

Mobile tip: downward movement on smiling.
Smiling tip: posterior movement on smiling, the tip is at a lower level than the dorsum.

Postoperative

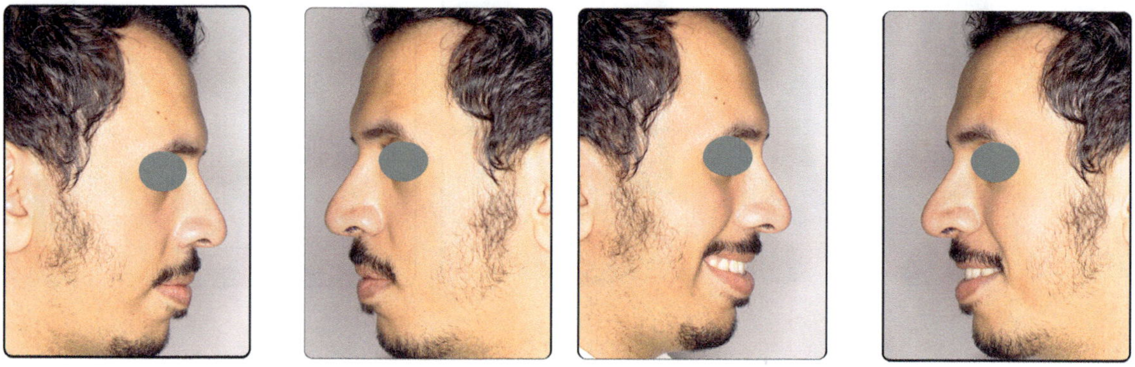

Right Lateral Middle Third | Left Lateral Middle Third

Preoperative

Postoperative

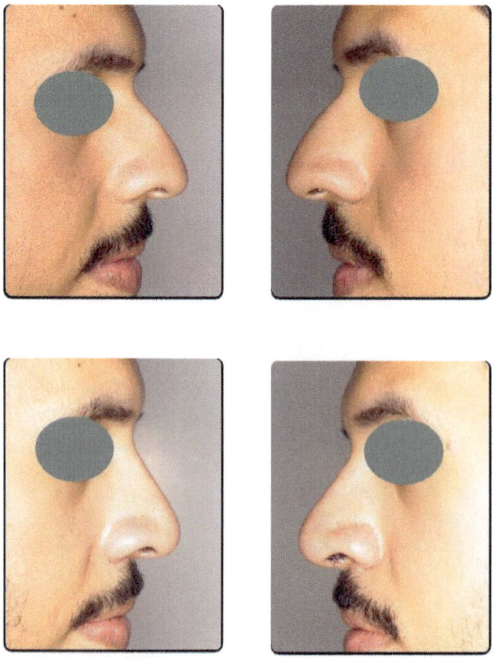

Part IV: Clinical Case 7

37

Preoperative Assessment

1. **Frontolateral walls**
   a. Large and bulky nasal tip overshadowing the alae nasi (Frontal and Direct Dorsal Views).
   b. The nasal tip is counter deviated to the left, as compared to the right deviation of the bony pyramid (Frontal, Direct Dorsal, and Backward Tilting Views).
2. **Medial Wall**
   Nil of note.
3. **Bony pyramid**
   a. Wide base of the boney pyramid (Direct Dorsal and Backward Tilting Views).
   b. Osteocartilaginous hump which is oblique and deviated to the right side due to bilateral maxillary asymmetry. The left cheek is wide and low and the right cheek is high and narrow (Backward Tilting Views).
4. **Alar base**
   Wide alar base due to long inferior segments of rim-sill folds (Basal and Nasal Aperture Views).

Aims of Surgery

a. Reduction of the bulk and size of the Nasal tip.
b. Correction of crookedness of the nose including the bony pyramid and deviated nasal septum with the nasal tip.

Surgical Plan

1. **Frontolateral walls**
   a. DDD including the weak triangle to reduce the bulk of the nasal tip and supratip area.
   b. Cephalic trim of the lateral crurae to reduce the size of the tip.
2. **Medial Wall**
   Nil of note.
3. **Bony pyramid**
   a. Excision of the Osteocartilaginous hump.
   b. Osteotomies and Kassanjian maneuver to the patient's left i.e. cross fracture of the bony pyramid after osteotomies (see Surgery of the Bony Pyramid in the Text).
4. **Alar base**
   Excision of the inferior segments of the rim sill folds.

Surgical Procedure

a. As per Surgical Plan.
b. There was no need to excise the posterior segments of the rim-sill folds. Nasal apertures looked satisfactory.

Post-Operative Analysis

1. **Frontolateral Wall**
   a. Tip Definition: nasal tip is smaller with thinner and smoother overlying skin. It is more prominent and well identified from the alae nasi on both sides. The alae nasi come into view to become clearly visible and share in nasal aesthetics (Frontal, Direct Dorsal, Overhead, Backward Tilting and Basal Views).
   b. Tip projection: The nasal tip is at the same level of the nasal dorsum with good aesthetic angle. This is coupled with good aesthetic nasolabial angle (lateral and oblique views).
   c. Tip light reflex is seen as one spot off the nasal tip. (Frontal and Backward Tilting Views).
2. **Medial Wall**
   Nil of Note.
3. **Bony Pyramid**
   a. Bony pyramid aesthetics improved: the nasal dorsum is straight in the midline and the sidewalls are smooth and narrow (all views except the Basal Views).

M. H. A. Shafy, *Atlas of Clinical Cases in Rhinoplasty*,
https://doi.org/10.1007/978-3-031-07504-9_37

b. Dorsal light reflex is seen as an uninterrupted line off the nasal dorsum (Direct Dorsal Views).

4. **Alar Base**
   a. Superior alar groove aesthetics improved by defatting. The grooves become longer and deeper (Oblique, Lateral and Direct Dorsal grooves).
   b. Posterior alar groove aesthetics improved. Defatting pulled the alae nasi medially widening the posterior alar groove angles. Aesthetics of alae nasi improved (Nasal Aperture and Oblique Views).
   c. Nasal aperture aesthetics improved after defatting and excision of inferior segments of rim-sill folds:
      i. The size is smaller.
      ii. The shapes are more elegantly better.
   d. Alae nasi aesthetics improved. They are pulled medially and become better seen, smaller and share in nasal aesthetics. (Nasal Aperture, Oblique and Lateral Views).
   e. Marginal light reflexes are clearly seen at:
      i. Inferior alar margins (Nasal Aperture Views).
      ii. Nasal sill bands (Oblique Views).
      iii. Lateral crural prominences (Lateral Views).

Commentary

a. The post-operative photographs were taken five years after the surgery.
b. The long term result of defatting, even though minimal fat was found, is quite impressive.
   His five year post-operative photos have shown that the size of the nose remained relatively small, i.e. no new fat deposition.
c. No tip graft was used for this patient because he had a naturally projecting, rounded tip which matched his large, rounded face.

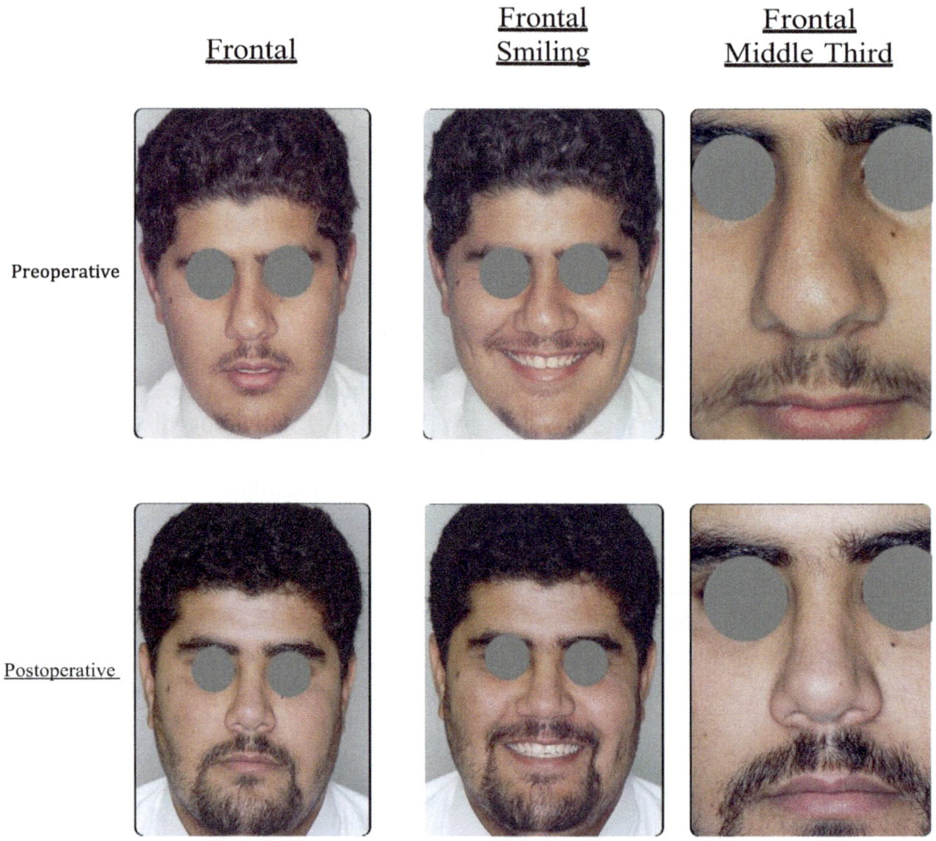

Direct Dorsal | Direct Dorsal Smiling

Preoperative

Postoperative

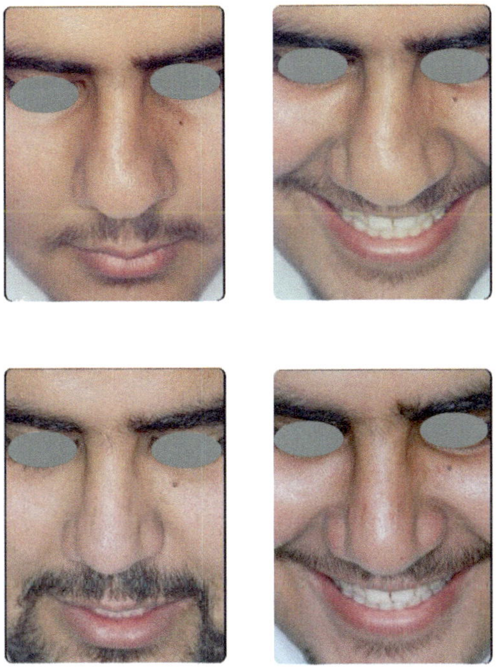

Backward Tilting | Steeper Backward Tilting | Basal | Basal Smiling

Preoperative

Postoperative

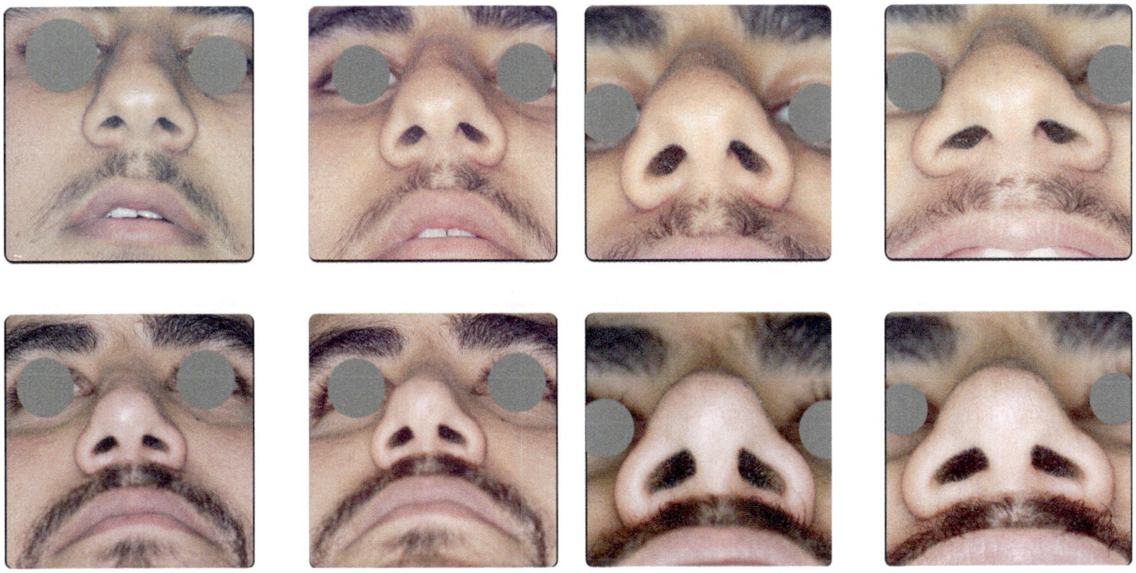

Right Nasal Aperture | Right Nasal Aperture Rim Sill Test | Left Nasal Aperture Rim Sill Test | Left Nasal Aperture

Preoperative

Postoperative

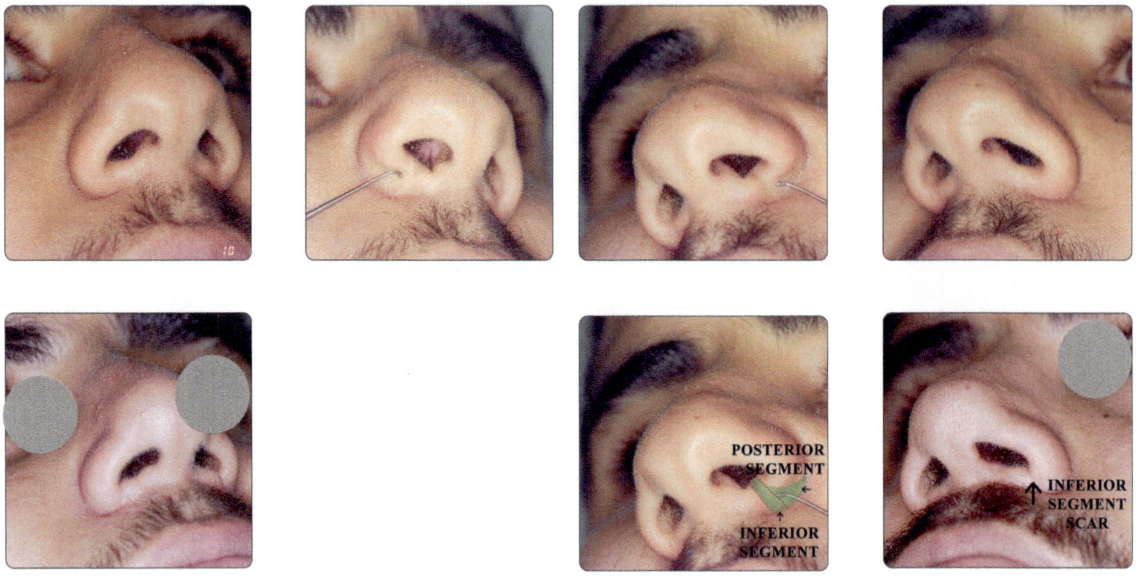

Right Oblique Mid Cheek Full Face | Left Oblique Mid Cheek Full Face | Right Oblique Mid Cheek Middle Third | Left Oblique Mid Cheek Middle Third

Preoperative

Postoperative

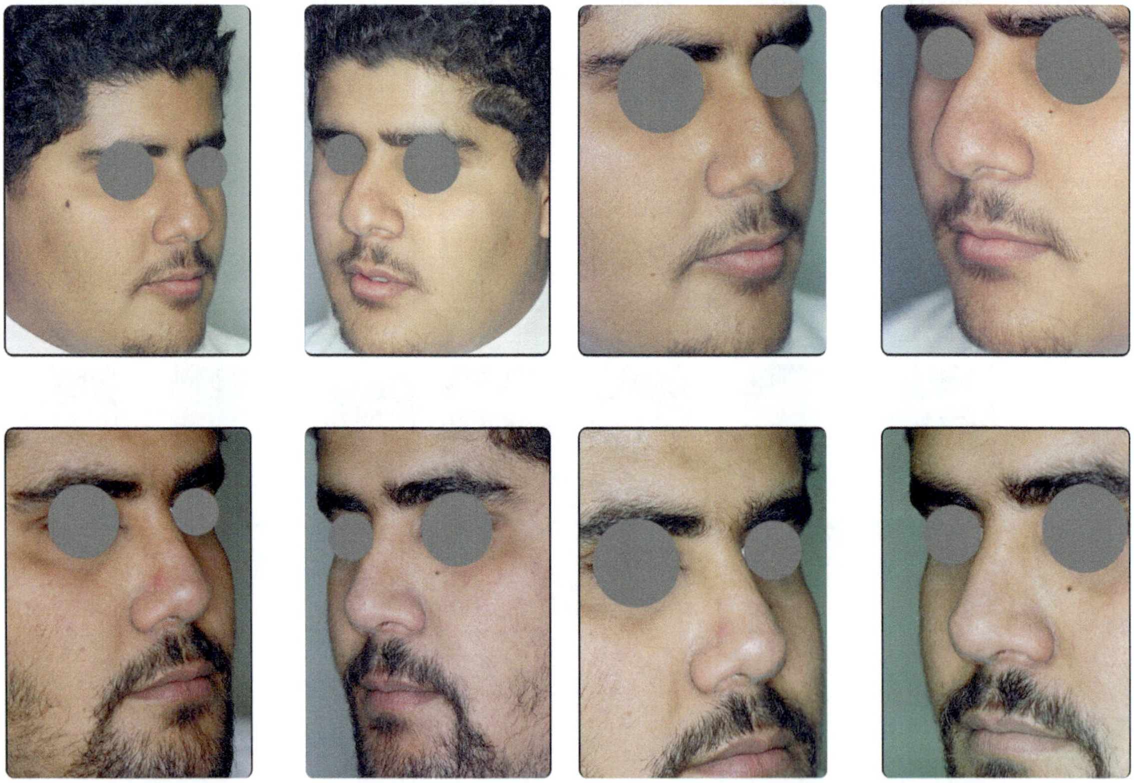

Right Oblique Cheek Margin Full Face | Left Oblique Cheek Margin Full Face | Right Oblique Cheek Margin Middle Third | Left Oblique Cheek Margin Middle Third

Preoperative

Postoperative

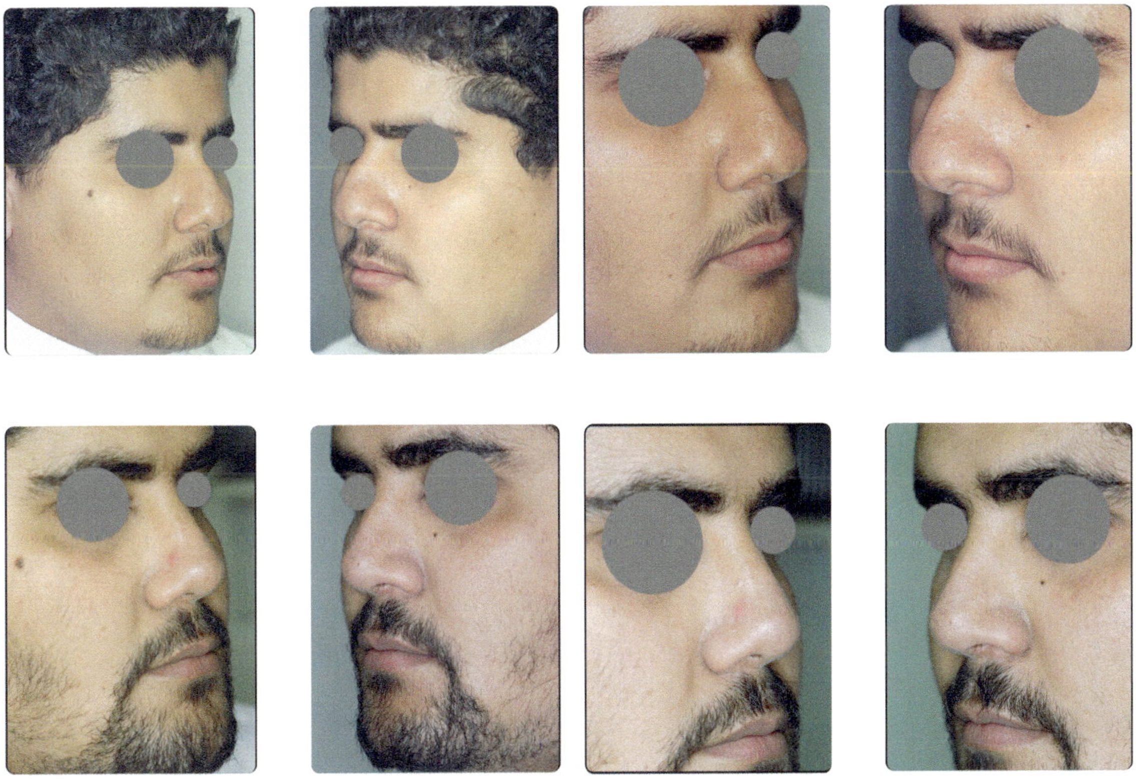

Right Lateral | Left Lateral

Preoperative

Postoperative

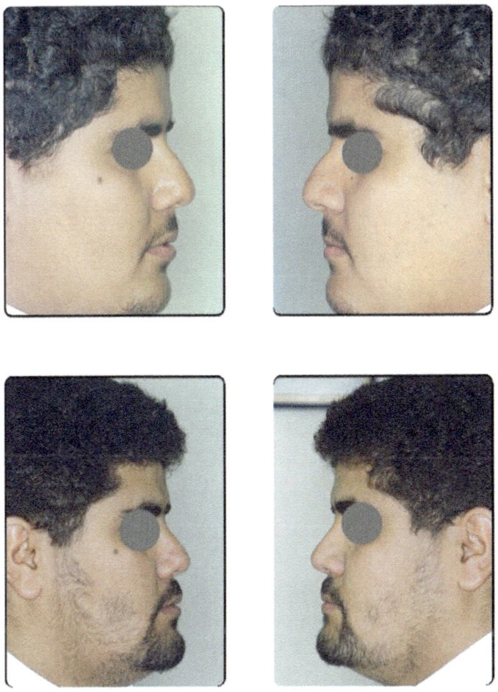

Right Lateral Middle Third | Left Lateral Middle Third

Preoperative

Postoperative

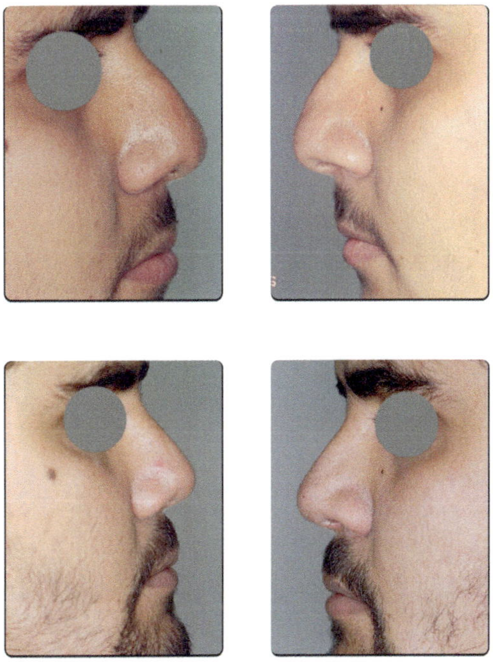

38 Part IV: Clinical Case 8

Preoperative Assessment

1. **Frontolateral walls**
   a. Large and bulky frontolateral walls that completely overshadowed the alae nasi. (Frontal, Direct Dorsal and Overhead Views).
   b. Nasal tip is counter-deviated to the right as compared to the left sided deviation of the bony pyramid. (Frontal, Overhead and Smiling Direct Dorsal Views).
2. **Medial Wall**
   a. Left deviation of the caudal cartilaginous septum (Backward Tilting, Basal and Left Nasal Aperture Views). The posterior septal angle is dislocated off the maxillary crest. There is lateralization of the left medial crus (Backward Tilting, and Basal Views). The left nasal sill band is displaced inferiorly (Frontal and Backward Tilting Views).
   b. Mobile tip i.e. the nasal tip moves inferiorly on smiling (Lateral Smiling Views).
3. **Bony pyramid**
   a. Wide base of the bony pyramid (Frontal, Direct Dorsal, Overhead and Backward Tilting Views).
   b. Osteocartilaginous hump. The hump is predominantly cartilaginous (Backward Tilting, Oblique and Lateral Views).
   c. The bony pyramid is deviated to the left due to bilateral maxillary asymmetry. The right cheek is wide and low while the left cheek is narrow and high. (Backward Tilting Views). The bony pyramid is only deviated to the left but not oblique.
4. **Alar base**
   a. The left nasal aperture was enchroached upon by the dislocated caudal septum leading to unpleasant distortion.
   b. The right nasal aperture look unpleasantly rounded and shifted upwards.
   c. The alae nasi are bowing laterally in acute angles with the upper lip.

Aims of Surgery

1. Reduce the size and bulk of the nasal tip.
2. Correction of the crookedness in the bony pyramid and the nasal tip.
3. Abolish the mobility of the nasal tip.

Surgical Plan

1. **Frontolateral walls**
   a. DDD including the weak triangle to reduce the bulk of the nasal tip and the mid vault.
   b. Cephalic trim of the lateral crurae to reduce the size of the nasal tip.
2. **Medial Wall**
   a. Septoplasty which includes 2 mm trim of the inferior and posterior margins of the cartilaginous septum.
   b. Division of the Depressor Septi muscles.
3. **Bony pyramid**
   a. Excision of the osteocartilaginous hump
   b. Osteotomies with Kassanjian maneuver to the right i.e. cross fracture of the bony pyramid after osteotomies (See Surgery of the Bony Pyramid in the Text).
4. **Alar base**
   Nil of note.

Surgical Procedure

1. As per Surgical Plan.
2. Skoog dorsal graft.
3. Augmentation graft over the left side of upper lateral cartilage, was necessary, using lateral crural cephalic trimmings.
4. Supratip depression developed during surgery. Cartilaginous graft from lateral crural trimmings was used.

M. H. A. Shafy, *Atlas of Clinical Cases in Rhinoplasty*,
https://doi.org/10.1007/978-3-031-07504-9_38

Post-Operative Analysis

1. **Frontolateral Wall**
   a. Tip definition improved: the nasal tip is smaller with thinner and smoother overlying skin. It is more prominent and well identified from the alae nasi on both sides. The alae nasi come into view to become clearly visible and share in nasal aesthetics (Frontal, Direct Dorsal, Overhead, Backward Tilting and Basal Views).
   b. Tip projection: The nasal tip at the same level of the nasal dorsum with good aesthetic angle. This is coupled with good aesthetic nasolabial angle (lateral and oblique views).
   c. Tip light reflex is seen as one spot off the nasal tip. (Frontal and Backward Tilting Views).
2. **Medial Wall**
   a. Left caudal septal deviation was corrected.
   b. Mobility of the tip was overcome.
3. **Bony Pyramid**
   a. Bony pyramid aesthetics improved: the nasal dorsum is straight in the midline and the sidewalls are smooth and narrow (all views except the Basal Views).
   b. Dorsal light reflex is seen as an uninterrupted line off the nasal dorsum (Direct Dorsal Views).
4. **Alar Base**
   a. Superior alar groove aesthetics improved eventhough she had a small alae nasi.
   b. Posterior alar groove aesthetics improved after defatting. The alae nasi pulled medially widening the posterior groove angles (backward Tilting, Basal, and Nasal Aperature views).
   c. Alae nasi aesthetics improved. They are pulled medially become better seen, smaller and share in nasal aesthetics. (Nasal Aperture, Oblique and Lateral Views).
   d. Nasal aperture aesthetics improved after defattingand correction of caudal dislocation.
      i. Both nasal apertures became closer to each other in size and shape.
      ii. Nasal apertures look more elegantly oval in shape.
   e. Marginal light reflexes are clearly seen at:
      i. Inferior alar margins (Nasal Aperture Views).
      ii. Nasal sill bands (Oblique Views).
      iii. Lateral crural prominences (Lateral Views).

Commentary

a. The Skoog graft, i.e. replacing the excised, osteo-cartilaginous hump over the lowered open roof deformity of the nasal dorsum. This was necessary as the resulting bony margins appeared sharp and irregular, through her extremely thin skin. The Skoog graft was perfect in producing a naturally, rounded dorsum.
b. After defatting, the left lateral crus was bulging laterally more than the right side. This was overcome by small pieces of crushed cartlidge graft over the left side of the upper lateral cartilage.
c. A unilateral bulge of the lateral crus may be due to:
   i. Bilateral, developmental variation in the size of the lateral crurae.
   ii. Bilateral, developmental variation in the size of the two sides of the upper lateral cartilage due to facial asymmetry. This is the case in this patient.
   iii. Secondary to a displaced cartilaginous septum.
   iv. Unilateral excess fat overlying a smaller lateral crus. Defatting discloses the larger lateral crus and therefore appears more bulging.
d. The supratip graft was necessary as there was a supratip depression after the excision of the severely deviated caudal cartilaginous septum.

Frontal | Frontal Smiling | Frontal Middle Third

Preoperative

Postoperative

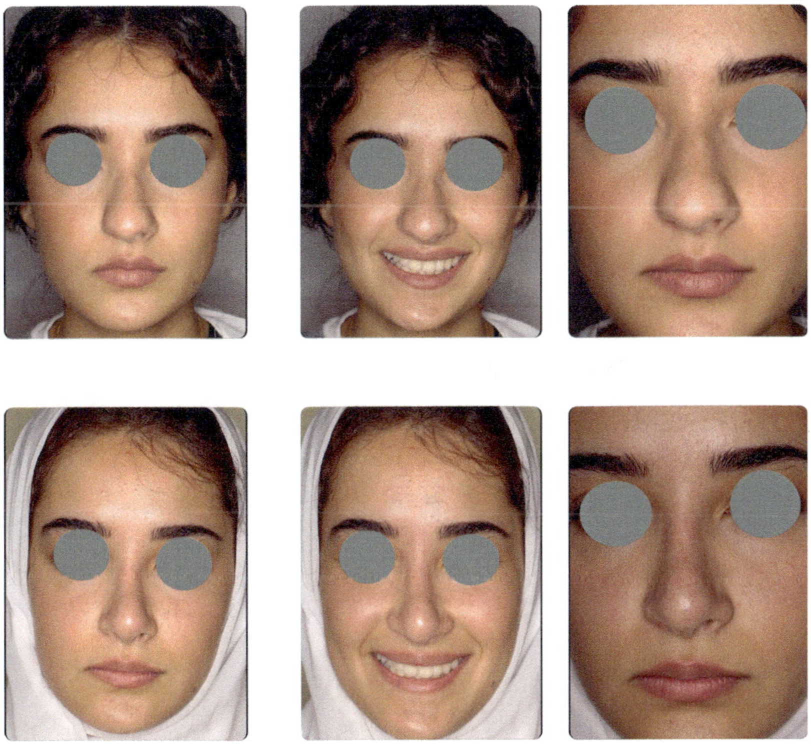

Direct Dorsal | Direct Dorsal Smiling | Overhead | Overhead Smiling

Preoperative

Postoperative

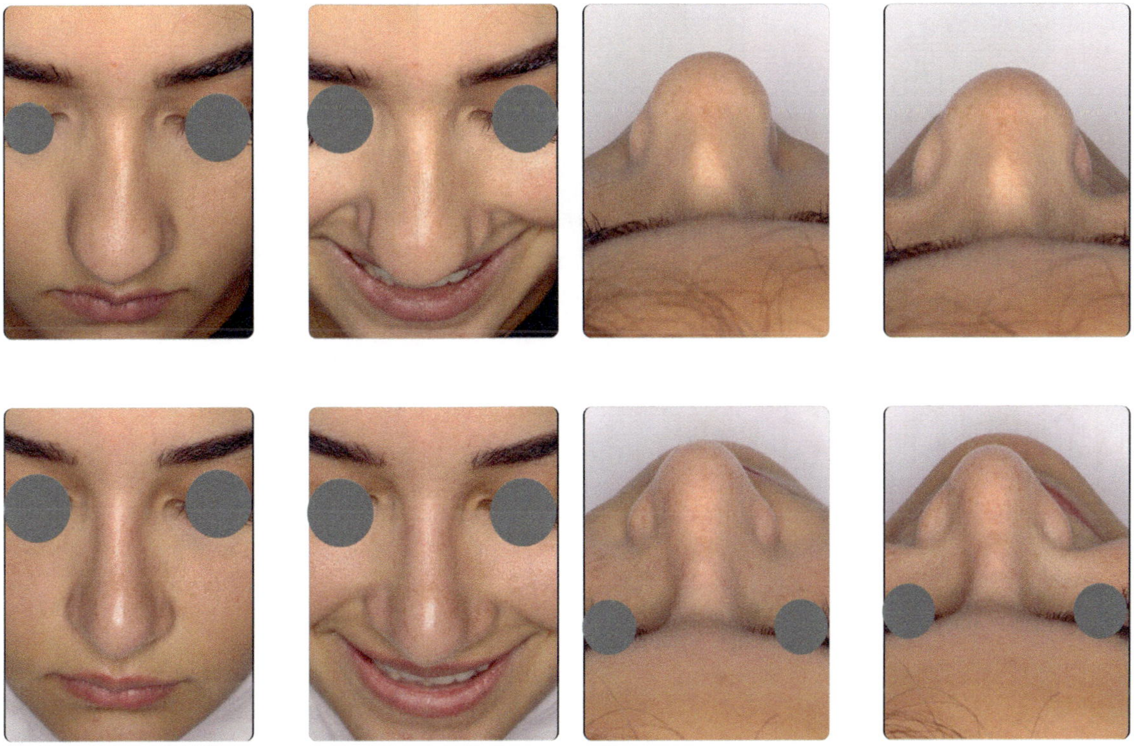

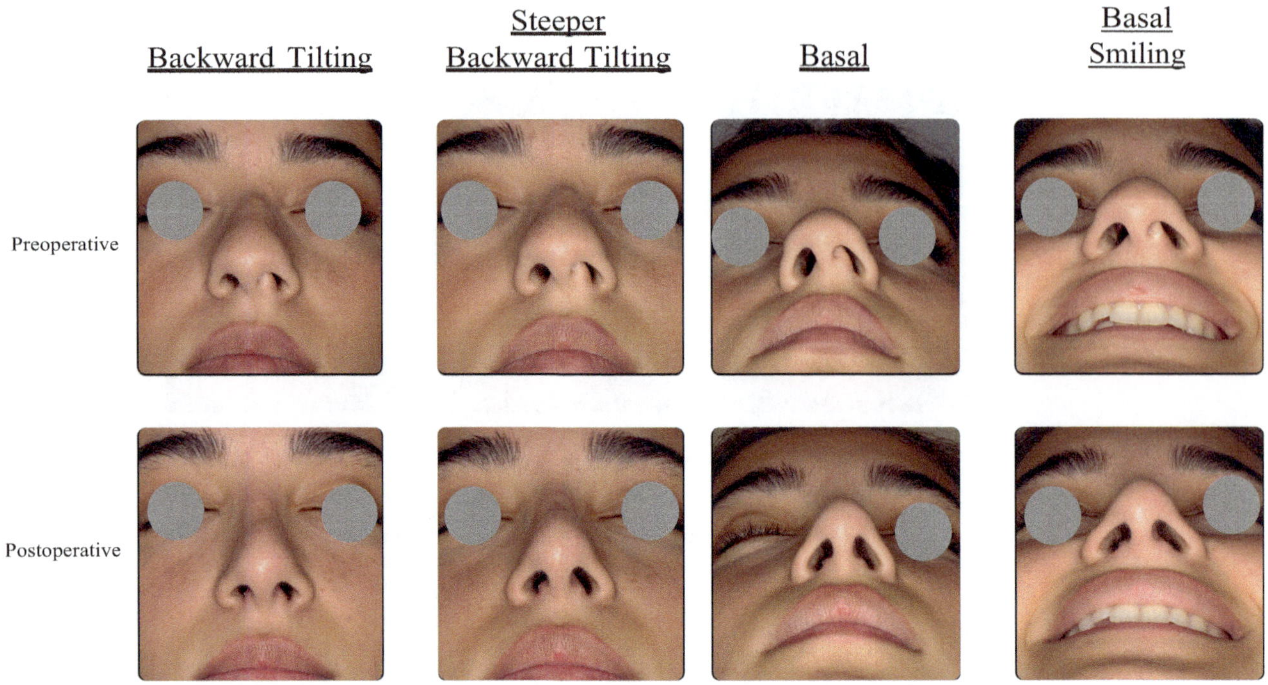
Backward Tilting
Steeper Backward Tilting
Basal
Basal Smiling
Preoperative
Postoperative

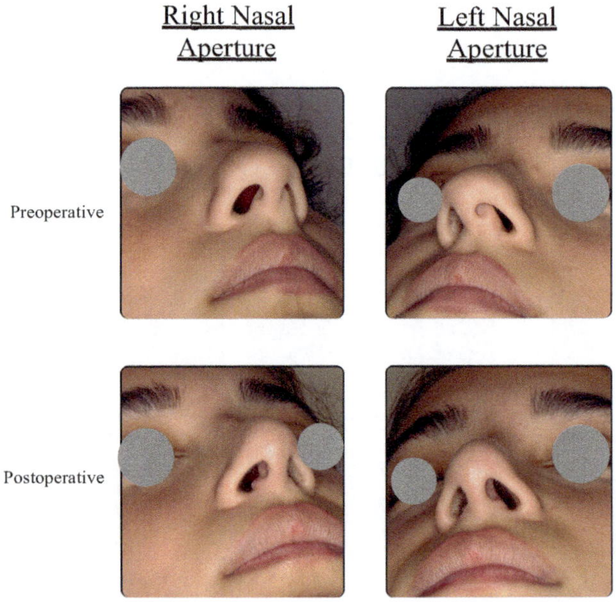
Right Nasal Aperture
Left Nasal Aperture
Preoperative
Postoperative

Right Oblique Mid Cheek Full Face	Left Oblique Mid Cheek Full Face	Right Oblique Mid Cheek Middle Third	Left Oblique Mid Cheek Middle Third

Preoperative

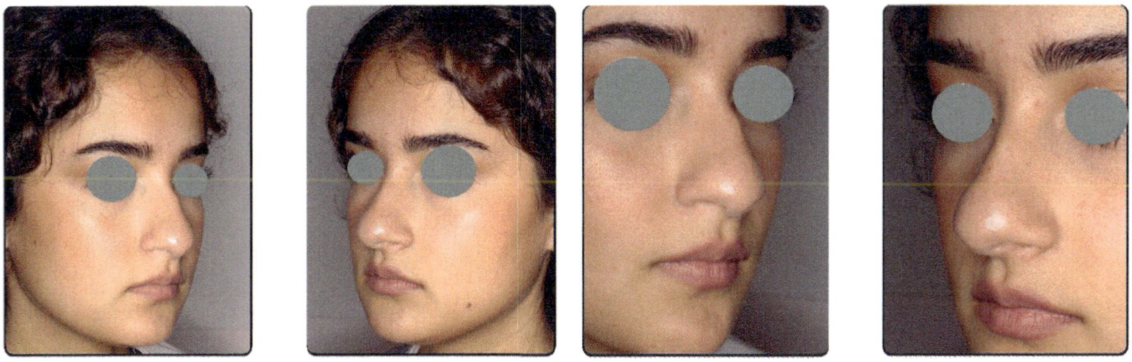

Postoperative

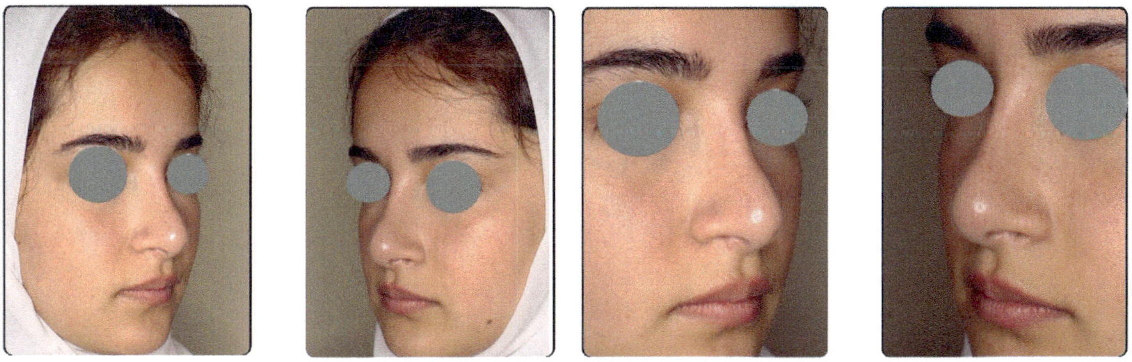

Right Oblique Cheek Margin Full Face	Left Oblique Cheek Margin Full Face	Right Oblique Cheek Margin Middle Third	Left Oblique Cheek Margin Middle Third

Preoperative

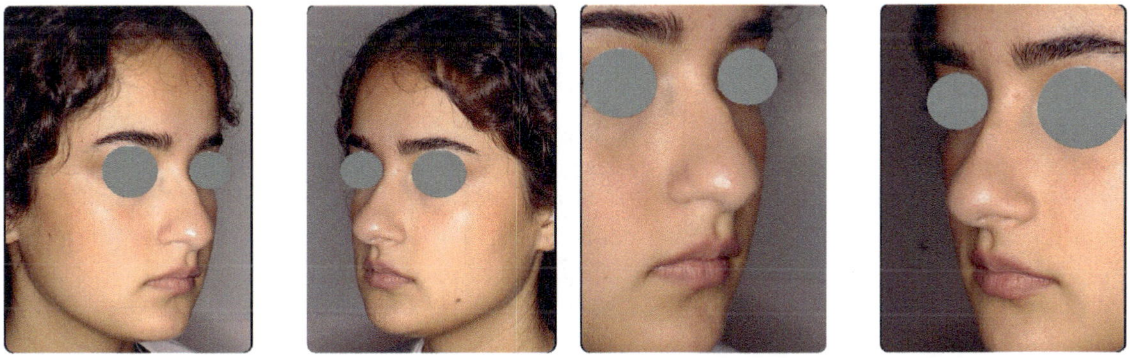

Postoperative

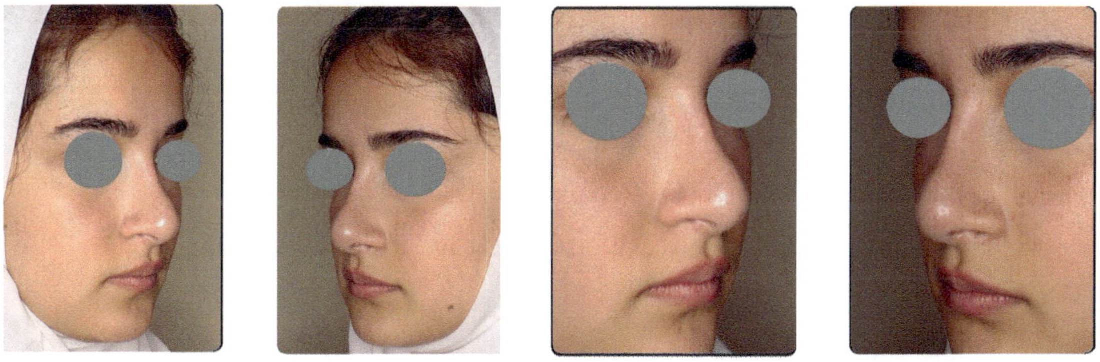

Right Lateral | Left Lateral | Right Lateral Smiling | Left Lateral Smiling

Preoperative

Postoperative

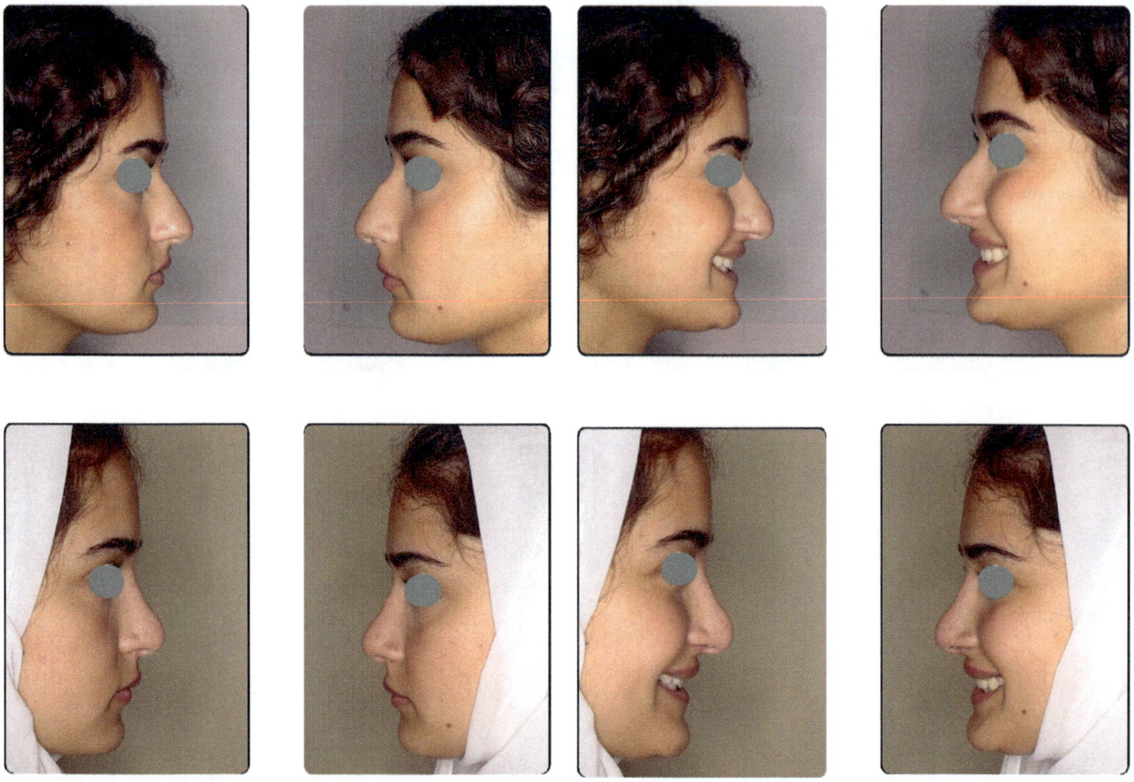

Right Lateral Middle Third | Left Lateral Middle Third

Preoperative

Postoperative

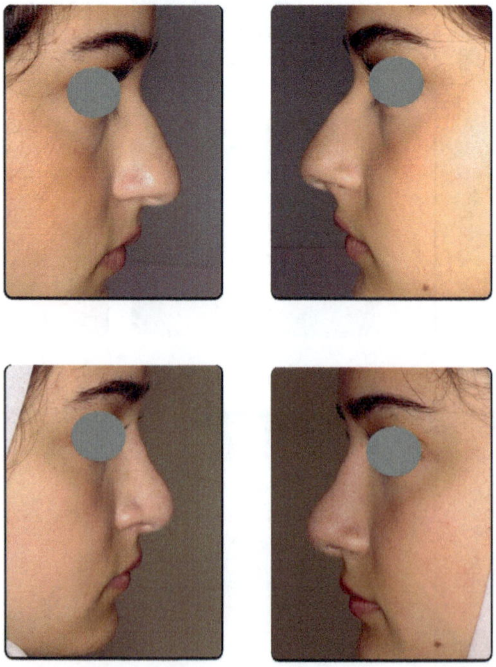

Part IV: Clinical Case 9

39

Preoperative Assessment

1. **Frontolateral walls**
   a. Large bulky tip, that is deviated to the left side. (Frontal, Direct Dorsal and Backward Tilting Views).
   b. The alae nasi are overshadowed by the large bulbous tip. The left ala nasi is larger than the right (Frontal and Direct Dorsal Views).
   c. Asymmetrical smile. The right cheek is larger and the left ala nasi was at a higher level on smiling.
2. **Medial Wall**
   Right caudal septal deviation (Right Nasal Aperture Views).
3. **Bony pyramid**
   a. Small osteocartilaginous hump which was mainly oblique and slightly deviated to the right side due to bilateral maxillary asymmetry (Backward Tilting, Oblique and Lateral Views). The right cheek is wide and low while the left cheek is narrow and high (Backward Tilting Views).
   b. Wide base of the bony pyramid (Frontal, Direct Dorsal, Overhead and Backward Tilting Views).
4. **Alar base**
   a. Wide nasal apertures. The left nasal opening is naturally wider than the right. (Backward Tilting and Basal view).
   b. Asymmetrical smile partly due to asymmetrical alae nasi. The left nasolabial fold and the left cheek ball were different from the right (preoperative Frontal Smiling View).

Aims of Surgery

1. Reduce the size and bulk of the frontolateral walls.
2. Excision of the osteocatilagenous hump.
3. Reduction of the size of the bony pyramids and centralise its deviation.
4. Reduction of the sizes of nasal apertures and equalising both sides.

Surgical Plan

1. **Frontolateral walls**
   a. DDD excluding the weak triangle. The area of the weak triangle is rich in fat. Any attempt of defatting this area will lead to supratip depression.
2. **Medial Wall**
   Septoplasty to correct the caudal septal deviation.
3. **Bony pyramid**
   a. Excision of the osteocartilaginous hump.
   b. Osteotomies, Kassanjian maneuver to the left i.e. cross fracture of the bony pyramid after osteotomies (see Surgery of the Bony Pyramid in the Text).
4. **Alar base**
   a. Bilateral excision of the inferior segments of the rim-still folds to reduce the size of the nasal openings. More to be resected from the left side as the segment is longer on this side.
   b. Bilateral resection of the posterior segments of the rim-sill folds to reduce the bulk of the alar base.

Surgical Procedure

1. As the surgical plan.
2. There was a supratip depression despite preserving the weak triangular fat. Cephalic trimmings of the lateral crurae were used as a supra-tip graft.

Post-Operative Analysis

1. **Frontolateral Wall**
   a. Tip definition: the nasal tip is smaller with thinner and smoother overlying skin. The tip is more prominent and well identified from the alae nasi on both sides. The alae nasi come into view to become clearly visible and share in nasal aesthetics (Frontal, Direct Dorsal, Overhead, Backward Tilting and Basal Views).

M. H. A. Shafy, *Atlas of Clinical Cases in Rhinoplasty*,
https://doi.org/10.1007/978-3-031-07504-9_39

   b. Tip projection: The nasal tip at the same level of the nasal dorsum with good aesthetic angle. This is coupled with good aesthetic nasolabial angle (lateral and oblique views).
   c. Tip light reflex is seen as one spot off the nasal tip. (Frontal and Backward Tilting Views).
2. **Medial Wall**
   a. The right caudal septal deviation is corrected.
   b. Mobile tip is abolished.
3. **Bony Pyramid**
   a. Bony pyramid aesthetics improved: the nasal dorsum is straight in the midline and the sidewalls are smooth and narrow (all views except the Basal Views).
   b. Dorsal light reflex is seen as an uninterrupted line off the nasal dorsum (Direct Dorsal Views).
4. **Alar Base**
   a. Superior alar groove aesthetics improved. They are longer, deeper and better seen.
   b. Posterior alar groove aesthetics improved by defatting as well as excising the posterior segments of the rim-sill folds. The flat tire appearance is no longer present. (Backward Tilting, Basal and Nasal Aperture Views).
   c. Alae nasi aesthetics improved. They are pulled medially become better seen, smaller and share in nasal aesthetics. (Nasal Aperture, Oblique and Lateral Views).
   d. Nasal aperture aesthetics improved after defatting and excision of the rim-sill folds:
      i. The sizes became equal and smaller.
      ii. The shapes became more elegantly oval in shape.
   e. Marginal light reflexes are clearly seen at:
      i. Inferior alar margins (Nasal Aperture Views).
      ii. Nasal sill bands (Oblique Views).
      iii. Lateral crural prominences (Lateral Views).

Commentary

a. The height of the nasal dorsum was carefully chosen to be slightly lower than she would have liked as an Arab in general. This height seemed to suit her face and overall small body. The relatively large size of the lower third, even after being reduced by defatting, provided a good tip projection with the sloping medium height nasal dorsum.
b. After resection of the Inferior segments of rim-sill folds, predominantly more on the left side, the patient now has better symmetrical smile than before the surgery.
c. It was not sufficient just to correct the crookedness of the nose. An overall care of the four areas of the nose was necessary to produce an attractive nose.
d. All goals of the surgery were achieved so that:
   i. The frontolateral walls were reduced in bulk and size.
   ii. Crookedness of the nose was straightened.
   iii. The size of the body pyramid was reduced.
   iv. The sizes of the nasal apertures were reduced and equalized.
   v. She has a postoperative symmetrical smile.
   vi. The overall result is an attractive small nose that suits her small body.

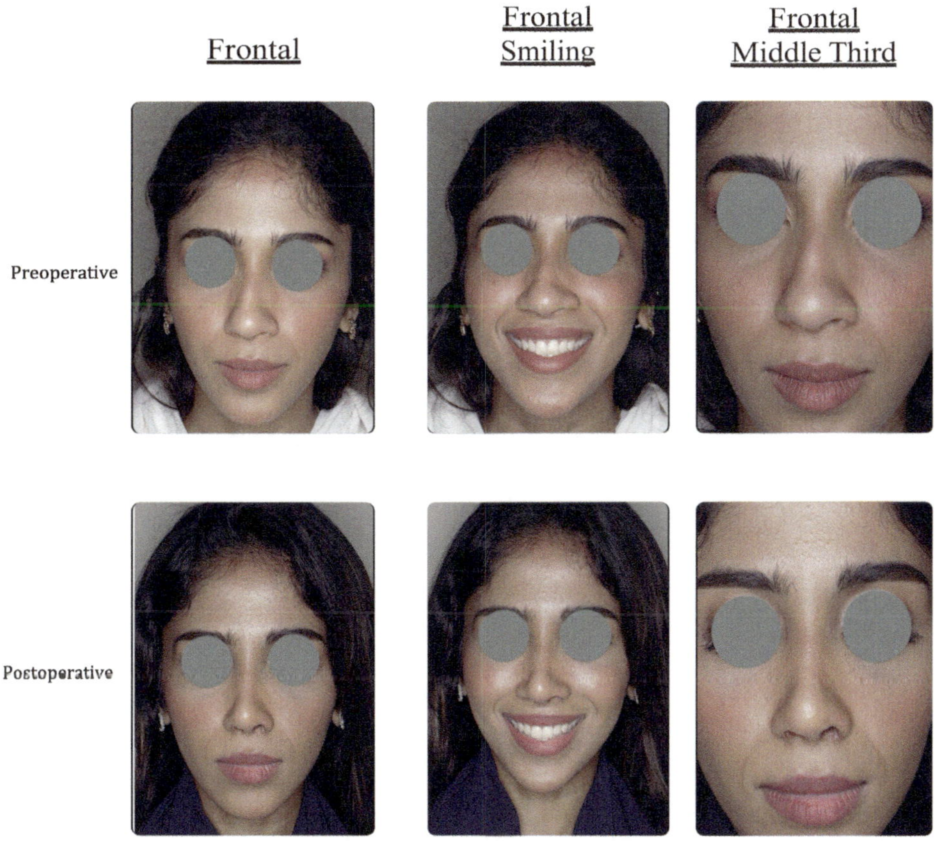
Frontal
Frontal Smiling
Frontal Middle Third
Preoperative
Postoperative

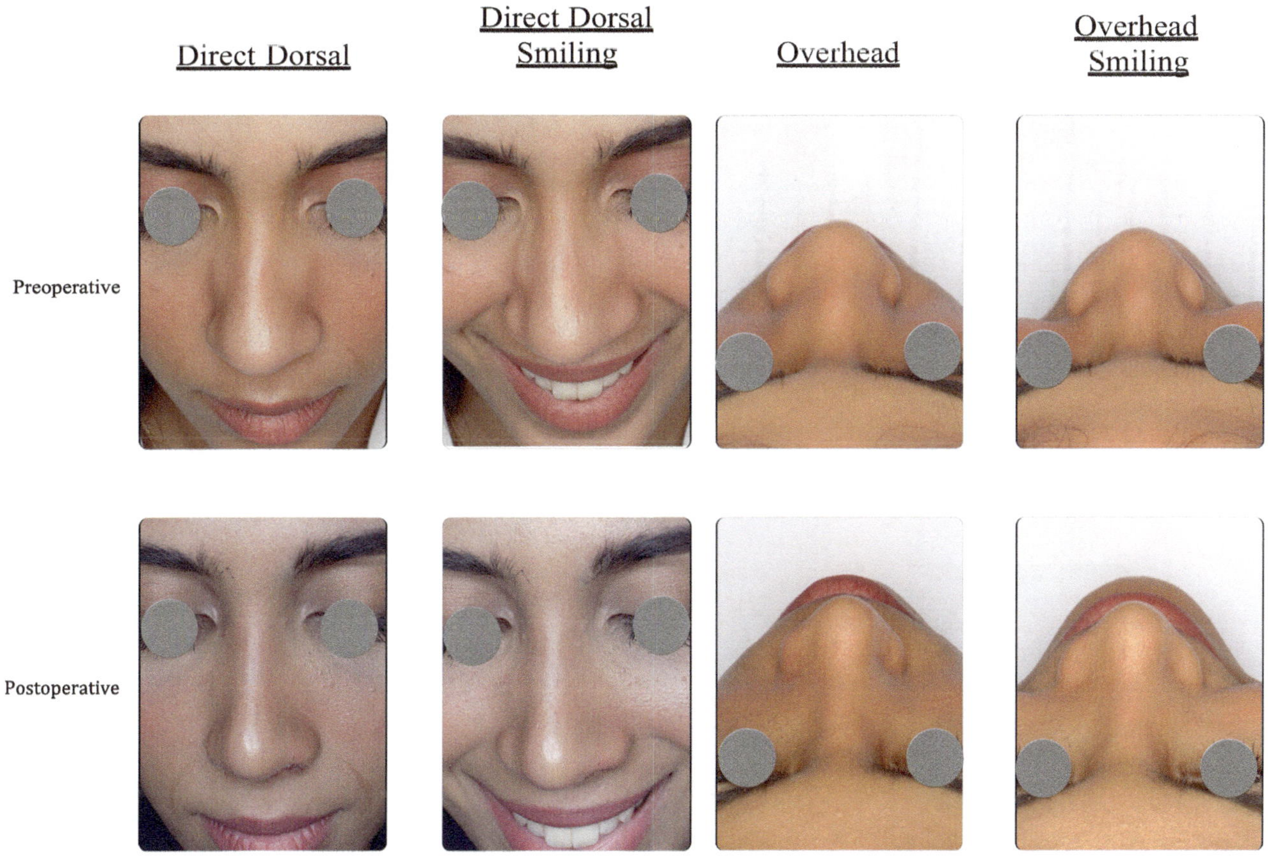
Direct Dorsal
Direct Dorsal Smiling
Overhead
Overhead Smiling
Preoperative
Postoperative

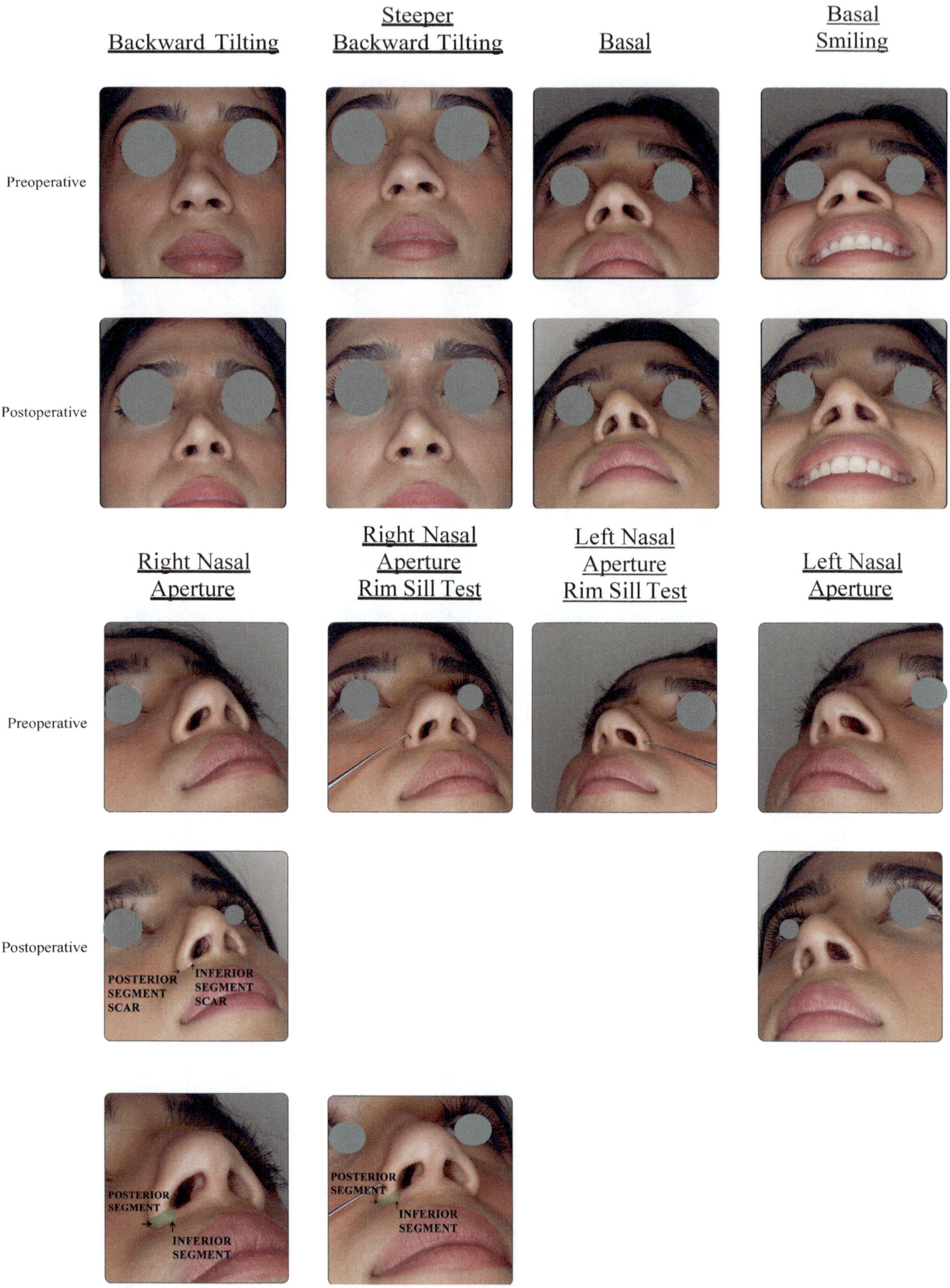
Backward Tilting
Steeper Backward Tilting
Basal
Basal Smiling
Preoperative
Postoperative
Right Nasal Aperture
Right Nasal Aperture Rim Sill Test
Left Nasal Aperture Rim Sill Test
Left Nasal Aperture
Preoperative
Postoperative
POSTERIOR SEGMENT SCAR
INFERIOR SEGMENT SCAR
POSTERIOR SEGMENT
INFERIOR SEGMENT
POSTERIOR SEGMENT
INFERIOR SEGMENT

Right Oblique Mid Cheek Full Face | Left Oblique Mid Cheek Full Face | Right Oblique Mid Cheek Middle Third | Left Oblique Mid Cheek Middle Third

Preoperative

Postoperative

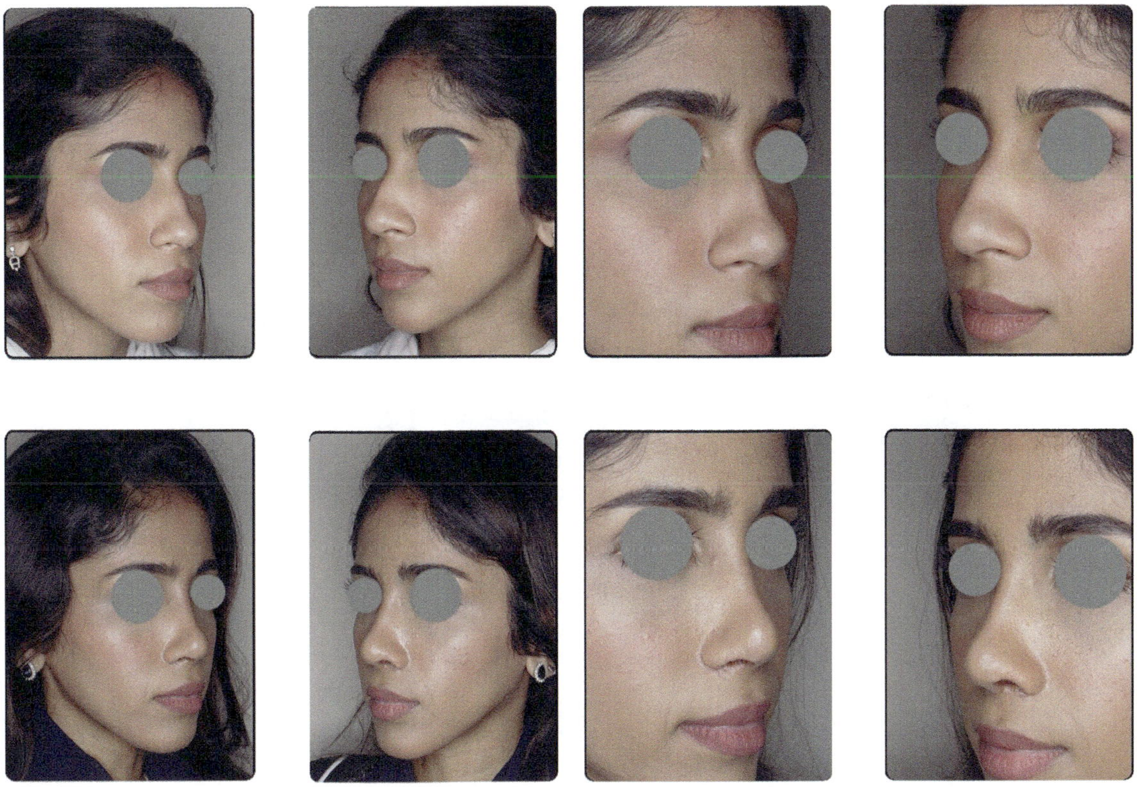

Right Oblique Cheek Margin Full Face | Left Oblique Cheek Margin Full Face | Right Oblique Cheek Margin Middle Third | Left Oblique Cheek Margin Middle Third

Preoperative

Postoperative

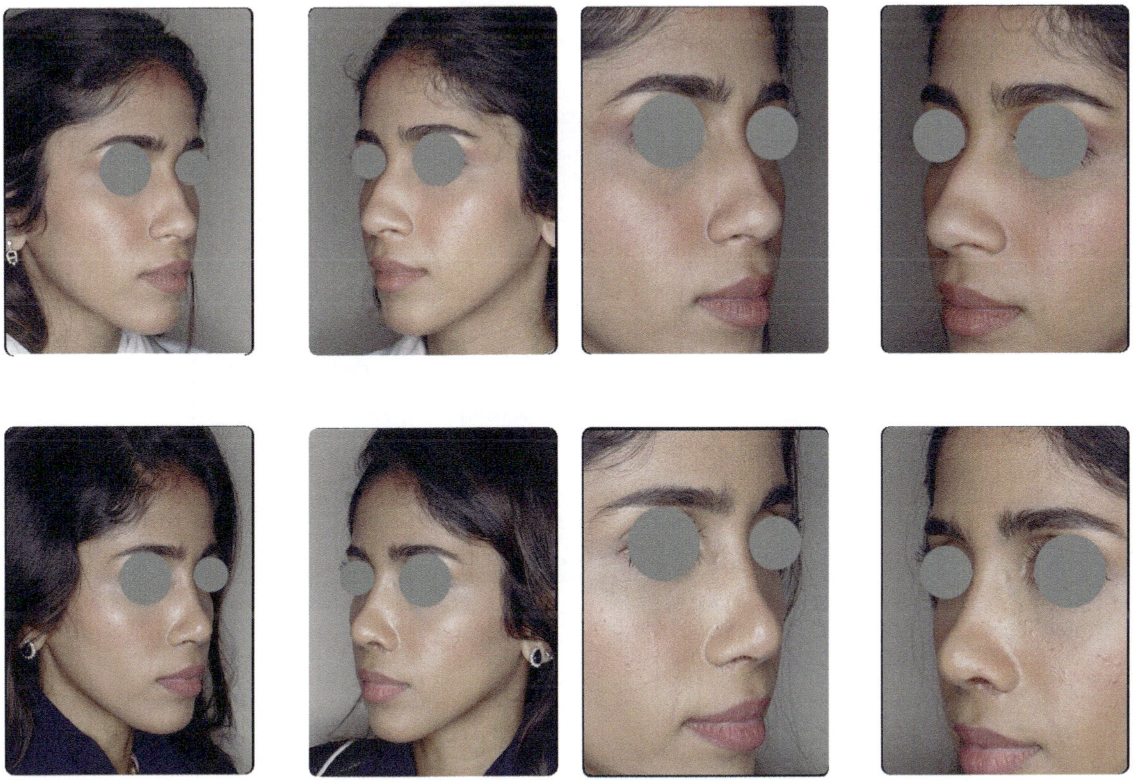

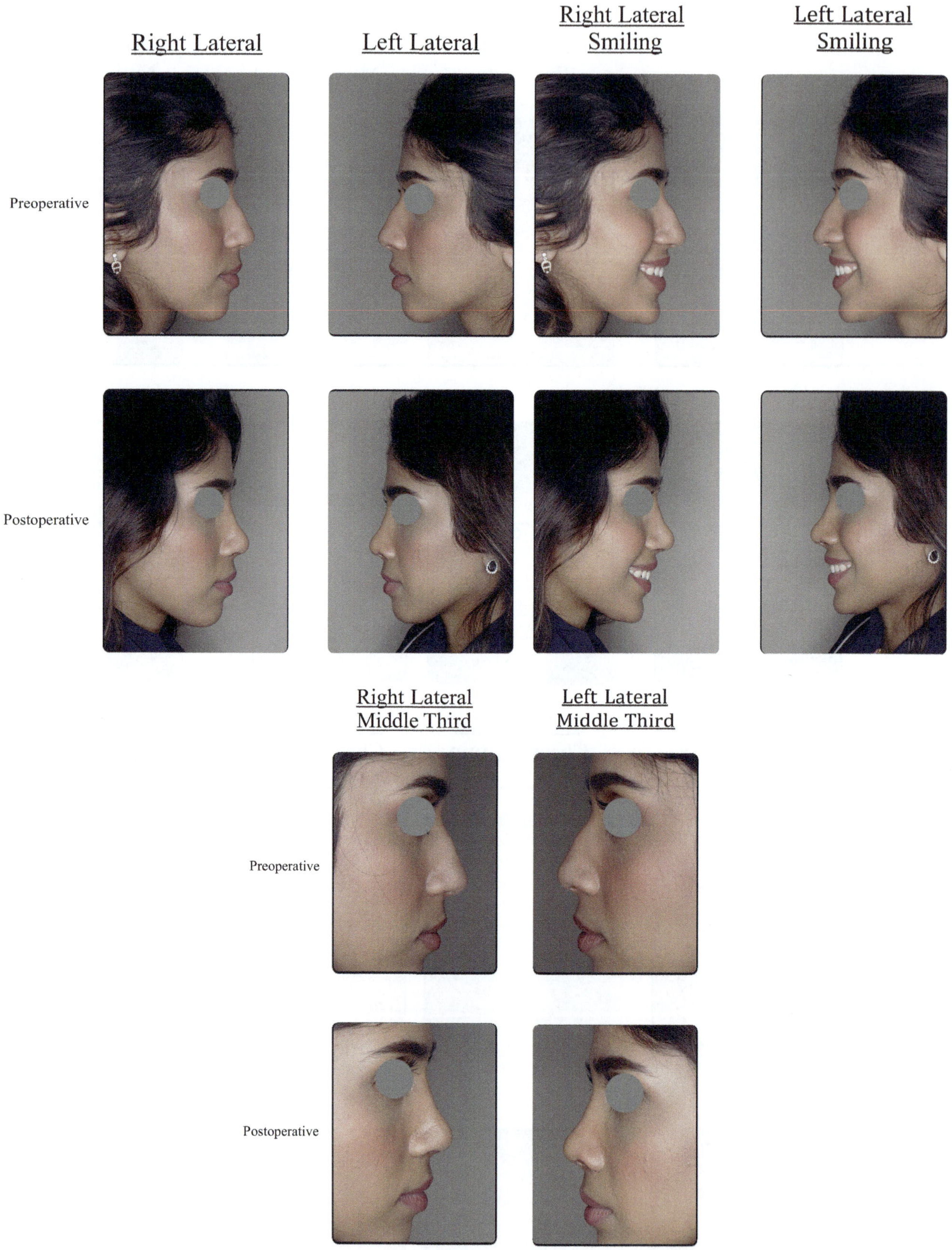
Right Lateral
Left Lateral
Right Lateral Smiling
Left Lateral Smiling
Preoperative
Postoperative
Right Lateral Middle Third
Left Lateral Middle Third
Preoperative
Postoperative

Part V

Deviated Nose and Oblique Nose Rhinoplasty

Part V: Clinical Case 1

40

Preoperative assessment

1. **Frontolateral walls**
   Bulky tip overshadowing the alae nasi (Frontal and Direct Dorsal views).
2. **Medial Wall**
   a. Sliding nasal tip i.e. the nasal tip moves posteriorly on smiling at a lower level than the anterior septal angle (Lateral Smiling Views).
   b. Mobile tip i.e. the nasal tip moves inferiorly on smiling (Lateral Smiling Views).
   c. Right caudal septal deviation (Basal, Backward Tilting and Right Nasal Aperture Views).
3. **Bony pyramid**
   a. Osteocartilaginous hump (Backward Tilting , Oblique and Lateral views).
   b. Flat nasofrontal angle (Lateral Views).
   c. Wide base of the bony pyramid (Direct Dorsal and Backward Tilting Views).
   d. The bony pyramid is slightly deviated (Frontal and Direct Dorsal views) but mainly oblique to the left due to bilateral maxillary asymmetry. The left cheek is narrow and high and the right cheek is wide and low (Backward tilting views). The bony pyramid is deviated to the left.
   e. The dorsal light reflex is irregular and distorted (Direct Dorsal Views).
4. **Alar base**
   a. Wide and bulky alar base due to long inferior and thick posterior segments of rim-sill folds producing the flat tire appearance.
   b. The right caudal deviation pushed the medial crus, with its surrounding inferior vestibular bend, laterally to encroach upon the right nasal aperture distorting its size and shape (Backward Tilting, Basal and Right Nasal Aperture Views). The right nasal sill band is pushed inferiorly (Frontal and Backward Tilting Views).

Aims of Surgery

1. Proportionate reduction of the size and bulk of the nasal tip.
2. Correction of the caudally displaced septum.
3. Correction of the sliding and mobile tip.
4. Creation of nasofrontal angle.
5. Reduction of the nasal hump.
6. Balancing of the boney pyramid to the mid line.
7. Reduction of the bulk and width of the alar base.

Surgical Plan

1. **Frontolateral walls**
   a. DDD including the weak triangle to reduce the bulk and size of the nasal tip, and supratip area.
   b. Bilateral cephalic trim of the lateral crurae to reduce the size of the nasal tip.
2. **Medial Wall**
   a. Septoplasty.
   b. Trim of the membranous septum to overcome the sliding tip.
   c. Transnasal division of the depressor septi muscles to overcome the mobile dip.
3. **Bony pyramid**
   a. Reduction of the osteocartilaginous hump, with more reduction of the right side of the boney pyramid.
   b. Osteotomies and Kassanjian maneuver to the patient's right i.e. cross fractural of the bony pyramid after osteotmies to centralize it.
4. **Alar base**
   Bilateral excision of the inferior and posterior segment of the rim sill folds.

Surgical Procedure

a. As per Surgical Plan.
b. Two millimeter trim of the membranous septum, followed by stitching the anterior septal angle to the

M. H. A. Shafy, *Atlas of Clinical Cases in Rhinoplasty*,
https://doi.org/10.1007/978-3-031-07504-9_40

superior margins of the medial crurae. This technique helps to elevate and fix the sliding tip.

c. Inter sill band stitch using two-zero prolene i.e. at the lateral ends of the nasal still bands as they turn superiorly behind the posterior margins of the medial crurae as the continuation of the inferior vestibular band (I.V.B., see the textbook, anatomy section).
d. Excision of the inferior as well as the posterior rim sill fold segments were necessary, to reduce the width and the bulk of the nasal aperture successively.

Post-Operative Analysis

1. **Frontolateral Wall**
   a. Tip definition: the nasal tip is slimmer with thinner overlying skin, more prominent and well identified from the alae nasi on both sides. The alae nasi become clearly visible and share in nasal aesthetics (Frontal, Direct Dorsal, Overhead, Backward Tilting and Basal Views).
   b. Tip projection: the nasal tip is at the same level of the nasal dorsum with good aesthetic angle. This is coupled with good aesthetic nasolabial angle (lateral and oblique views).
   c. Tip light reflex is seen as one spot off the nasal tip (Frontal and Backward Tilting Views).
2. **Medial Wall**
   The sliding and mobile tip disappeared.
3. **Bony Pyramid**
   a. Bony pyramid aesthetics improved: the nasal dorsum is in the midline, straight and the sidewalls are smooth and narrow (all views except the Basal Views).
   b. Dorsal light reflex is seen as a regular one line off the nasal dorsum (Direct Dorsal Views).
4. **Alar Base**
   a. Superior alar groove aesthetics improved by defatting. The grooves become longer and deeper (Oblique, Lateral and Direct Dorsal grooves).
   b. Posterior alar groove aesthetics improved by defatting as well as excising of the rim-sill folds. The flat tire appearance is no longer present (Backward Tilting, Basal and Nasal Aperture Views).
   c. Alae nasi aesthetics improved. They are pulled medially widening the posterior angles. They became more visible and look smaller in size.
   d. Nasal aperture aesthetics improved by defatting and resection of the rim-sill folds:
      i. The size of the nasal openings are reduced.
      ii. The shape of nasal openings become more elegantly oval (Backward Tilting, Basal and Nasal Aperture views).
   e. Marginal light reflex is seen at:
      i. Inferior alar margins light reflex (Nasal Aperture Views).
      ii. Nasal sill light reflex (Oblique Views).
      iii. Lateral crural prominence (Lateral Views).

Commentary

a. This man was mainly concerned about his deviated nose which caused him social embarrassment. Additionally he could not wear eye glasses due to the obliquity of the nasal bridge. Clinical assessment revealed numerous other unaesthetic features of the nose which if overlooked it would have resulted in an unsatisfactory result. The nose will continue to exhibit other unpleasant parts e.g. bulbous tip, sliding and mobile tip, wide alar base, caudal dislocation and elongation of the cartilaginous septum and finally the unpleasant large hump.
b. The patient has a flat frontal bone unlike the usual male prominent frontal region. The hump was not completely reduced to give the impression of a nasofrontal angle. This was seen to be more aesthetic than rasping a deep angle under the flat frontal bone.

Frontal | Frontal Smiling | Frontal Middle Third

Preoperative

Postoperative

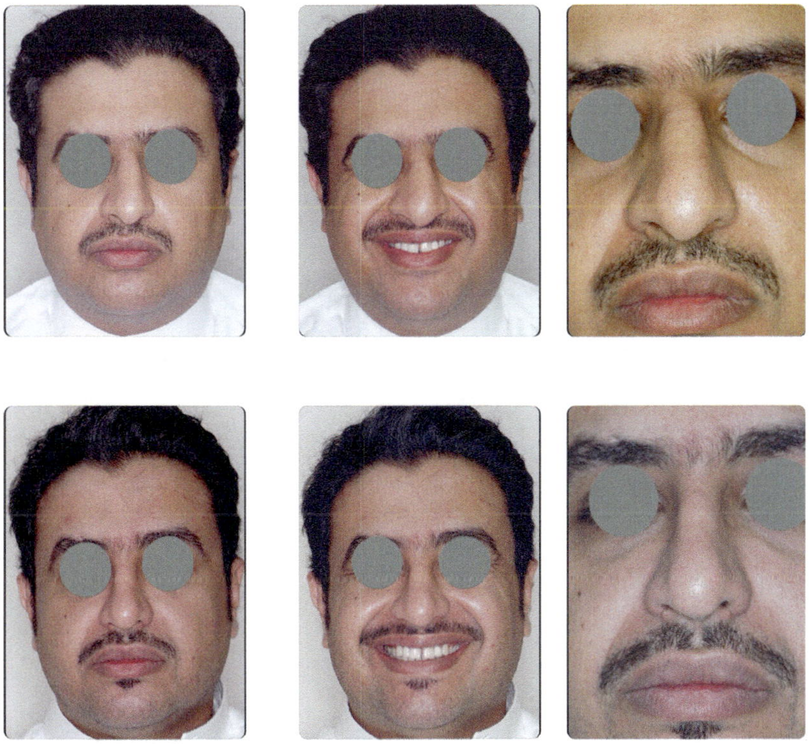

Direct Dorsal | Direct Dorsal Smiling

Preoperative

Postoperative

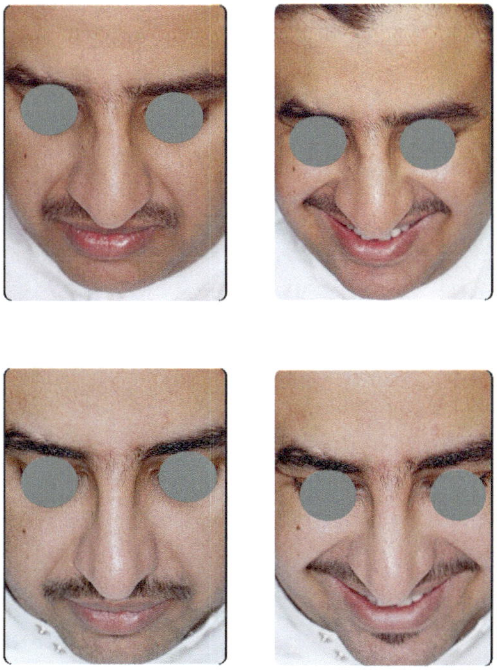

	Backward Tilting	Steeper Backward Tilting	Basal	Basal Smiling
Preoperative	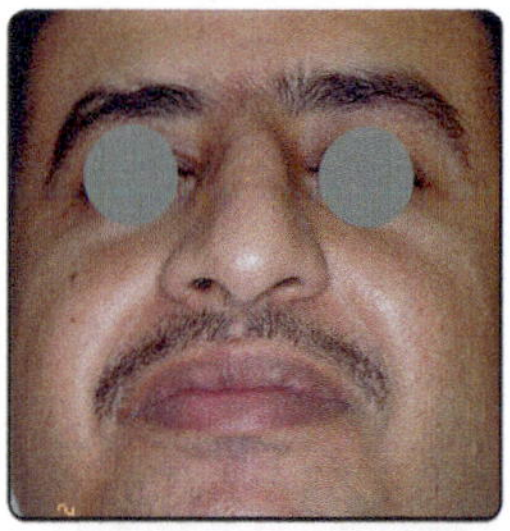	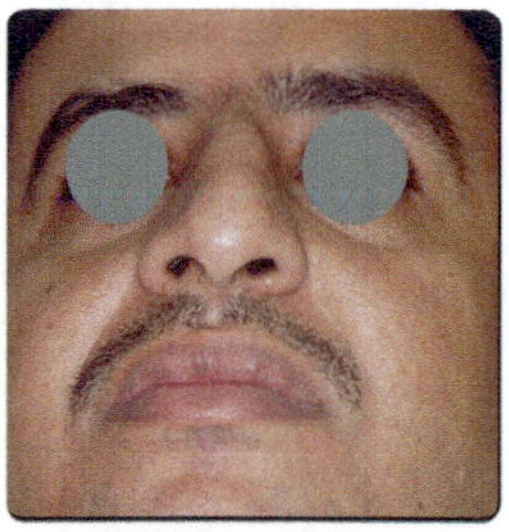	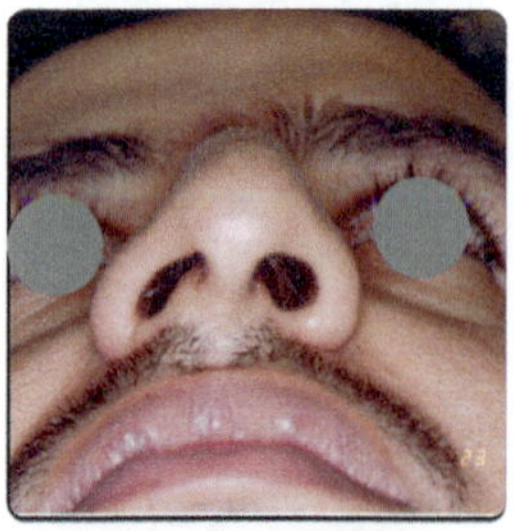	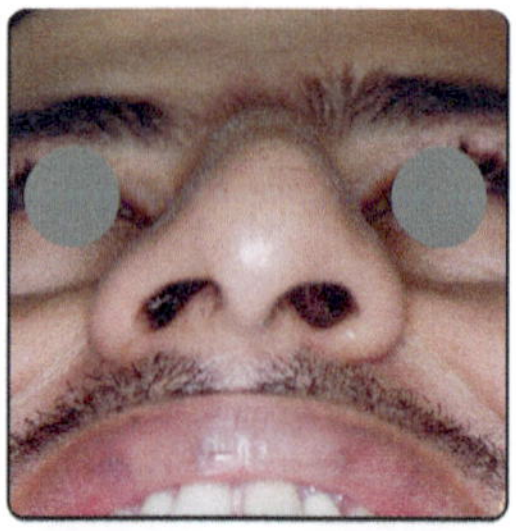
Postoperative	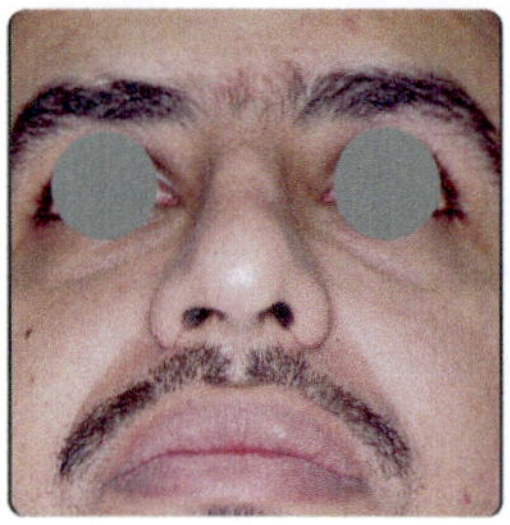	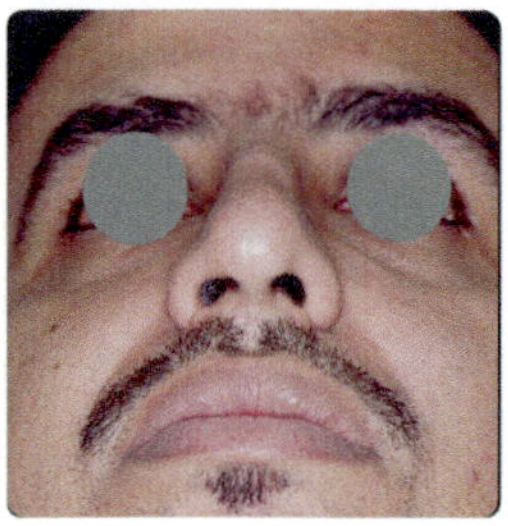	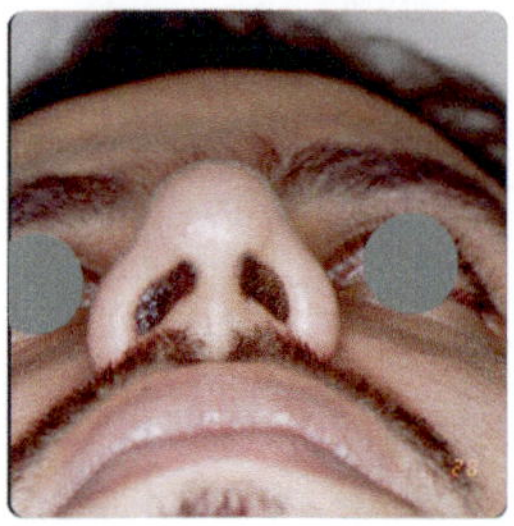	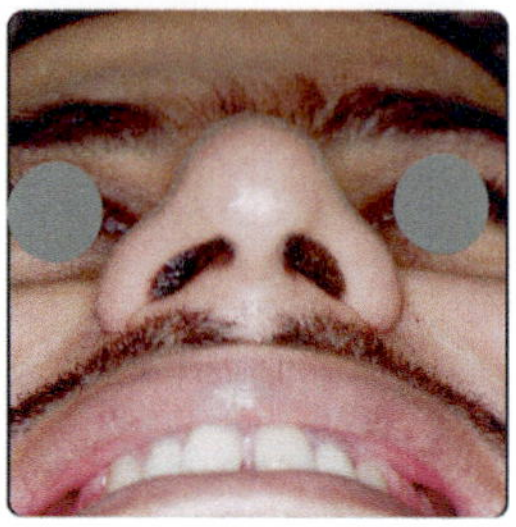

	Right Nasal Aperture	Right Nasal Aperture Rim Sill Test	Left Nasal Aperture Rim Sill Test	Left Nasal Aperture
Preoperative	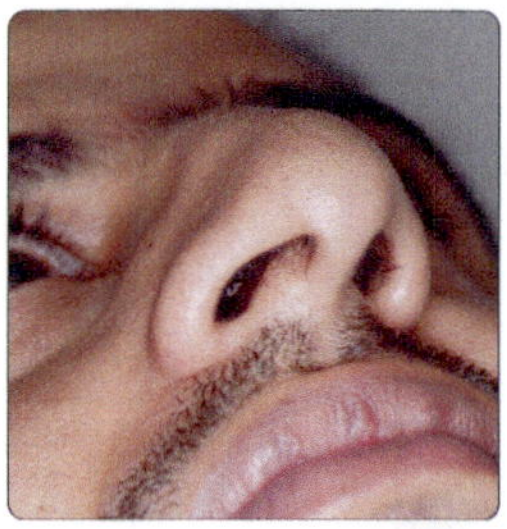	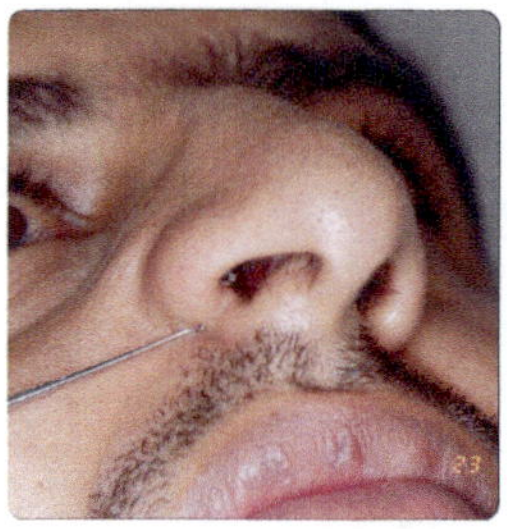	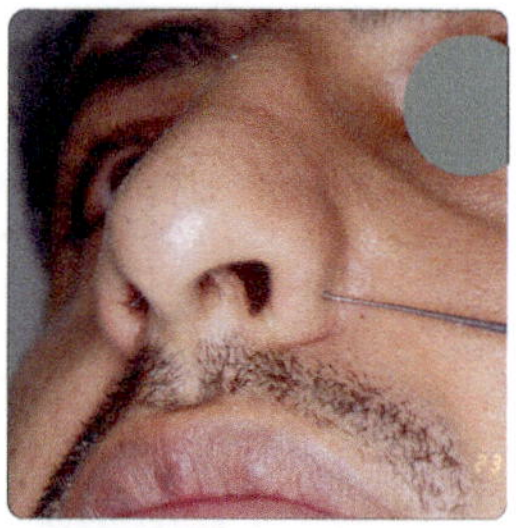	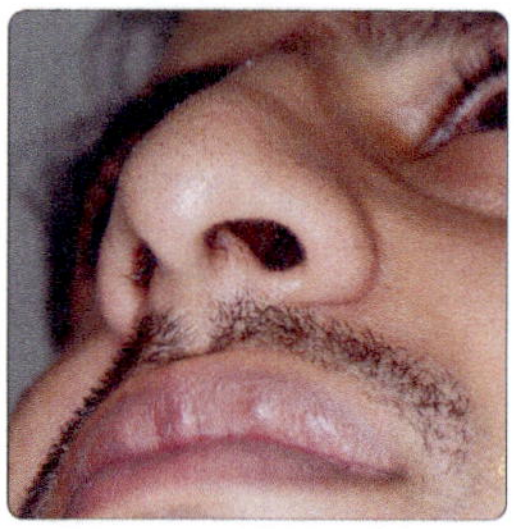
Postoperative	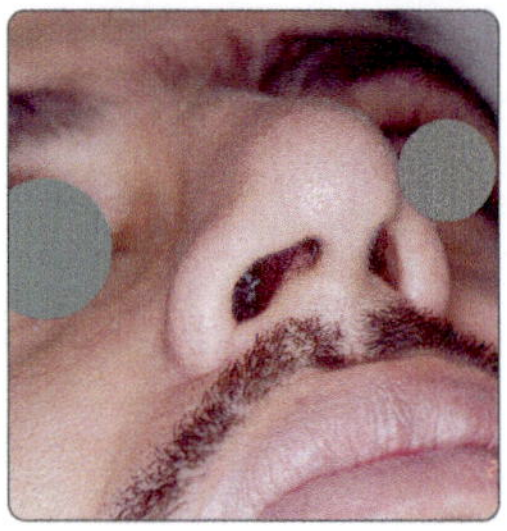		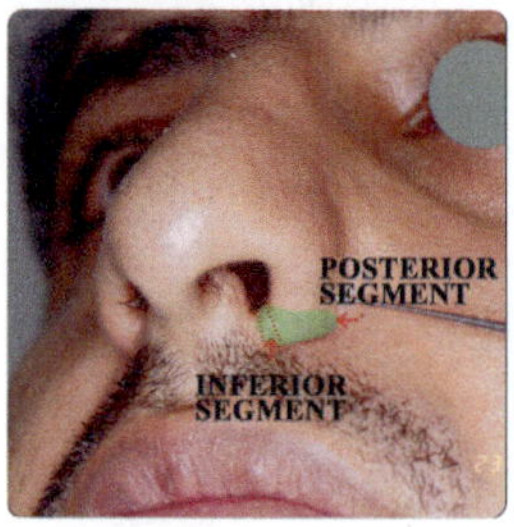	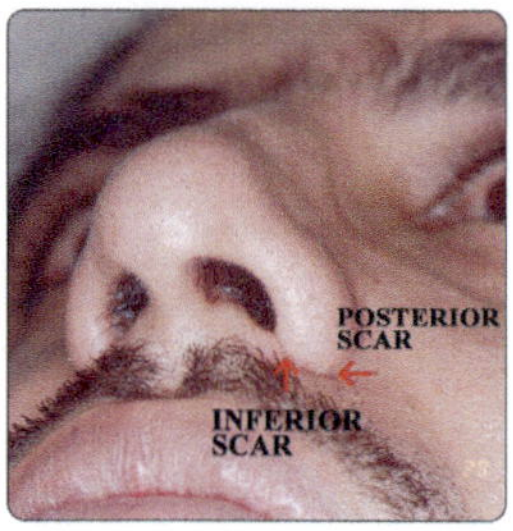

Right Oblique Mid Cheek Full Face	Left Oblique Mid Cheek Full Face	Right Oblique Mid Cheek Middle Third	Left Oblique Mid Cheek Middle Third

Preoperative

Postoperative

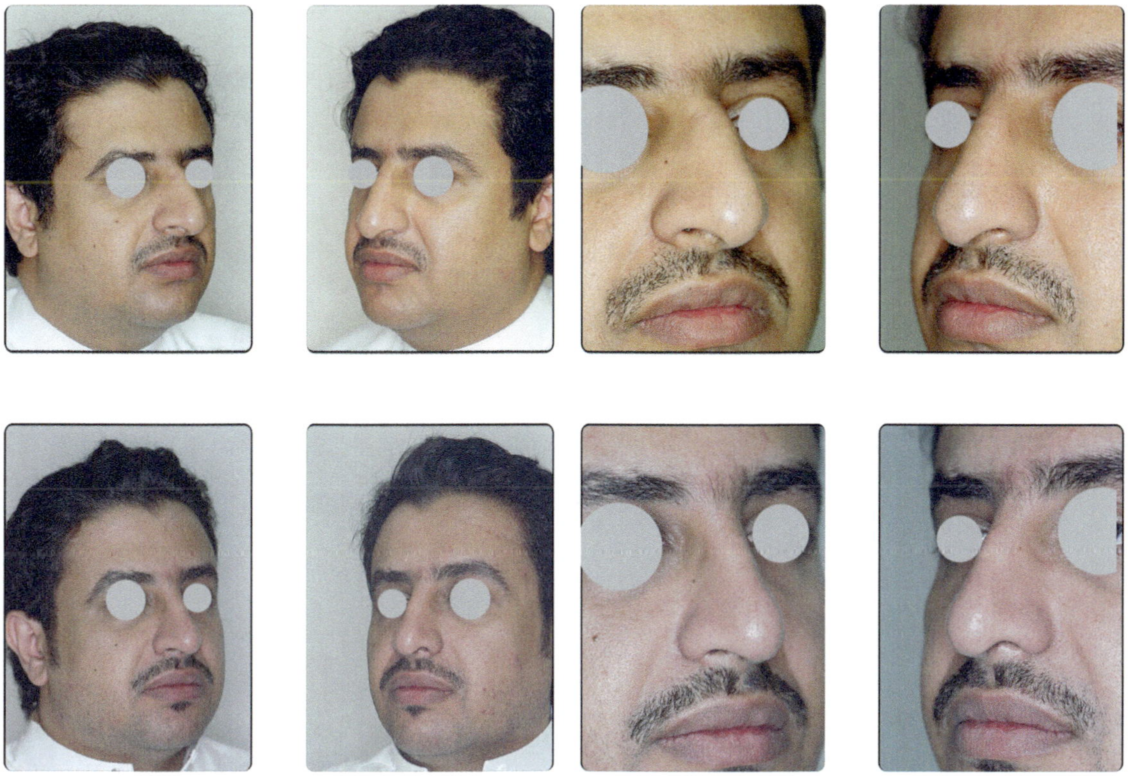

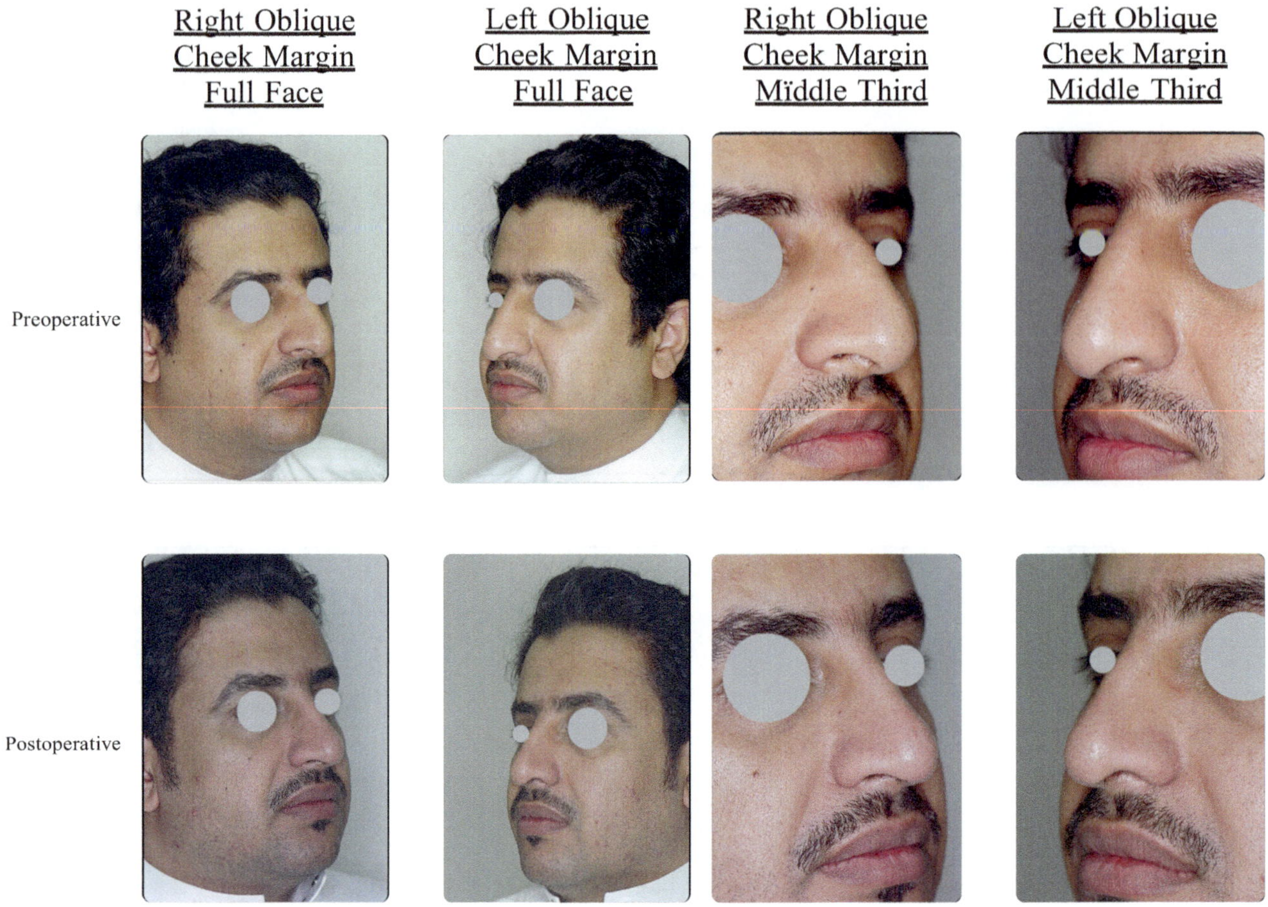
Right Oblique
Cheek Margin
Full Face
Left Oblique
Cheek Margin
Full Face
Right Oblique
Cheek Margin
Middle Third
Left Oblique
Cheek Margin
Middle Third
Preoperative
Postoperative

Right Lateral | Left Lateral | Right Lateral Smiling | Left Lateral Smiling

Preoperative

Postoperative

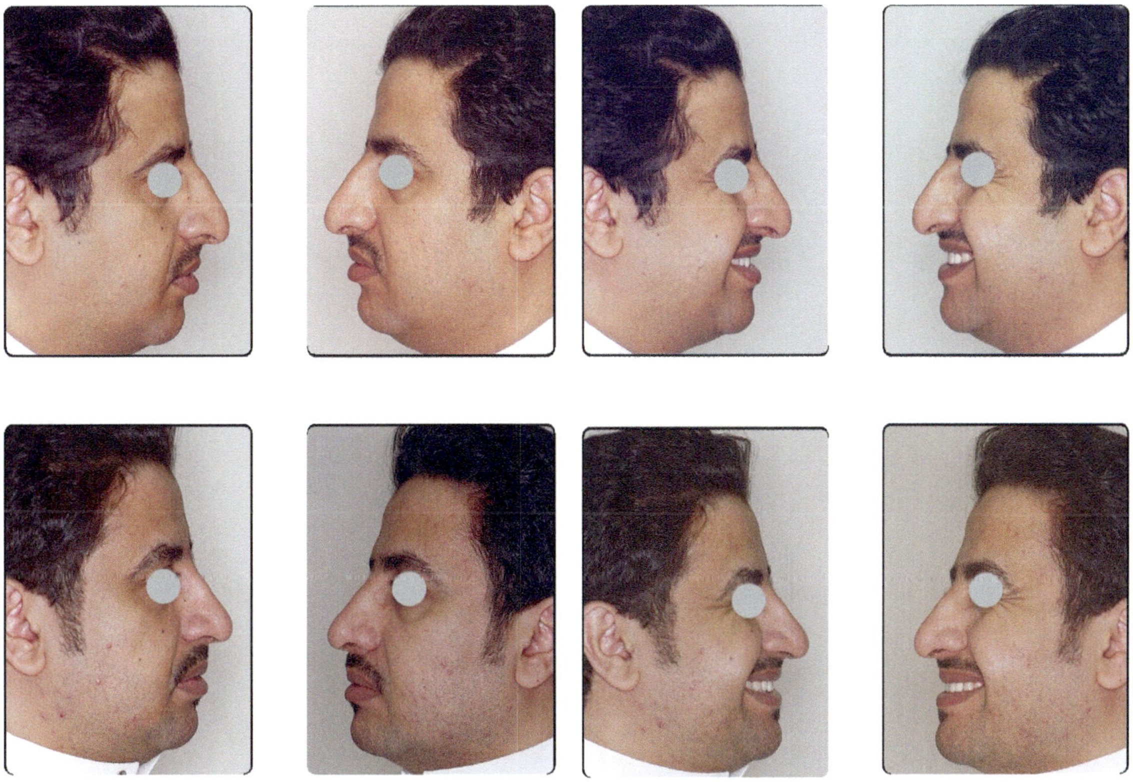

Right Lateral Middle Third | Left Lateral Middle Third

Preoperative

Postoperative

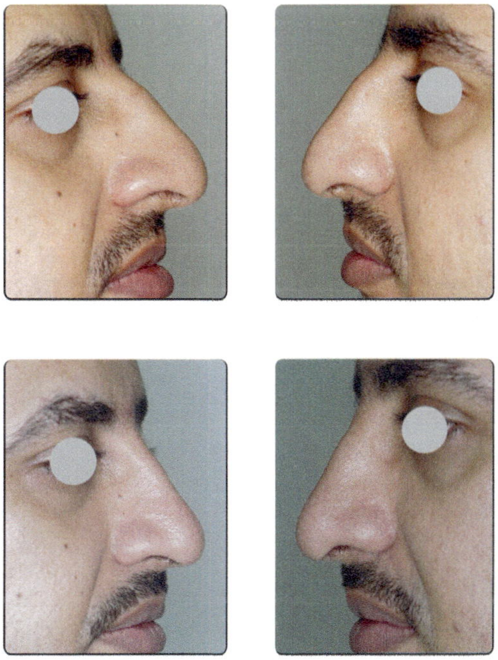

Part V: Clinical Case 2

41

Preoperative assessment

1. **Frontolateral walls**
   a. Large bulbous tip overshadowing the alae nasi (Frontal and Direct Dorsal Views).
   b. Nasal tip deviated to the right due to deviation of the bony pyramid, and cartilagenous septum (Frontal and Right Nasal Aperture Views).
2. **Medial Wall**
   a. Caudal septal deviation to the right (Right Nasal Aperture Views).
   b. Mobile tip (Lateral Smiling Views).
3. **Bony pyramid**
   a. Osteocartilaginous hump predominantly oblique (Backward Tilting Views) and slightly deviated (Frontal and Direct Dorsal) to the patient's right due to bilateral maxillary asymmetry. The right cheek wide and low and the left cheek is narrow and high (Backward Tilting Views).
   b. Wide base of the bony pyramid (Direct Dorsal and Backward Tilting Views).
   c. The dorsal light reflex is irregular and defuse (preoperative, Direct Dorsal Views).
4. **Alar base**
   Nasal apertures are thick walled heavy rounded in shape. The posterior segments of the rim-sill folds are thick with acute angles with the upper lip giving the flat tire appearance (Backward Tilting Views).

Aims of Surgery

1. Overall reduction of the size of the nose.
2. Abolish mobility of the tip.
3. Correct the nasal deviation.

Surgical Plan

1. **Frontolateral walls**
   a. DDD including the weak triangle to reduce the bulk and size of the nasal tip and supra tip area.
   b. Cephalic trim of the lateral crurae to reduce the size of the nasal tip.
2. **Medial Wall**
   a. Septoplasty.
   b. Division of the Depressor Septi muscles.
3. **Bony pyramid**
   a. Excision of the osteocartilaginous hump.
   b. Osteotomies and Kassanjean maneuver to the left i.e. cross fracture of the bony pyramid after osteotomies (refer to Surgery of the Bony Pyramid Section).
4. **Alar base**
   Nil of note.

Surgical Procedure

As per Surgical Plan.

Post-Operative Analysis

1. **Frontolateral Wall**
   a. Tip definition: the nasal tip is slimmer with thinner overlying skin, more prominent and well identified from the alae nasi on both sides. The alae nasi become clearly visible and share in nasal aesthetics (Frontal, Direct Dorsal, Overhead, Backward Tilting and Basal Views).
   b. Tip projection: the nasal tip at the same level of the nasal dorsum with good aesthetic angle. This is

M. H. A. Shafy, *Atlas of Clinical Cases in Rhinoplasty*,
https://doi.org/10.1007/978-3-031-07504-9_41

coupled with good aesthetic nasolabial angle (lateral and oblique views).

c. Tip light reflex is seen as one spot off the nasal tip (Frontal, Backward Tilting and Basal Views).

2. **Medial Wall**
   a. Caudal septal deviation was corrected.
   b. Mobile tip abolished.
3. **Bony Pyramid**
   a. Bony pyramid aesthetics improved: the nasal dorsum is straight in the midline and the sidewalls are smooth and narrow (all views except the Basal Views).
   b. Dorsal light reflex is seen as a regular one line off the nasal dorsum (Direct Dorsal Views).
4. **Alar Base**
   a. Superior alar groove aesthetics improved by defatting. The grooves become longer and deeper (Oblique, Lateral and Direct Dorsal grooves).
   b. Posterior alar groove aesthetics improved by defatting alone (Backward Tilting, Basal and Nasal Aperture Views).
   c. Alae nasi aesthetics improved. They were pulled medially, became more visible and smaller in size (Backward Tilting and Nasal Aperture Views).
   d. Nasal aperture aesthetics enhanced by defatting:
      i. The size of the nasal openings are reduced (Backward Tilting and Nasal Aperture Views).
      ii. The shape of the nasal openings: they become more elegantly oval (Backward Tilting and Nasal Aperture views).
   e. Marginal light reflexes are clearly seen at:
      i. Inferior alar margins (Nasal Aperture Views).
      ii. Nasal sill bands (Oblique Views).
      iii. Lateral crural prominences (Lateral Views).

Commentary

a. The post-operative photographs were taken 9 years after surgery, hence the change in the patients facial features.
b. Middle Eastern ladies commonly prefer an extremely narrow tip in contrast to the ethnically prevalent large or bulky tip.

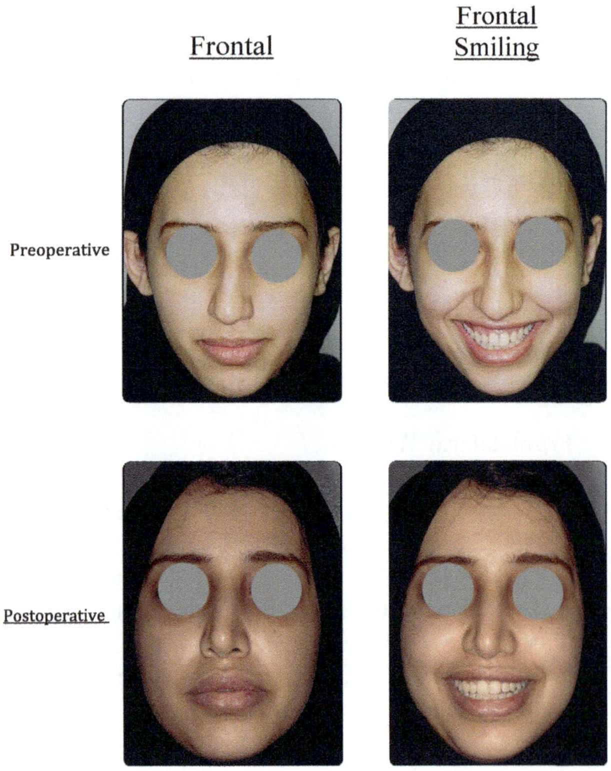

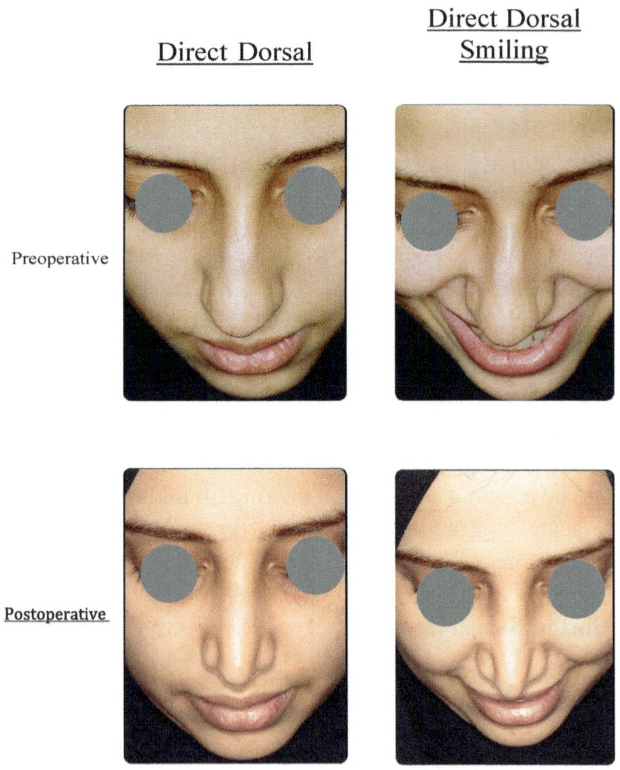

Backward Tilting | Steeper Backward Tilting

Preoperative

Postoperative

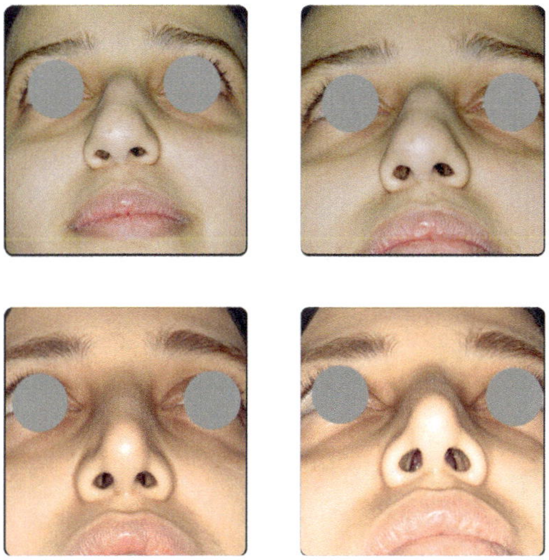

Right Oblique Mid Cheek Full Face | Left Oblique Mid Cheek Full Face

Preoperative

Postoperative

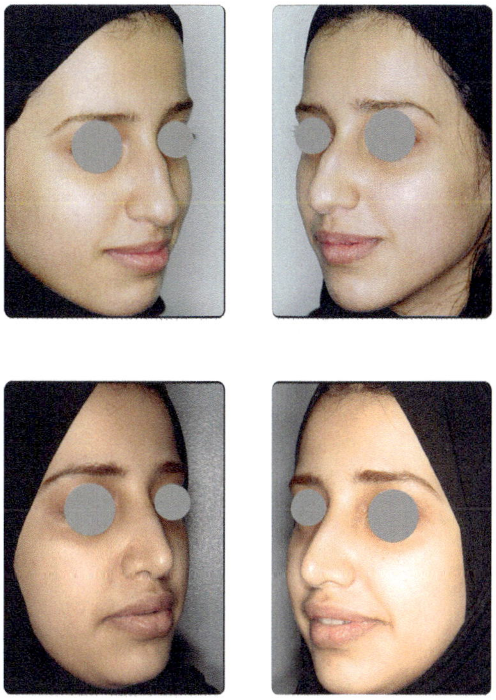

Right Nasal Aperture | Left Nasal Aperture

Preoperative

Postoperative

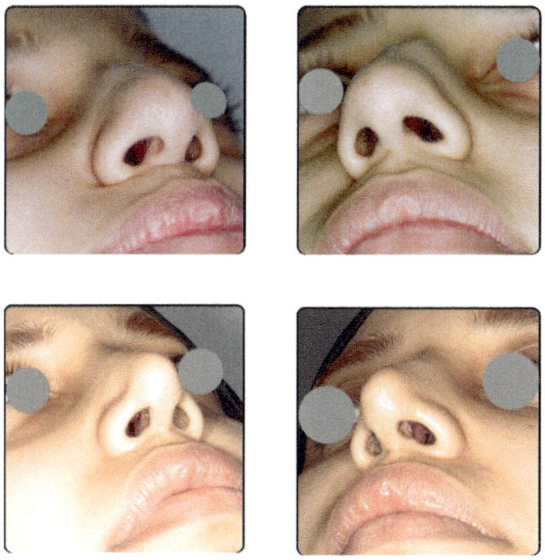

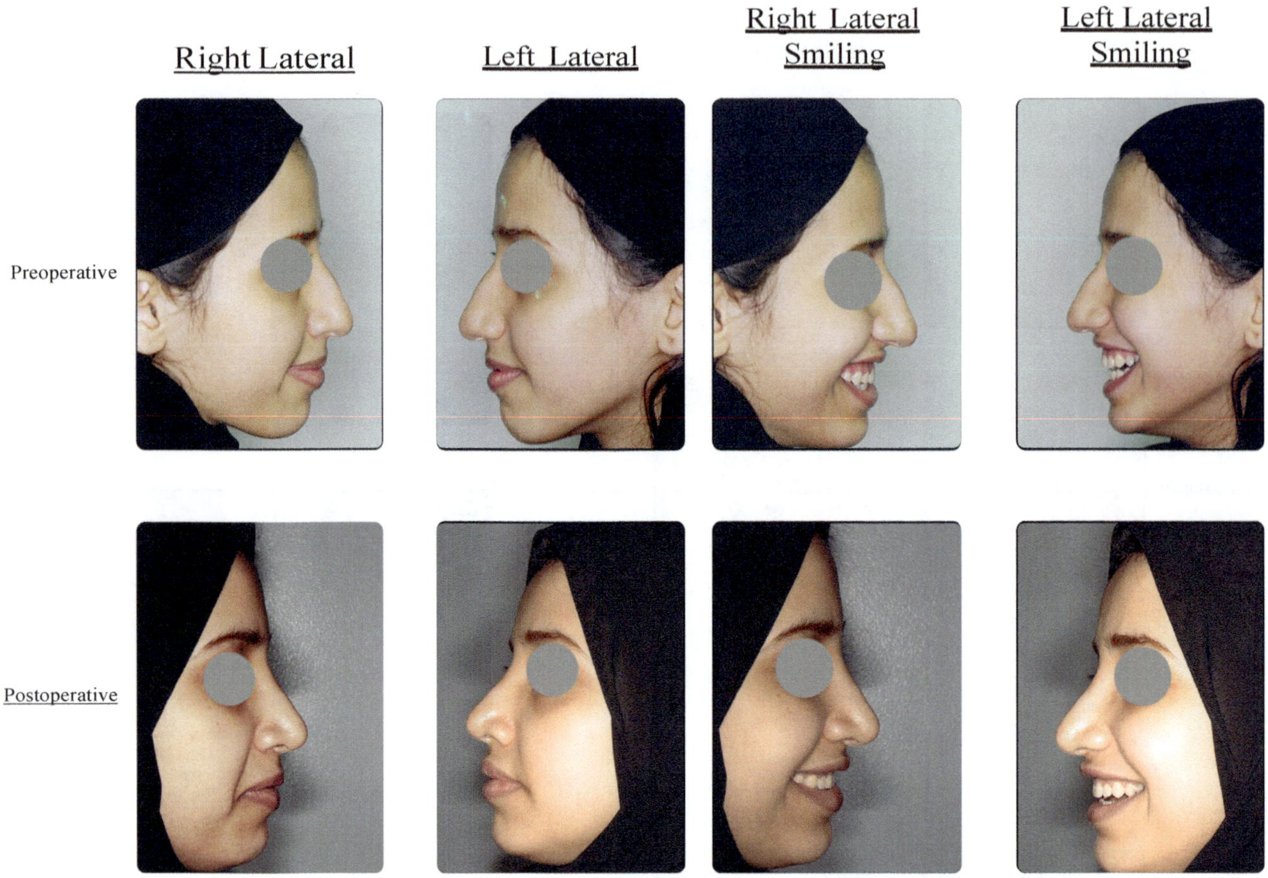
Right Lateral
Left Lateral
Right Lateral Smiling
Left Lateral Smiling
Preoperative
Postoperative

Part V: Clinical Case 3

42

Preoperative Assessment

1. **Frontolateral walls**
   a. The nasal tip is small but bulky due to its thick skin cover. The right dome is high and pushed forward and to the right by the deviated caudal septum (Frontal and Back, Tilting and Basal Views).
   b. The right ala nasi is almost totally overshadowed by the deviated bulky right dome (Frontal and Direct Dorsal Views).
2. **Medial Wall**
   a. High "C" shaped septal deviation to the left.
   b. There is caudal septal dislocation to the right side pushing the ipsilateral medial crus laterally (Backward Tilting and Basal Views). The right nasal sill band is pushed and displaced inferiorly by the elongated displaced septum (Frontal Views). The right dome is displaced forward and to the right (Frontal, Backward Tilting and Basal Views).
3. **Boney pyramid**
   a. The boney pyramid and the nose are severely oblique (Backward Tilting Views) and deviated (Frontal, Overhead and Direct Dorsal Views) to the right due to severe bilateral maxillary asymmetry. The right cheek is wide and low and the left cheek is narrow and high (backward tilting views).
   b. Osteocartilaginous hump (Oblique and Lateral Views).
   c. The dorsal light reflex is distorted (preoperative Direct Dorsal Views).
4. **Alar base**
   The right nasal aperture is apparently smaller than the left due to deviation of the caudal cartilagenous septum which could be seen through the right opening (Backward Tilting and Basal Views).

Aims of Surgery

1. Proportionate reduction of the bulk and size of the lower third of the nose including the nasal tip.
2. Correction of the deviated septum.
3. Excision of the osteo-cartilaginous hump and balancing of the boney pyramid to the mid line.

Surgical Plan

1. **Frontolateral walls**
   a. DDD including the weak triangle to reduce the bulk of nasal tip and supratip area.
   b. Bilateral cephalic trim of lateral crurae to reduce the size of the nasal tip.
2. **Nasal Septum**
   Septoplasty.
3. **Boney pyramid**
   a. Excision of the osteocartilaginous hump.
   b. Osteotomies and Kassanjian maneuver to the left side of the patient i.e. fracture of the bony pyramid after osteotomies (Refer to Surgery of the Bony Pyramid Section).
4. **Alar base**
   Nil of note.

Surgical Procedure

a. As per Surgical Plan.
b. Cephalic trim of the left lateral crus only.

M. H. A. Shafy, *Atlas of Clinical Cases in Rhinoplasty*,
https://doi.org/10.1007/978-3-031-07504-9_42

Post-Operative Analysis Commentary

1. **Frontolateral Wall**
   a. Tip definition: the nasal tip is slimmer, with thinner overlying skin, more prominent and well identified from the alae nasi on both sides. The alae nasi become clearly visible and share in nasal aesthetics (Frontal, Direct Dorsal, Overhead, Backward Tilting and Basal Views).
   b. Tip projection: the nasal tip at the same level of the nasal dorsum with good aesthetic angle. This is coupled with good aesthetic nasolabial angle (lateral and oblique views).
   c. Tip light reflex is seen as one spot off the nasal tip (Frontal and Backward Tilting Views).
2. **Medial Wall**
   Correction of caudal septal deviation have resulted in the following:
   a. The right lateral protrusion of the medial crus disappeared (post-operative Backward Tilting, Basal and Right Nasal Aperture Views).
   b. The inferior displacement of the right nasal sill band leveled with the left side (Post-operative Frontal Views).
3. **Bony Pyramid**
   a. Bony pyramid aesthetics improved: nasal deviation is corrected. The nasal dorsum as well as the rest of the nose are straight in midline and the sidewalls are smooth and narrow (all views except the Basal Views).
   b. Dorsal light reflex appears as uninterrupted line of light (postoperative Direct Dorsal Views).
4. **Alar Base**
   a. Superior alar groove aesthetics improved by defatting. The grooves become longer and deeper (Oblique, Lateral and Direct Dorsal grooves).
   b. Posterior alar groove aesthetics improved. The angles with the upper lip are wider and look aesthetically better (Nasal Aperture Views).
   c. Aesthetics of the alae nasi are better. They moved medially after defatting and are better seen (Nasal Aperture and Oblique Views).
   d. Nasal apertures became equal in size and shape after correction of the caudal septal deviation and defatting.
   e. Marginal light reflexes are clearly seen at:
      i. Inferior alar margins (Nasal Aperture Views).
      ii. Nasal sill bands (Oblique Views).
      iii. Lateral crural prominences (Lateral Views).

Commentary

a. There is a compensatory larger left lateral crus in these cases of severe bilateral maxillary asymmetry with deviation to the right. Hence cephalic trim was only done on the left side.
b. The bulge in the left dome of nasal tip was secondary to the left caudal deviation pushing the dome forward. The bulge disappeared after correction of the septal deviation.

Frontal | Frontal Smiling | Frontal Middle Third

Preoperative

Postoperative

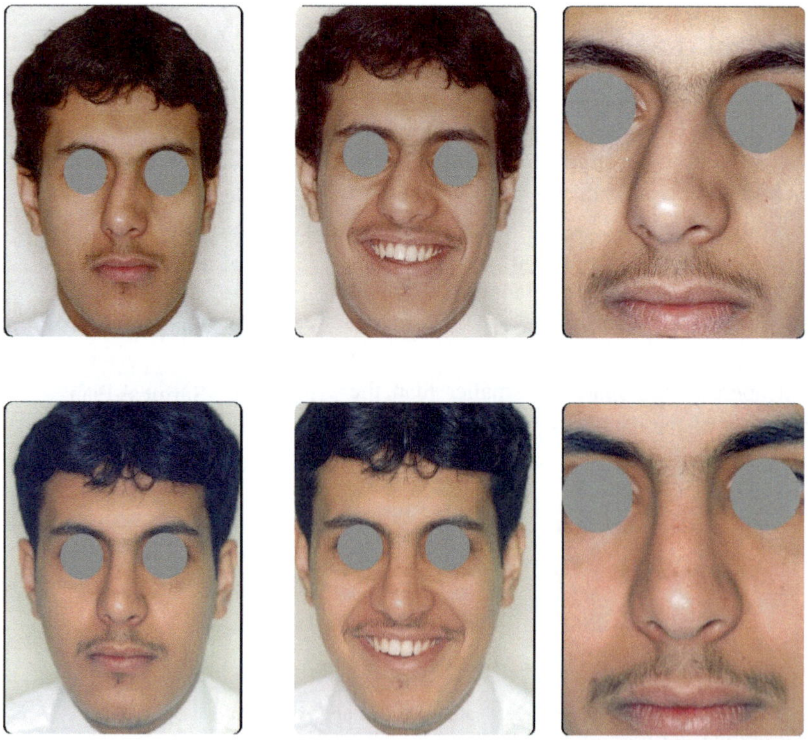

Direct Dorsal | Direct Dorsal Smiling | Overhead | Overhead Smiling

Preoperative

Postoperative

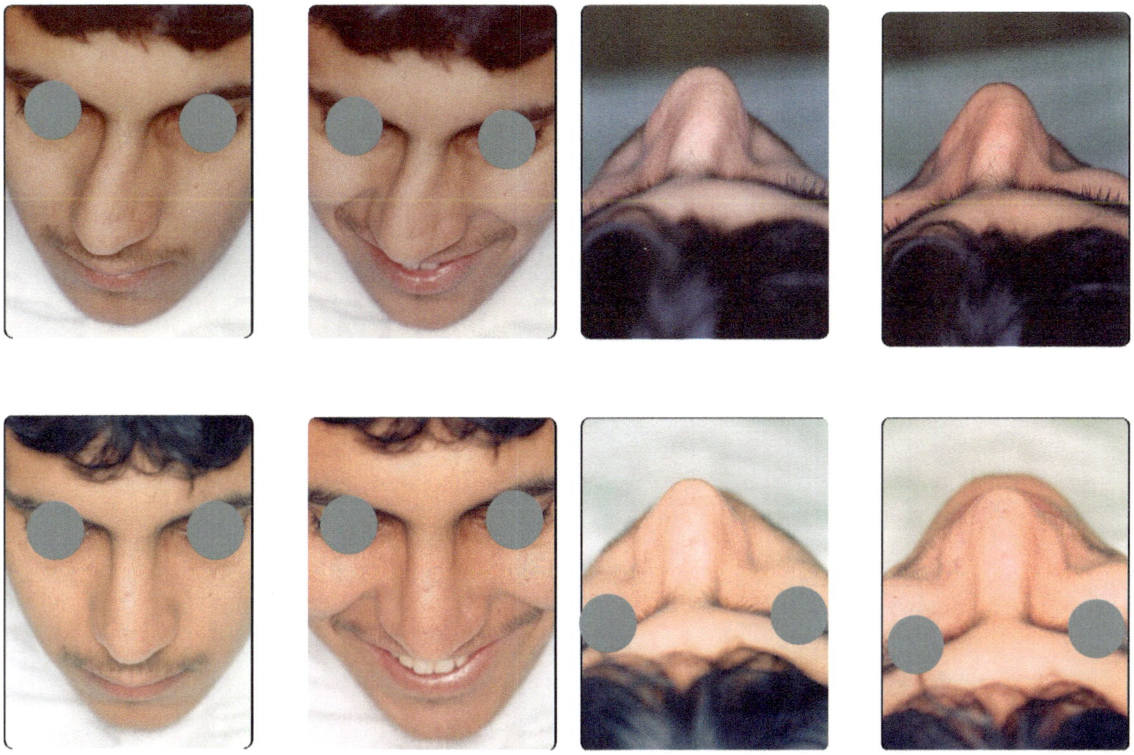

Backward Tilting | Steeper Backward Tilting | Basal

Preoperative

Postoperative

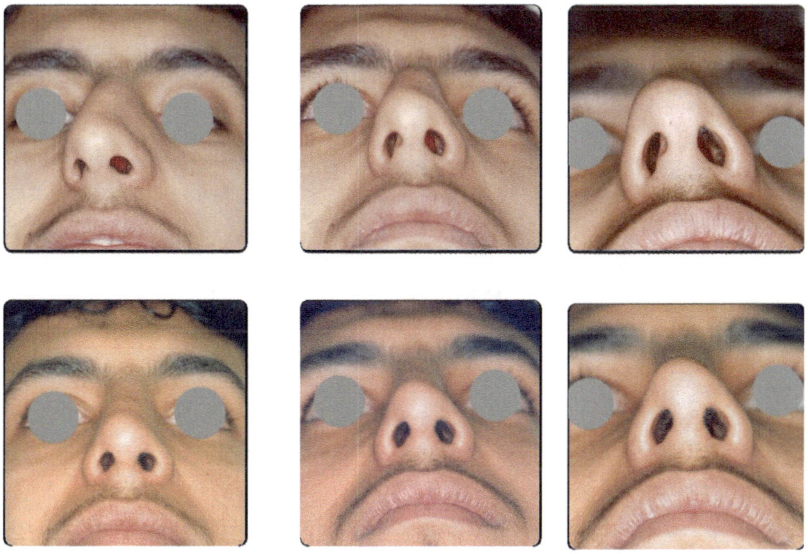

Right Nasal Aperture | Left Nasal Aperture

Preoperative

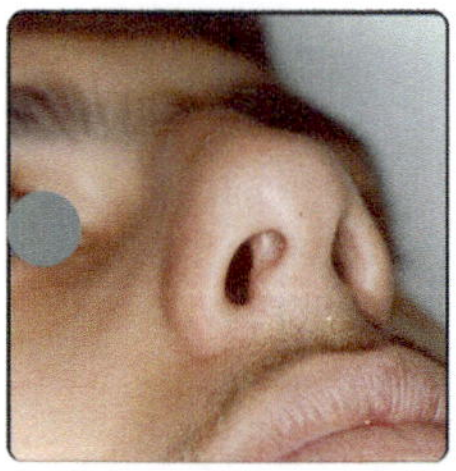

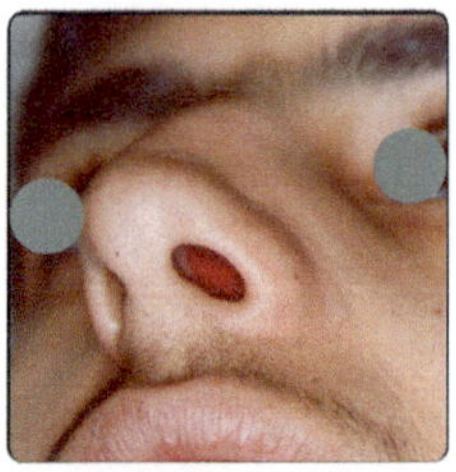

Postoperative

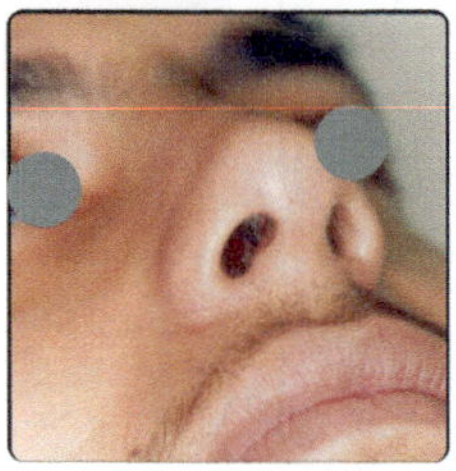

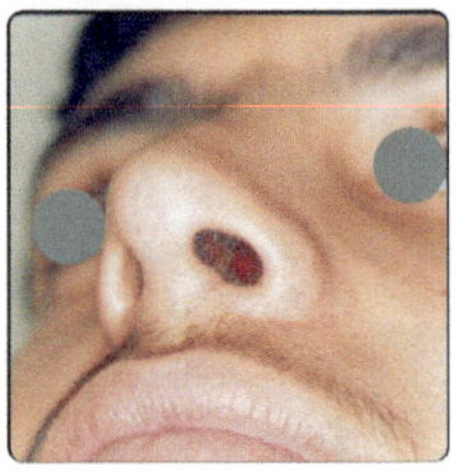

Right Oblique Mid Cheek Full Face | Left Oblique Mid Cheek Full Face | Right Oblique Mid Cheek Middle Third | Left Oblique Mid Cheek Middle Third

Preoperative

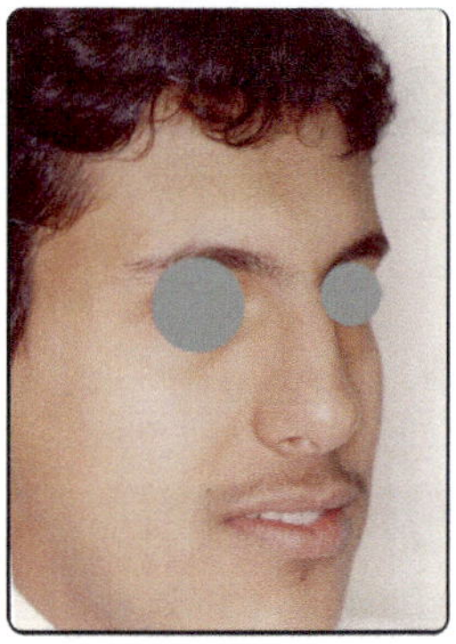

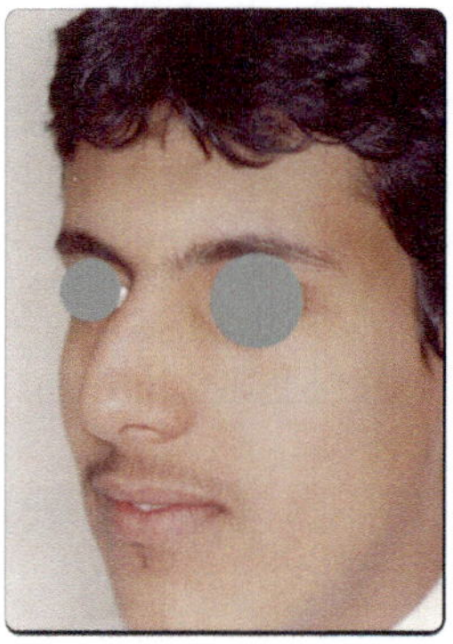

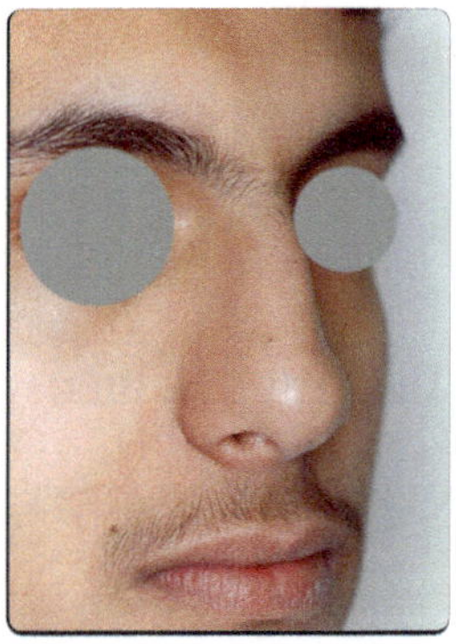

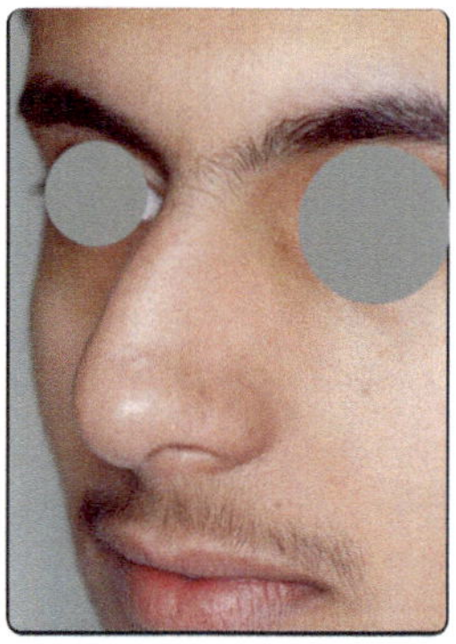

Postoperative

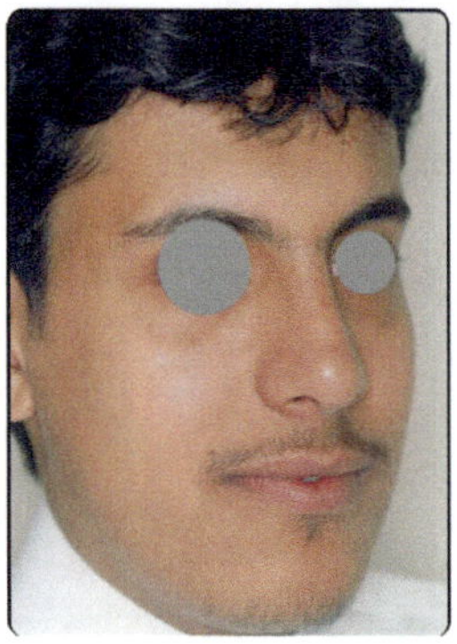

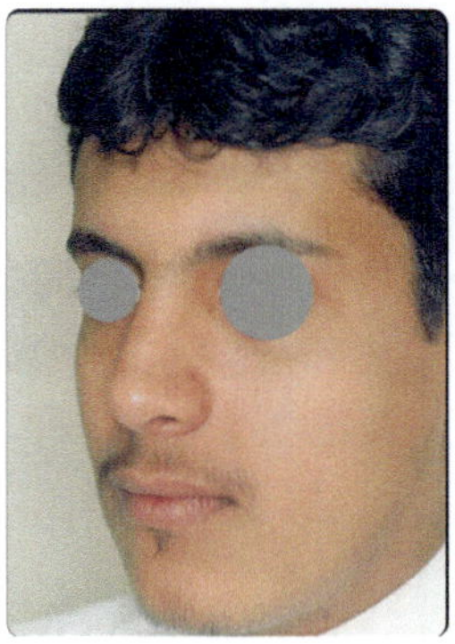

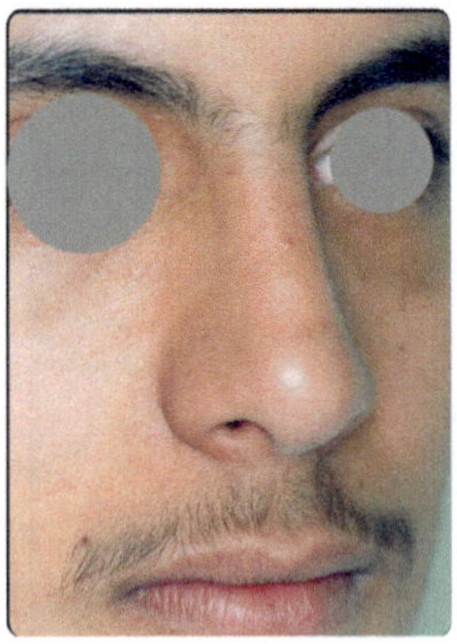

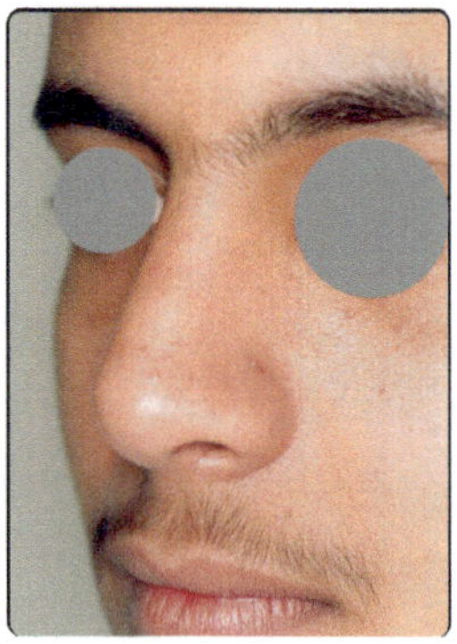

Right Oblique Cheek Margin Full Face	Left Oblique Cheek Margin Full Face	Right Oblique Cheek Margin Middle Third	Left Oblique Cheek Margin Middle Third

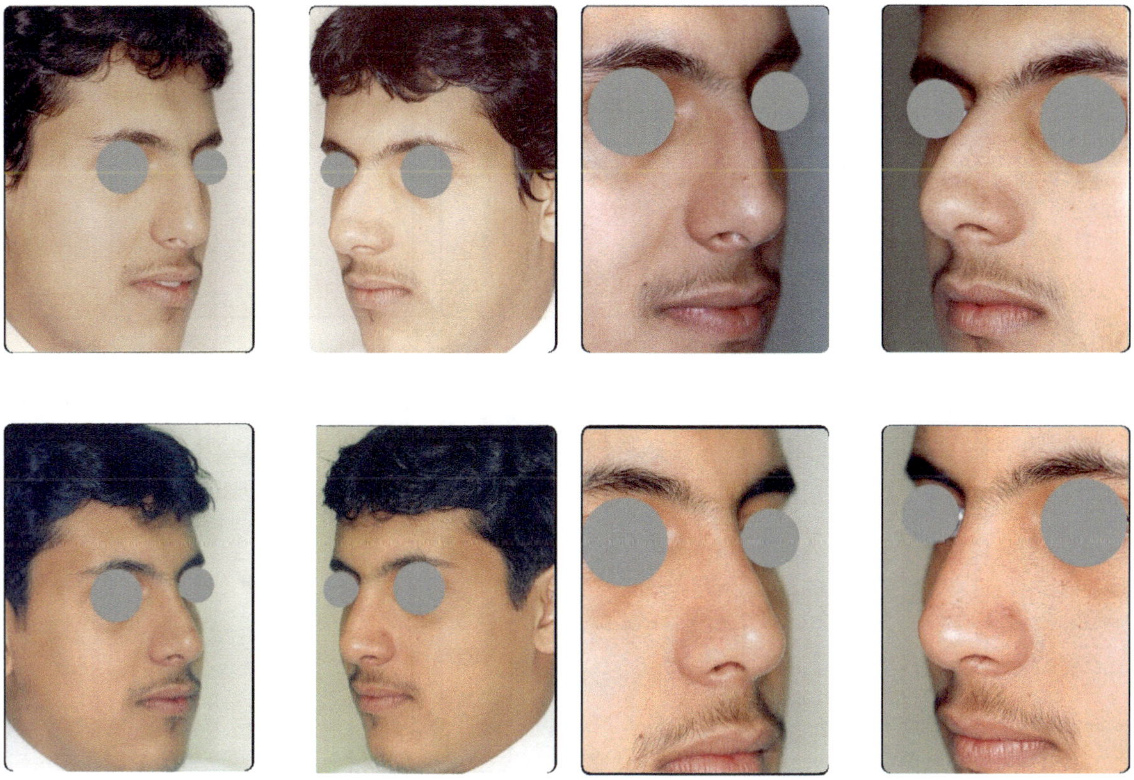

Preoperative

Postoperative

Right Lateral | Left Lateral | Right Lateral Smiling | Left Lateral Smiling

Preoperative

Postoperative

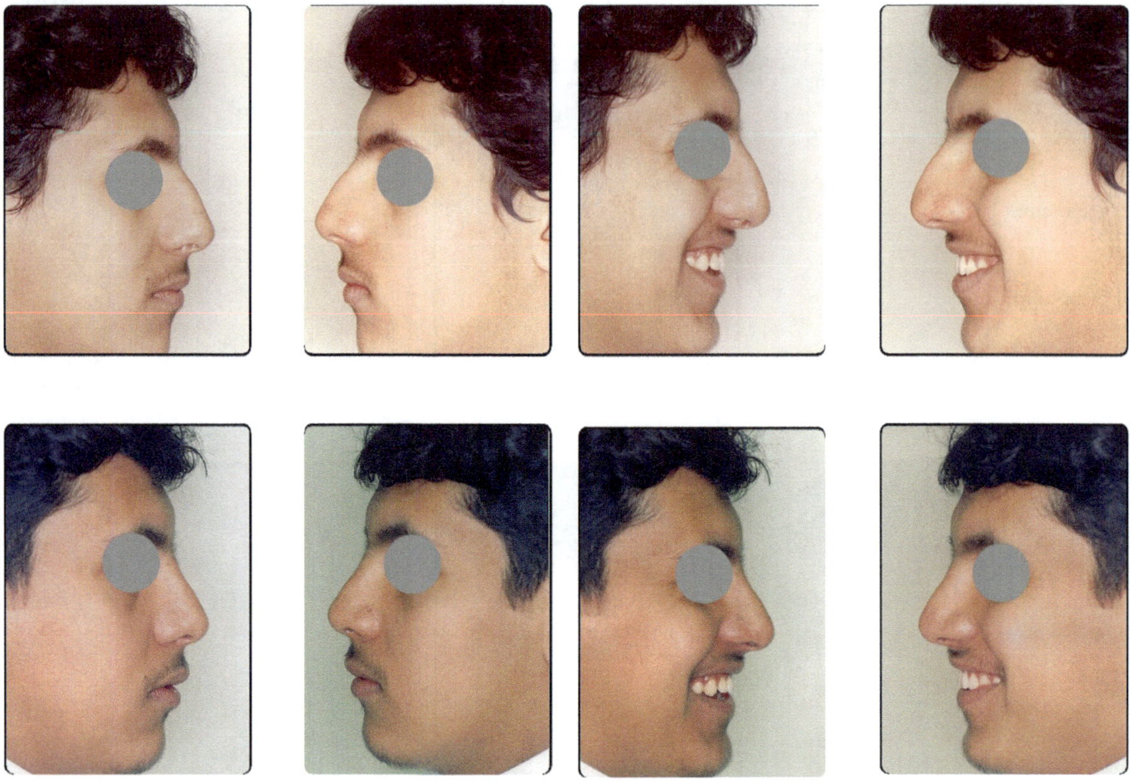

Right Lateral Middle Third | Left Lateral Middle Third

Preoperative

Postoperative

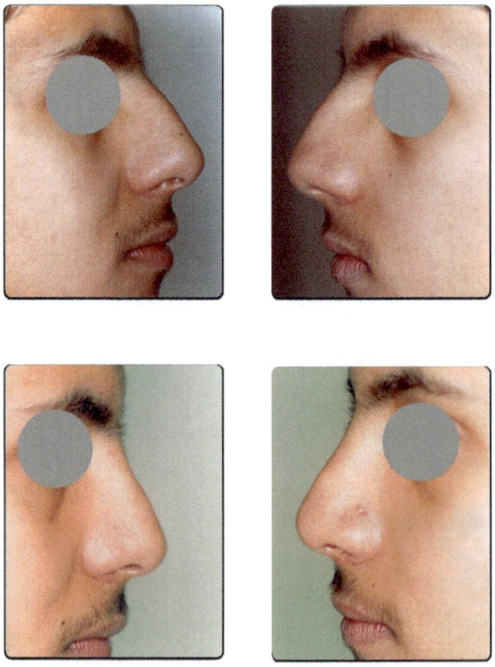

43 Part V: Clinical Case 4

Preoperative Assessment

1. **Frontolateral walls**
   A medium sized bulky tip overshadowing the alae nasi, predominantly the right side (Frontal and Overhead Views).
2. **Medial Wall**
   a. Mobile tip (Lateral Smiling Views).
   b. Caudal septal deviation to the right (Right Nasal Aperture View).
3. **Boney pyramid**
   a. Osteocartilaginous hump, which is deviated (Frontal, Direct Dorsal and Overhead View) and Oblique to the right (Backward Tilting Views).
   b. Bilateral Maxillary asymmetry. The left cheek is wide and low and the right cheek is narrow and high (Backward Tilting Views).
   c. The light reflex of nasal dorsum is irregularly distorted (Preoperative Direct Dorsal View).
4. **Alar base**
   a. Asymmetrical smile due to asymmetrical alae nasi and deviated nose (Pre-operative Frontal Smiling View). The nasal tip and left ala nasi deviated to the left.
   b. The nasal apertures are wide, thick walled and rounded (Basal Views).

Aims of Surgery

1. Reduction of the size and bulk of the nasal tip.
2. Abolish mobility of nasal tip.
3. Excision of the osteocartilaginous hump.
4. Correction of nasal deviation and obliquity.

Surgical Plan

1. **Frontolateral walls**
   a. DDD including the weak triangle to reduce the bulk of nasal tip and supratip area.
   b. Cephalic trim of the lateral crurae to reduce the size of the nasal tip.
2. **Medial Wall**
   a. Septoplasty with minimal trim of the membranous septum.
   b. Division of the Depressor Septi muscles.
3. **Boney pyramid**
   a. Excision of the Osteocartilaginous hump.
   b. Osteotomies and Kasanjian manoeuvre to the left i.e. cross fracture of the bony pyramid after osteotomies (See text Chapter of Surgery of the Bony Pyramid).
4. **Alar base**
   Nil of note.

Surgical Procedure

As per Surgical Plan.

Post-Operative Analysis

1. **Frontolateral Wall**
   a. Tip definition: nasal tip is smaller with thinner and smoother overlying skin. It is more prominent and well identified from the alae nasi on both sides. The alae nasi come into view to become clearly visible and share in nasal aesthetics (Frontal, Direct Dorsal, Overhead, Backward Tilting and Basal Views).

M. H. A. Shafy, *Atlas of Clinical Cases in Rhinoplasty*,
https://doi.org/10.1007/978-3-031-07504-9_43

   b. Tip projection: the nasal tip is at the same level of the nasal dorsum with good aesthetic angle. This is coupled with good aesthetic nasolabial angle (lateral and oblique views).
   c. Tip light reflex is seen as one spot off the nasal tip (Frontal and Backward Tilting Views).
2. **Medial Wall**
   Caudal septal deviation was corrected.
3. **Bony Pyramid**
   a. Bony pyramid aesthetics improved: the nasal dorsum is in the midline, straight and the sidewalls are smooth and narrow (all views except the Basal Views).
   b. Dorsal light reflex is seen as an uninterrupted line off the nasal dorsum (Post operative Direct Dorsal View).
4. **Alar Base**
   a. Superior alar groove aesthetics improved by defatting. The grooves became longer and deeper (Oblique, Lateral and Direct Dorsal Views).
   b. Nasal aperture aesthetics:
      i. The size of the nasal openings are reduced by defatting alone (Backward Tilting, Basal and Nasal Aperture views).
      ii. The shape: defatting enhanced aesthetics of the nasal openings, they become thin walled and elegantly oval in shape (Backward Tilting, Basal and Nasal Aperture Views).
   c. Alae nasi aesthetics improved. They were pulled medially after defatting and became better seen.
   d. The smile became symmetrical post-operatively after equalizing the alae nasi and correction of deviation of the bony pyramid including the nasal septum.
   e. Marginal light reflexes are clearly seen at:
      i. Inferior alar margins (Nasal Aperture Views).
      ii. Nasal sill bands (Oblique Views).
      iii. Lateral crural prominences (Lateral Views).

Commentary

Three of the four areas of Rhinoplasty were addressed in this case in order to transform her nose from an ordinary looking into an attractive nose and face:

i. The nasal tip was bulky, large, mobile and deviated. Post operatively nasal tip becomes small, slim, immobile and centrally midline.
ii. The caudal septum was deviated to the right. Postoperatively the septal deviation is corrected.
iii. The bony pyramid was deviated, oblique with a hump. Postoperatively the bony pyramid is slim, central, and Strait.
iv. Alar base aesthetics consequently improved after defatting and caudal septal correction.

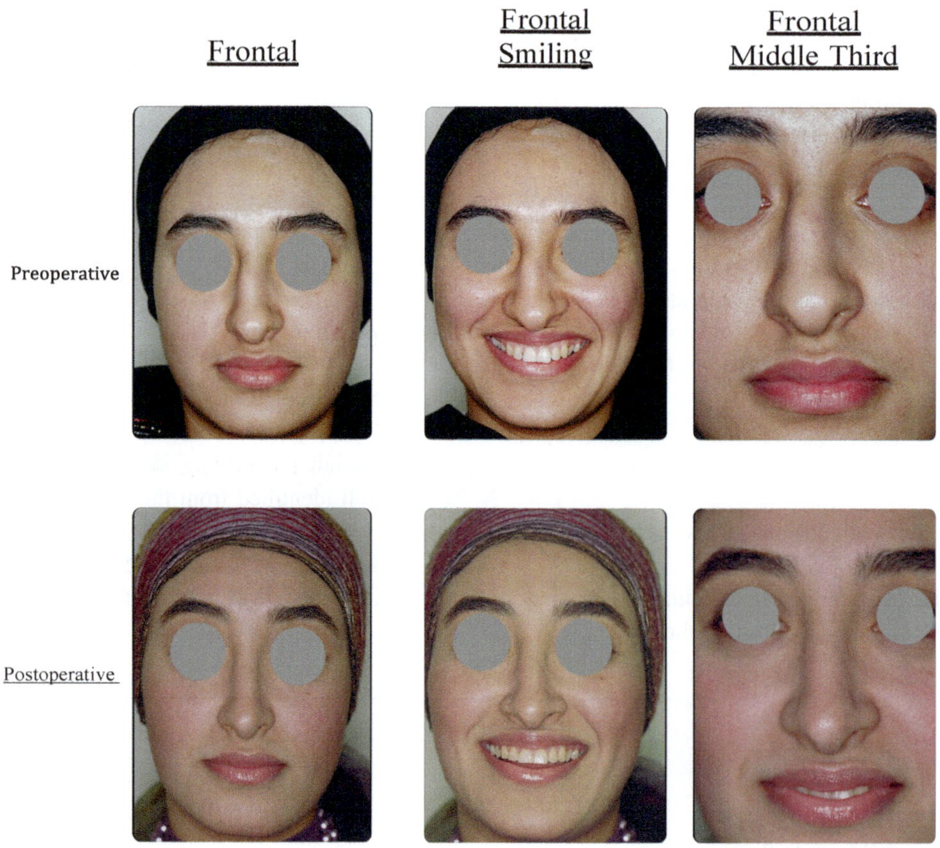

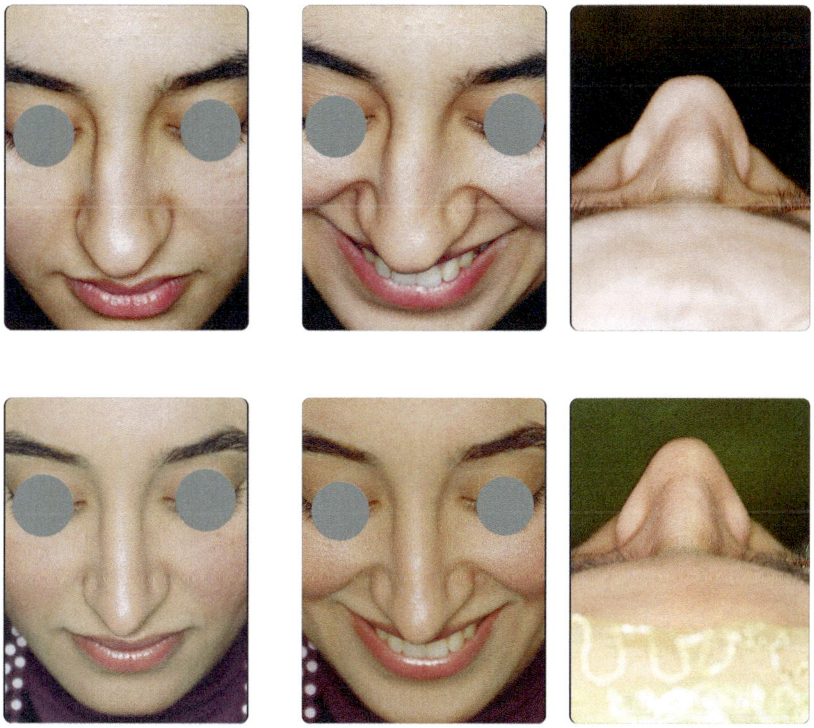
Direct Dorsal
Direct Dorsal Smiling
Overhead
Preoperative
Postoperative

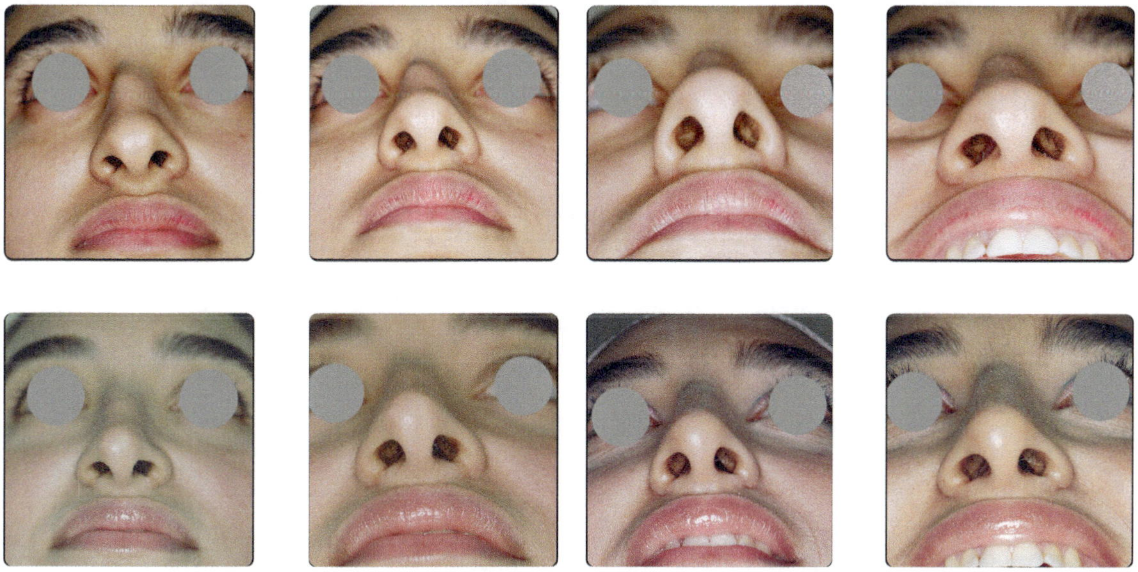
Backward Tilting
Steeper Backward Tilting
Basal
Basal Smiling
Preoperative
Postoperative

Right Nasal Aperture | Right Nasal Aperture Rim Sill Test | Left Nasal Aperture Rim Sill Test | Left Nasal Aperture

Preoperative

Postoperative

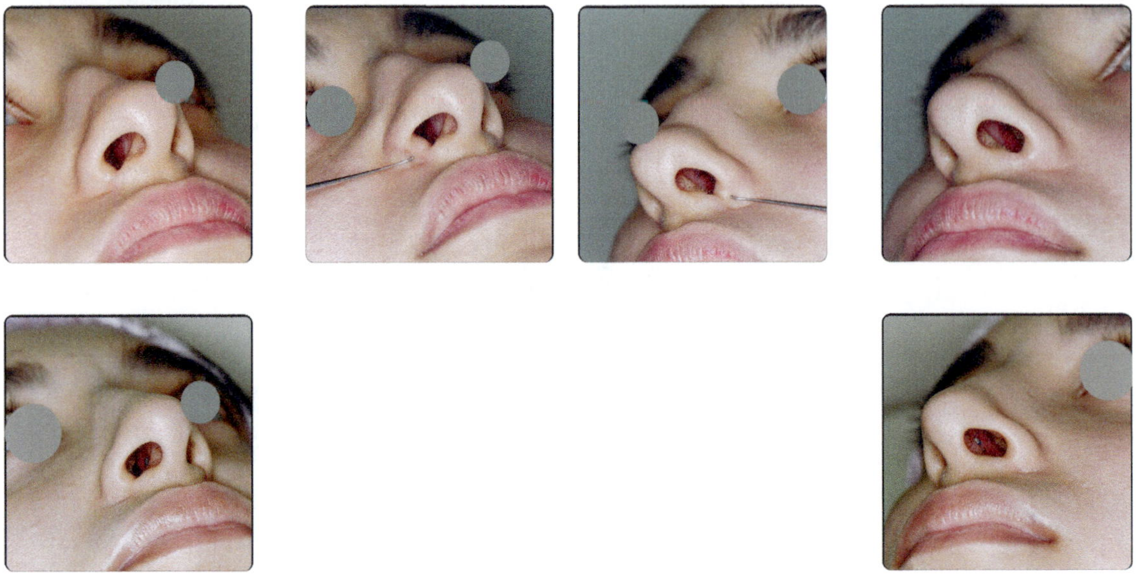

Right Oblique Mid Cheek Full Face | Left Oblique Mid Cheek Full Face | Right Oblique Mid Cheek Middle Third | Left Oblique Mid Cheek Middle Third

Preoperative

Postoperative

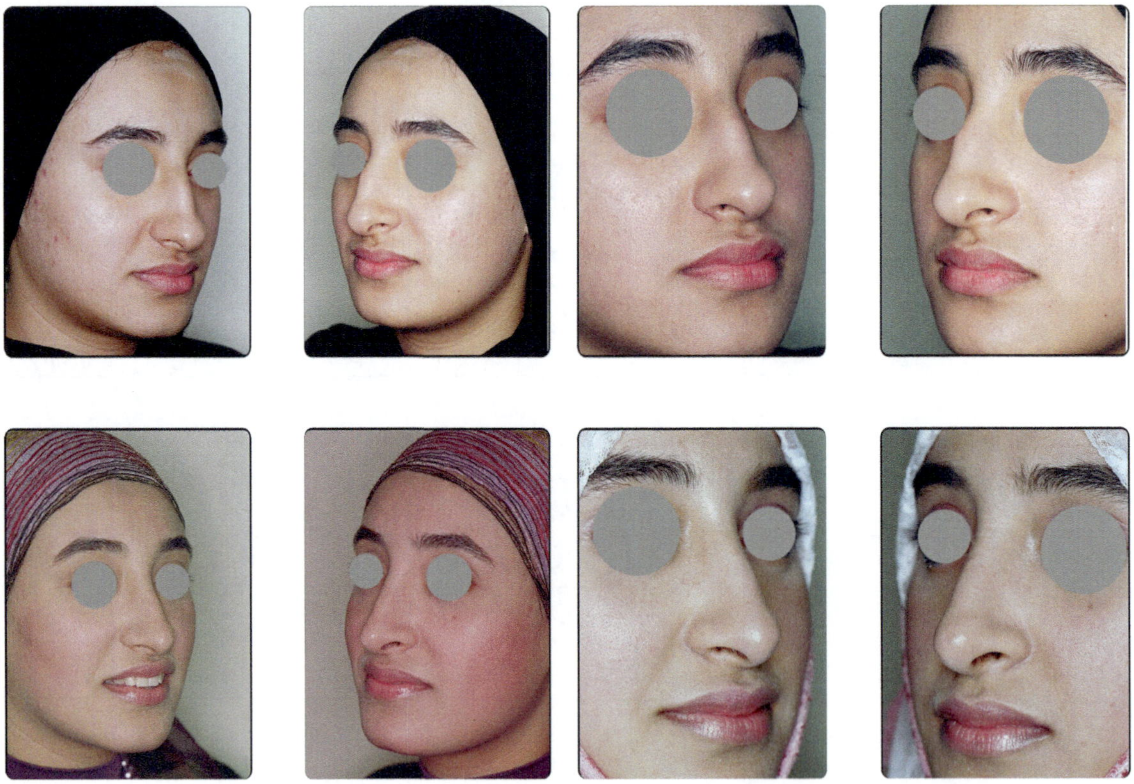

Right Oblique Cheek Margin Full Face	Left Oblique Cheek Margin Full Face	Right Oblique Cheek Margin Middle Third	Left Oblique Cheek Margin Middle Third

Preoperative

Postoperative

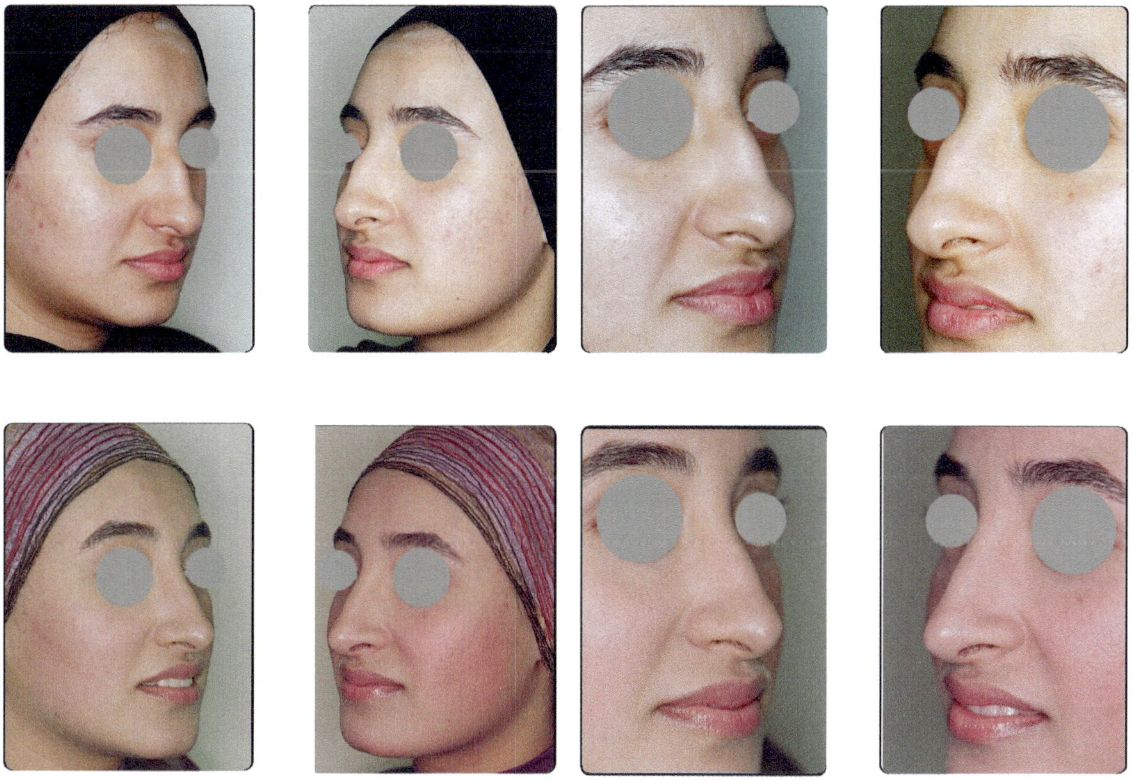

Right Lateral | Left Lateral | Right Lateral Smiling | Left Lateral Smiling

Preoperative

Postoperative

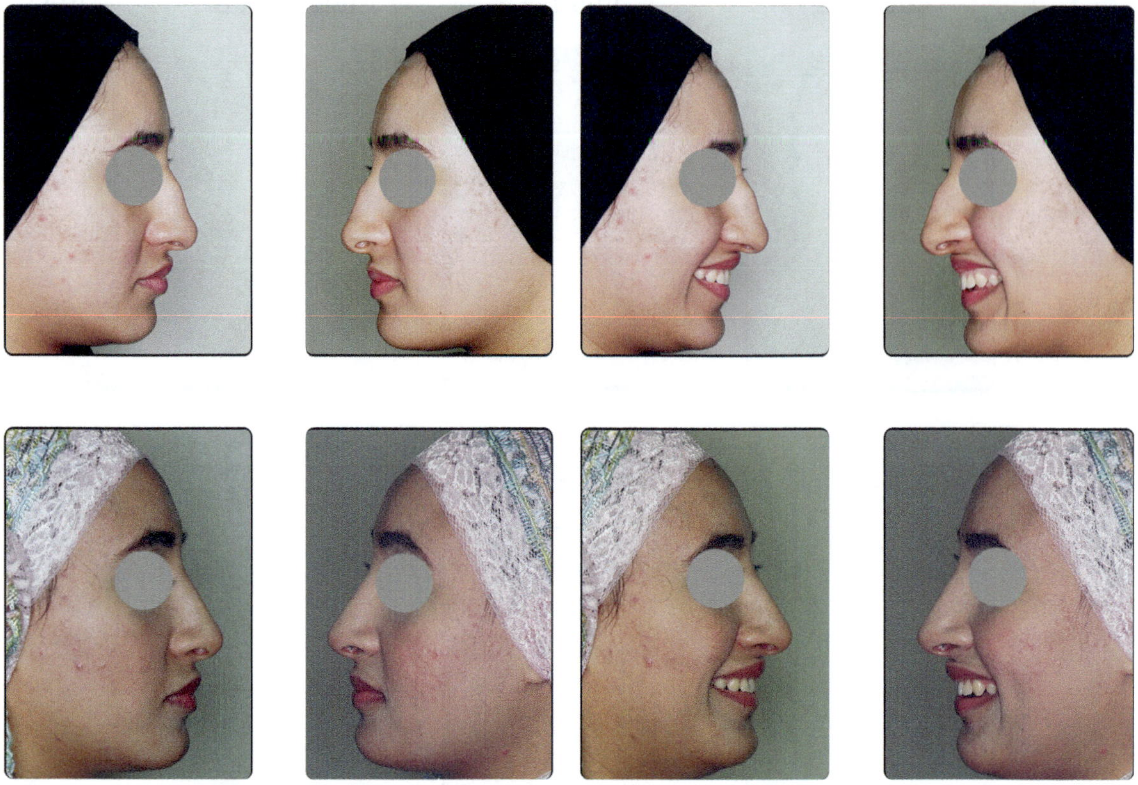

Right Lateral Middle Third | Left Lateral Middle Third

Preoperative

Postoperative

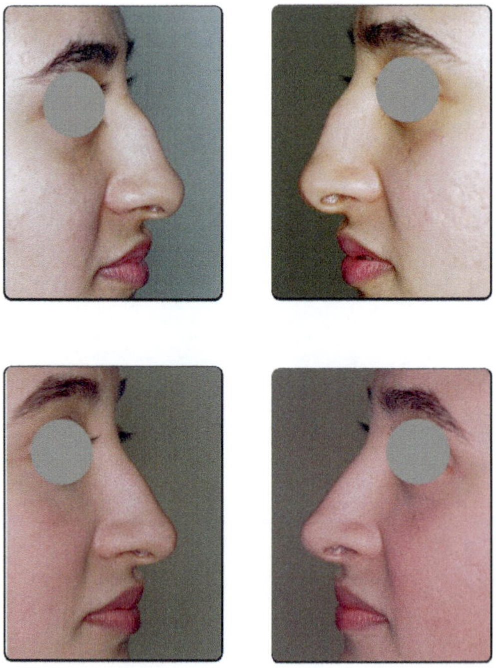

Part V: Clinical Case 5

44

Preoperative Assessment

1. **Frontolateral walls**
   a. Flat, small but bulky and ill defined nasal tip overshadowing the alae nasi (Frontal, Direct Dorsal and Overhead Views).
   b. The nasal tip is ill defined due to the flat middle crurae.
2. **Media Wall**
   a. Acute nasolabial angle (Lateral Views).
   b. Mobile tip (Lateral Smiling Views).
   c. Severe internal right residual septal deviation.
3. **Boney pyramid**
   a. Wide base of the bony pyramid (Direct Dorsal and Backward Tilting Views).
   b. Supra tip saddle deformity, as well as collapse of the lower 2/3rds of the nose secondary to previous surgery (Oblique and Lateral Views).
   c. The bony pyramid deviated and oblique to the right (deviation seen in the Overhead, Direct Dorsal and Frontal Views, Obliquity is seen in the Backward Tilting Views). There is bilateral maxillary asymmetry—the left cheek is high and narrow while the right cheek is low and wide (Backward Tilting Views).
   d. The dorsal light reflex is distorted (preoperative Direct Dorsal Views).
4. **Alar base**
   a. Wide nasal apertures with transverse long axes. This is secondary to the collapse of the lower third (Basal Views).

Aims of Surgery

1. Reduce the bulk and size of the nasal tip to match the new reduced size of the bony pyramid.
2. Elevation of the nasal tip.
3. Abolish mobility of nasal tip.
4. Elevating the saddle deformity and the collapsed lawer 2/3rds of the nose.
5. Reduce the size of the bony pyramid and correct its deviation and obliquity.

Surgical Plan

1. **Frontolateral walls**
   DDD not including the weak triangle to reduce the bulk of nasal tip only.
2. **Media Wall**
   a. Septoplasty.
   b. Division of the Depressor Septi muscles.
   c. Trim of the caudal end of the membranous septum.
3. **Boney pyramid**
   a. Reduction of the height of the bony pyramid.
   b. Osteotomies as well as Kassanjian maneuver to the left i.e. cross fracture of the bony pyramid after osteotomies (Refer to Surgery of the Bony Pyramid).
4. **Alar base**
   Nil of note.

Surgical Procedure

a. As per Surgical Plan.
b. Cephalic trim of the lateral crurae, before defatting, in order to salvage some needed supratip cartilaginous grafts.
c. The supra tip depression was filled in with the trimmings of the lateral crurae including their overlying fatty tissues.

Post-Operative Analysis

1. **Frontolateral Wall**
   a. Tip definition: nasal tip is slimmer with thinner overlying skin, more prominent and well identified from the alae nasi on both sides. The alae nasi become clearly visible and share in nasal aesthetics (Frontal,

M. H. A. Shafy, *Atlas of Clinical Cases in Rhinoplasty*,
https://doi.org/10.1007/978-3-031-07504-9_44

Direct Dorsal, Overhead, Backward Tilting and Basal Views).

b. Tip projection: the nasal tip at the same level of the nasal dorsum with good aesthetic angle. This is coupled with good aesthetic nasolabial angle (lateral and oblique views).

c. Tip light reflex is seen as one spot off the nasal tip (Anterior and Backward Tilting Views).

2. **Medial Wall**

Nil of Note.

3. **Bony Pyramid**

a. Bony pyramid aesthetics improved: the nasal dorsum is straight and the sidewalls are smooth and narrow (all views except the Basal Views).

b. Dorsal light reflex is seen as a regular one line off the nasal dorsum (postoperative Direct Dorsal Views).

4. **Alar Base**

a. Superior alar groove aesthetics improved by defatting. The grooves become longer and deeper (Oblique, Lateral and Direct Dorsal grooves).

b. Posterior alar groove aesthetics improved by defatting alone (Backward Tilting and Basal Views).

c. Alae nasi aesthetics improved. They are pulled medially become better seen, smaller and share in nasal aesthetics (Oblique and Lateral Views).

d. Nasal aperture aesthetics improved by defatting:

i. The sizes of nasal apertures became smaller.

ii. The shape of nasal apertures became elegantly oval.

e. Marginal light reflexes are clearly seen at:

i. Inferior alar margins (Nasal Aperture Views).

ii. Nasal sill bands (Oblique Views).

iii. Lateral crural prominences (Lateral Views).

Commentary

a. There was extensive removal of septal cartilage in the primary surgery. The supra tip depression was mild at first, then became steadily worse for almost two years after the surgery so that the depression extended to affect the lower 2/3rds of the nose.

b. The saddle deformity was automatically corrected after rasping the hump, osteotomies and medialization of the sidewalls of the bony pyramid. He only needed minimal supportive graft.

c. Having a better nasal respiration as well as appearance, his general attitude, behavior and mood had greatly improved. He regained his normal natural bubbling personality.

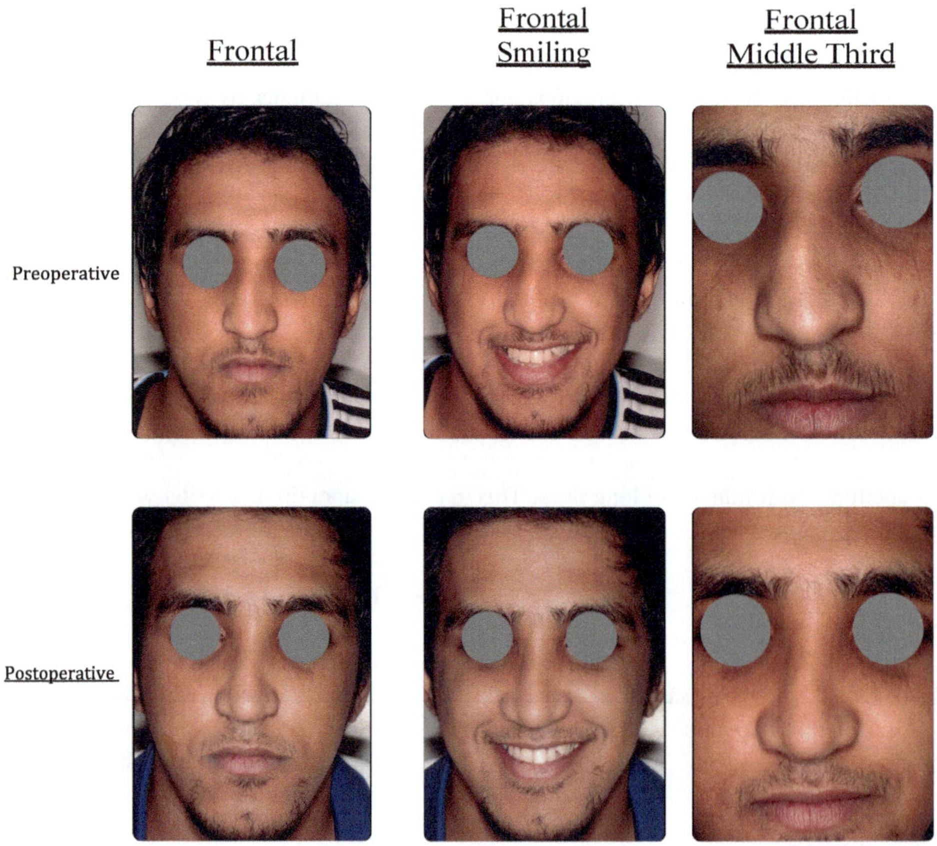

Direct Dorsal | Direct Dorsal Smiling | Overhead | Overhead Smiling

Preoperative

Postoperative

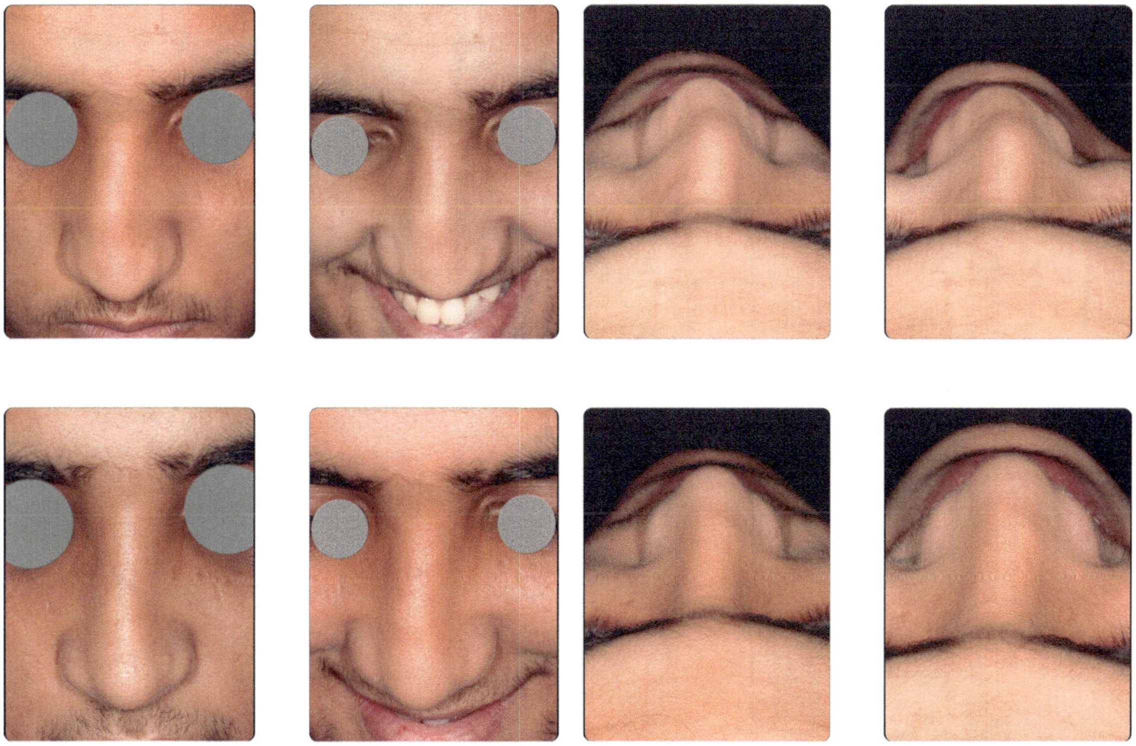

Backward Tilting | Steeper Backward Tilting | Basal | Basal Smiling

Preoperative

Postoperative

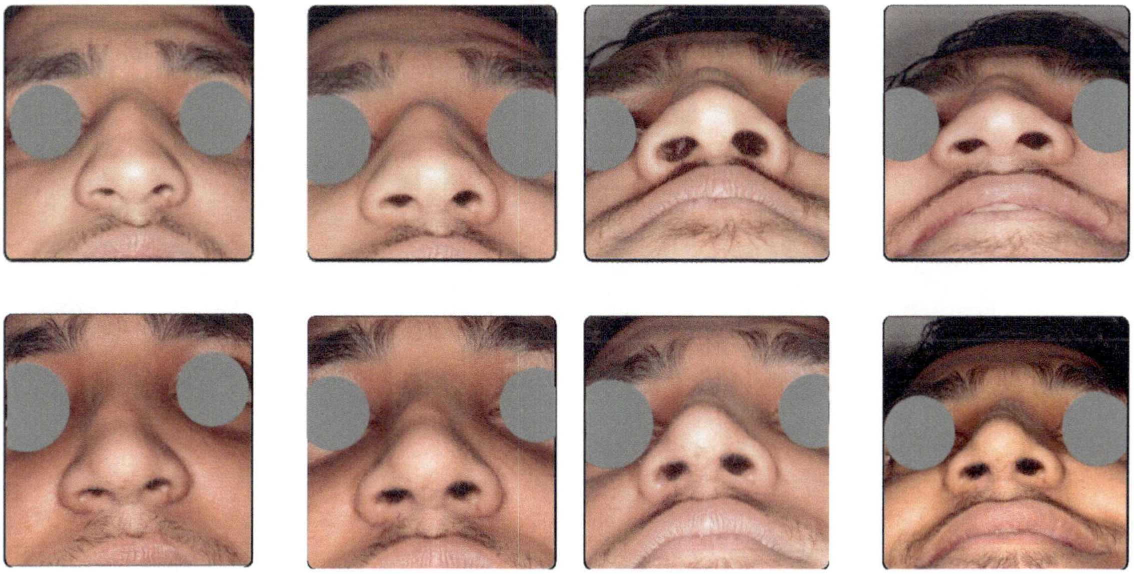

Right Oblique Mid Cheek Full Face | Left Oblique Mid Cheek Full Face | Right Oblique Mid Cheek Middle Third | Left Oblique Mid Cheek Middle Third

Preoperative

Postoperative

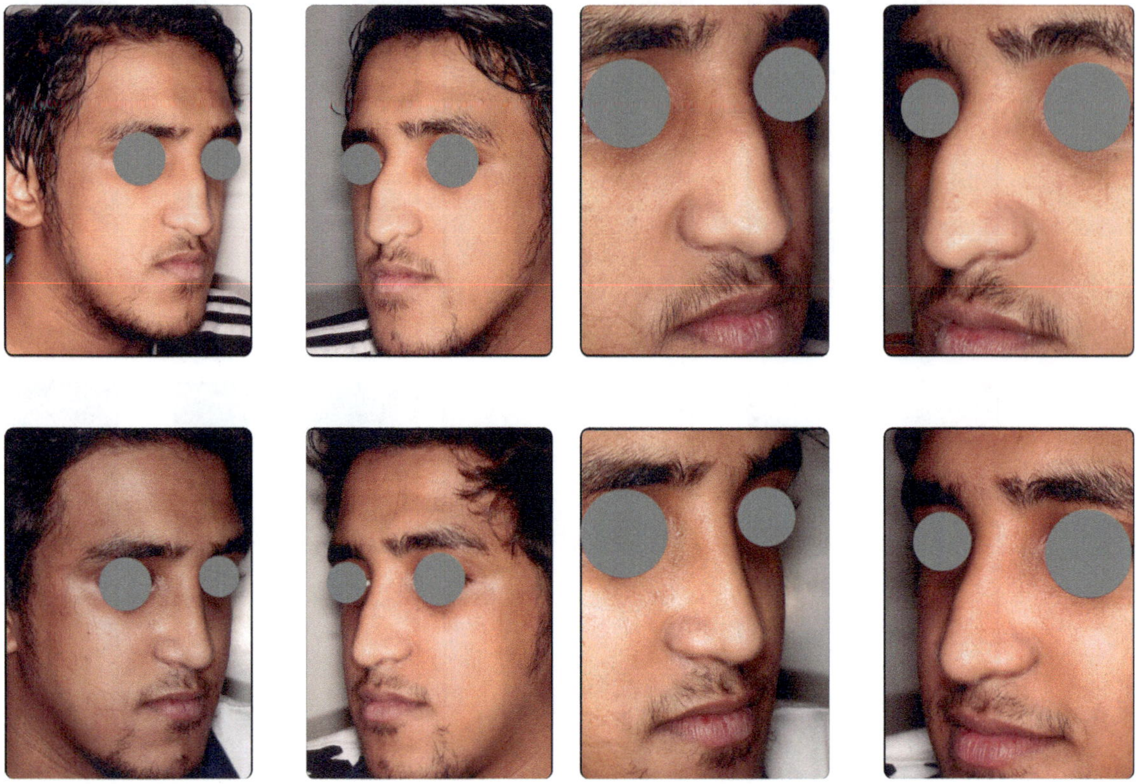

Right Oblique Cheek Margin Full Face | Left Oblique Cheek Margin Full Face | Right Oblique Cheek Margin Middle Third | Left Oblique Cheek Margin Middle Third

Preoperative

Postoperative

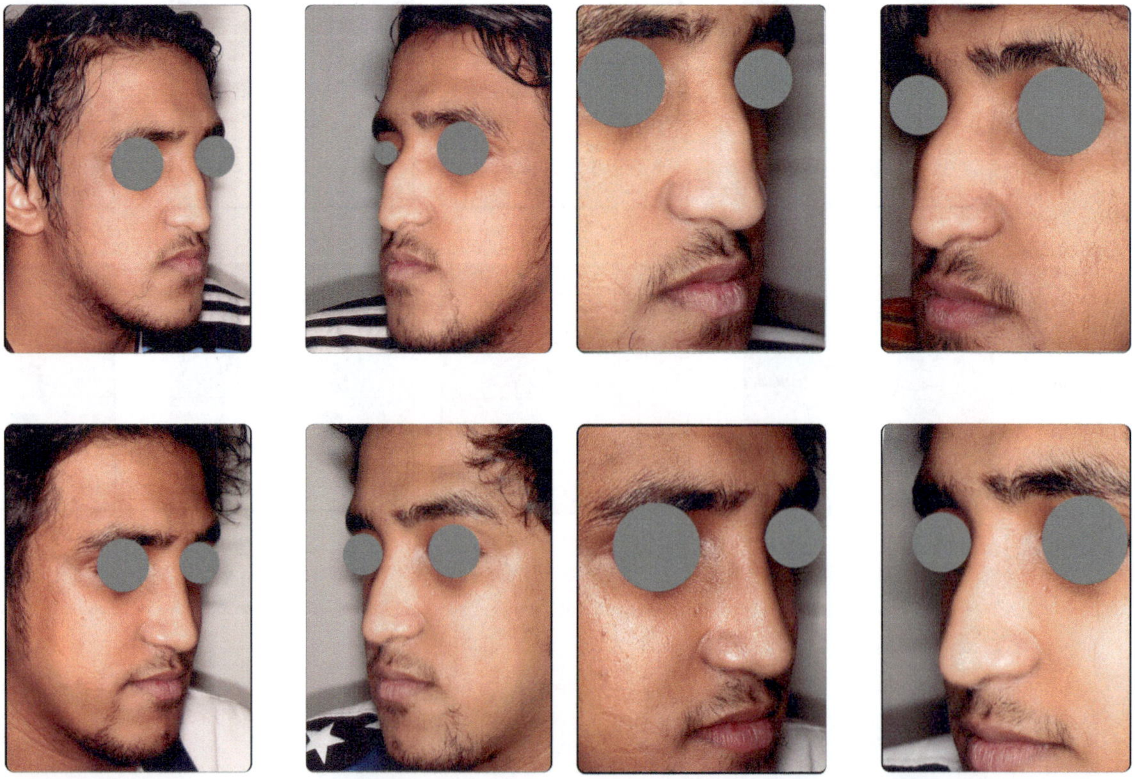

Right Lateral | Left Lateral | Right Lateral Smiling | Left Lateral Smiling

Preoperative

Postoperative

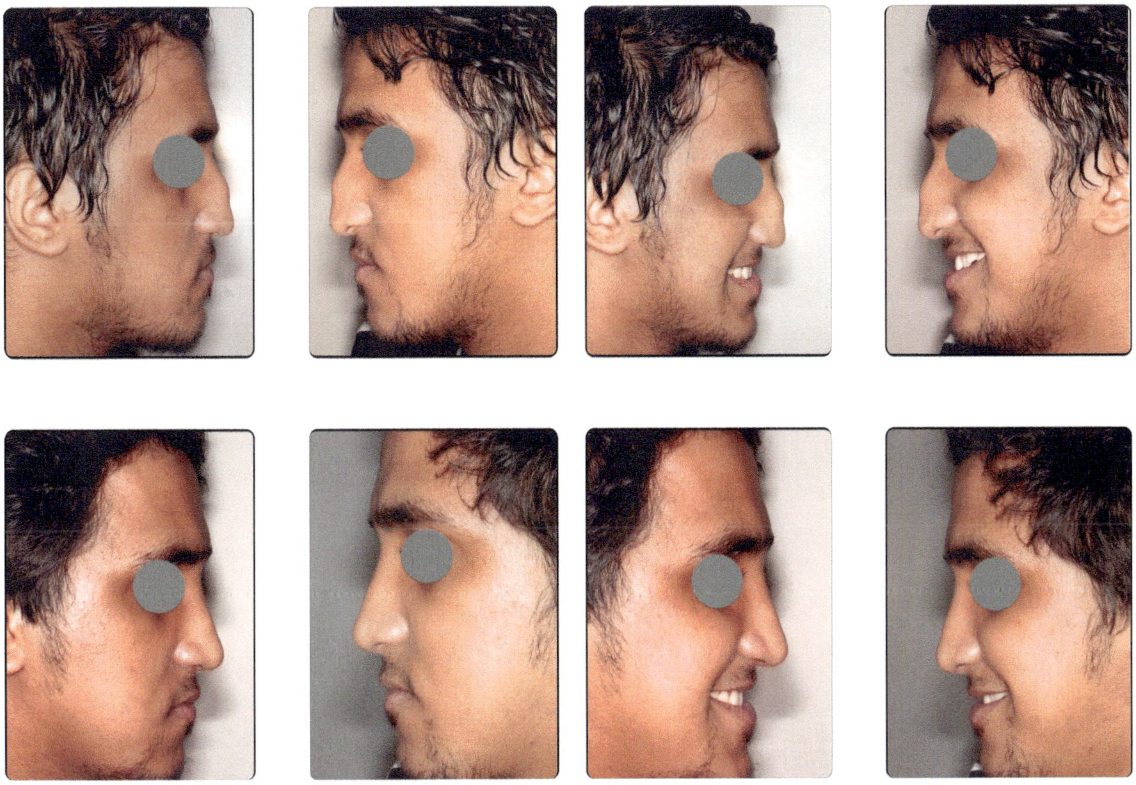

Right Lateral Middle Third | Left Lateral Middle Third

Preoperative

Postoperative

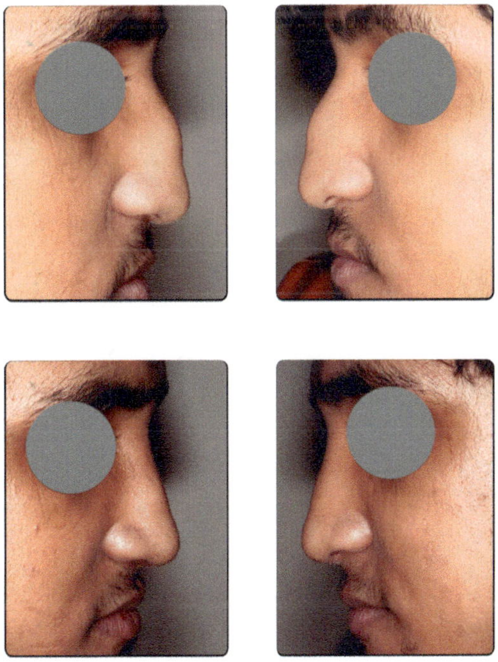

45 Part V: Clinical Case 6

Preoperative Assessment

1. **Frontolateral walls**
   a. A medium sized bulky frontolateral walls that overshadows the alae nasi, predominantly the left one (Frontal and Direct Dorsal Views).
   b. Asymmetrical smile, the left cheek ball is smaller than the right (Frontal and Lateral Smiling Views). There is bilateral maxillary asymmetry.
2. **Medial Wall**
   Right caudal septal deviation. The right medial crus is pushed literally encroaching upon the right nasal aperture that consequently looks smaller than the left (Basal Backward Tilting and Nasal Aperture Views). The right nasal sill band is pushed inferiorly (Frontal and Backward Tilting Views).
3. **Bony pyramid**
   a. Osteocartilaginous hump that is only oblique to the left side due to bilateral maxillary symmetry. The right cheek is wide and low while the left cheek is narrow and high (Backward Tilting Views) The nose is not deviated (Frontal, Direct Dorsal And Overhead Views).
   b. Wide base of bony pyramid (Direct Dorsal and Backward Tilting Views).
   c. The dorsal light reflex is irregular and distorted (preoperative Directed Dorsal Views).
4. **Alar base**
   Apparent asymmetrical nasal opening due to right caudal septal deviation. The right nasal aperture looked smaller (preoperative Backward Tilting, Basal and Nasal Aperture Views).

Aims of Surgery

1. Reduce the size and the bulk of the frontolateral walls.
2. Correct the deviation in the caudal septum to improve aesthetics of the columella.
3. To reduce the size and correct the obliquity of the bony pyramid.

Surgical Plan

1. **Frontolateral walls**
   a. DDD including the weak triangle to reduce the bulk and size of the nasal tip and supratip area.
   b. Cephalic trim of the lateral crurae to reduce the size of the frontolateral walls.
2. **Medial Wall**
   Septoplasty and trim the distal 2 mm of the caudal septum to improve the aesthetics of the columella.
3. **Bony pyramid**
   a. Excision of the osteocartilaginous hump down to the level of the anterior septal angle.
   b. Osteotomies and Kassanjean maneuver to the right i.e. cross fracture of the bony pyramid after osteotomies (see Surgery of the Bony Pyramid).
4. **Alar base**
   Nil of Note.

Surgical Procedure

As per surgical plan.

M. H. A. Shafy, *Atlas of Clinical Cases in Rhinoplasty*,
https://doi.org/10.1007/978-3-031-07504-9_45

Post-Operative Commentary

1. **Frontolateral Wall**
   a. Tip definition: the nasal tip is slimmer, more prominent and well identified from the alae nasi on both sides. The alae nasi become clearly visible and share in nasal aesthetics (Frontal, Direct Dorsal, Overhead, Backward Tilting and Basal Views).
   b. Tip projection: the nasal tip is at the same level of the nasal dorsum with good aesthetic angle. This is coupled with good aesthetic nasolabial angle (lateral and oblique views).
   c. Tip light reflex is seen as one spot off the nasal tip (Frontal and Backward Tilting Views).
2. **Medial Wall**
   Aesthetics of the columella improved after correction of the caudal septal deviation. Nasal apertures became similar in size (Backward Tilting and Basal Views).
3. **Bony Pyramid**
   a. Bony pyramid aesthetics improved: the nasal dorsum is straight in the midline and the sidewalls are smooth and narrow (all views except the Basal Views).
   b. Dorsal light reflex is seen as an uninterrupted line off the nasal dorsum (postoperative Direct Dorsal Views).
4. **Alar Base**
   a. Superior alar groove aesthetics improved by defatting. The grooves become longer and deeper (Oblique, Lateral and Direct Dorsal Views).
   b. Posterior alar groove aesthetics improved after defatting. They have wider angles with the upper lip (Backward Tilting, Basal and Nasal Aperture Views).
   c. Alae nasi aesthetics improved after defatting. They are pulled medially, become better seen and look more elegant (Nasal aperture and Oblique Views).
   d. Nasal apertures are equal in size and the shapes are elegantly oval.
   e. Marginal light reflexes are clearly seen at:
      i. Inferior alar margins (Nasal Aperture Views).
      ii. Nasal sill bands (Oblique Views).
      iii. Lateral crural prominences (Lateral Views).

Commentary

1. This patient maintained his exact features post-operatively as he wished. The nose print is the same.
2. The postoperative smaller nose matches the sizes of the eyes, lips and chin.
3. Post-operative photographs were one month after surgery. The nose and nasal skin continue to become thinner and better shaped in the long term result.
4. Symmetrical post-operative smile after defatting and the near equal alae nasi.

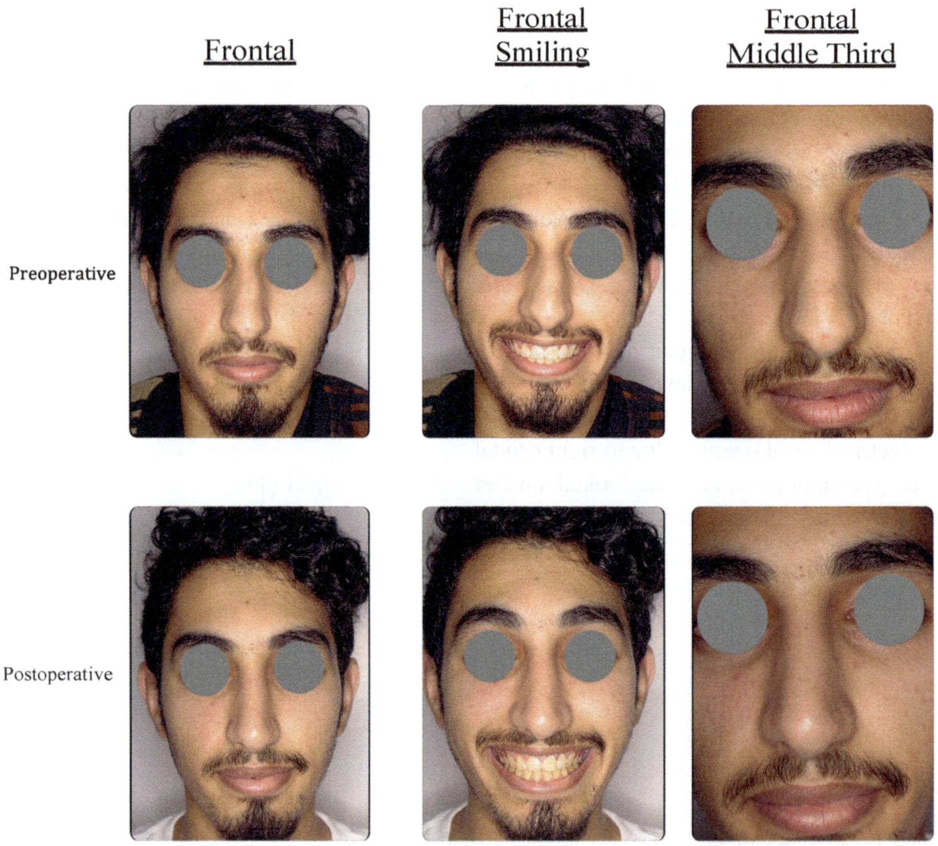

Direct Dorsal | Direct Dorsal Smiling | Overhead | Overhead Smiling

Preoperative

Postoperative

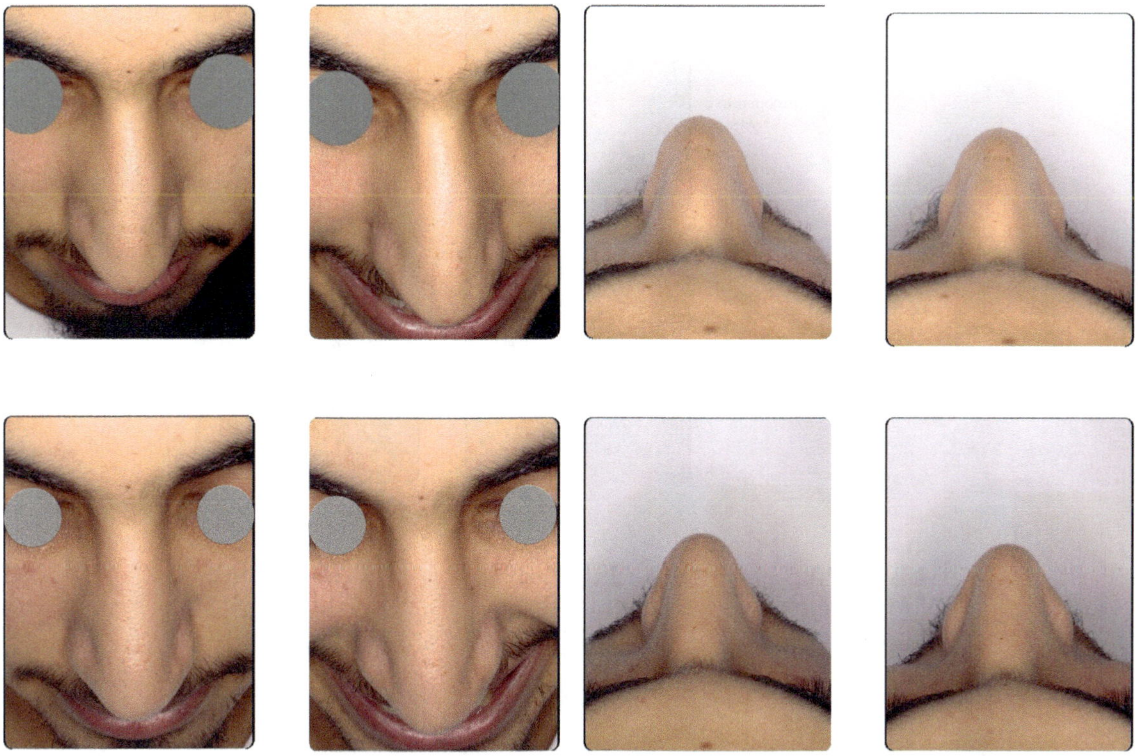

Backward Tilting | Steeper Backward Tilting | Basal | Basal Smiling

Preoperative

Postoperative

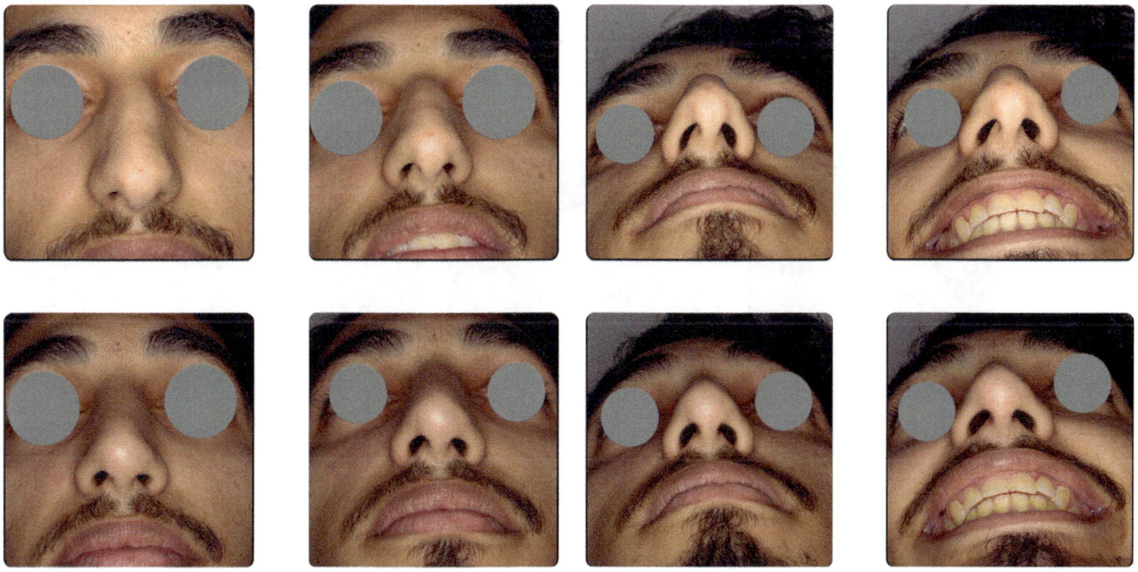

Right Nasal Aperture | Left Nasal Aperture

Preoperative

Postoperative

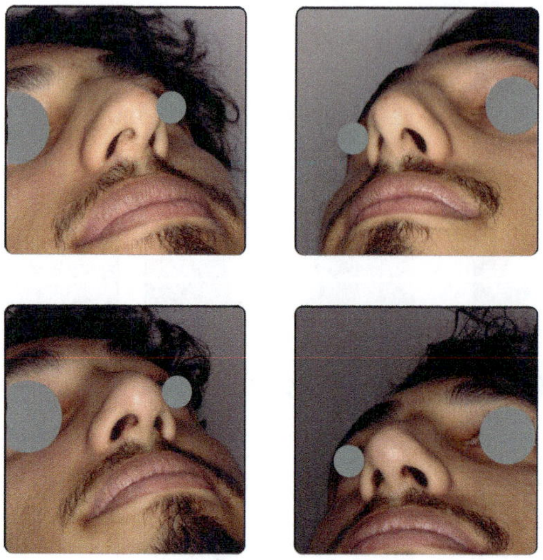

Right Oblique Mid Cheek Full Face | Left Oblique Mid Cheek Full Face | Right Oblique Mid Cheek Middle Third | Left Oblique Mid Cheek Middle Third

Preoperative

Postoperative

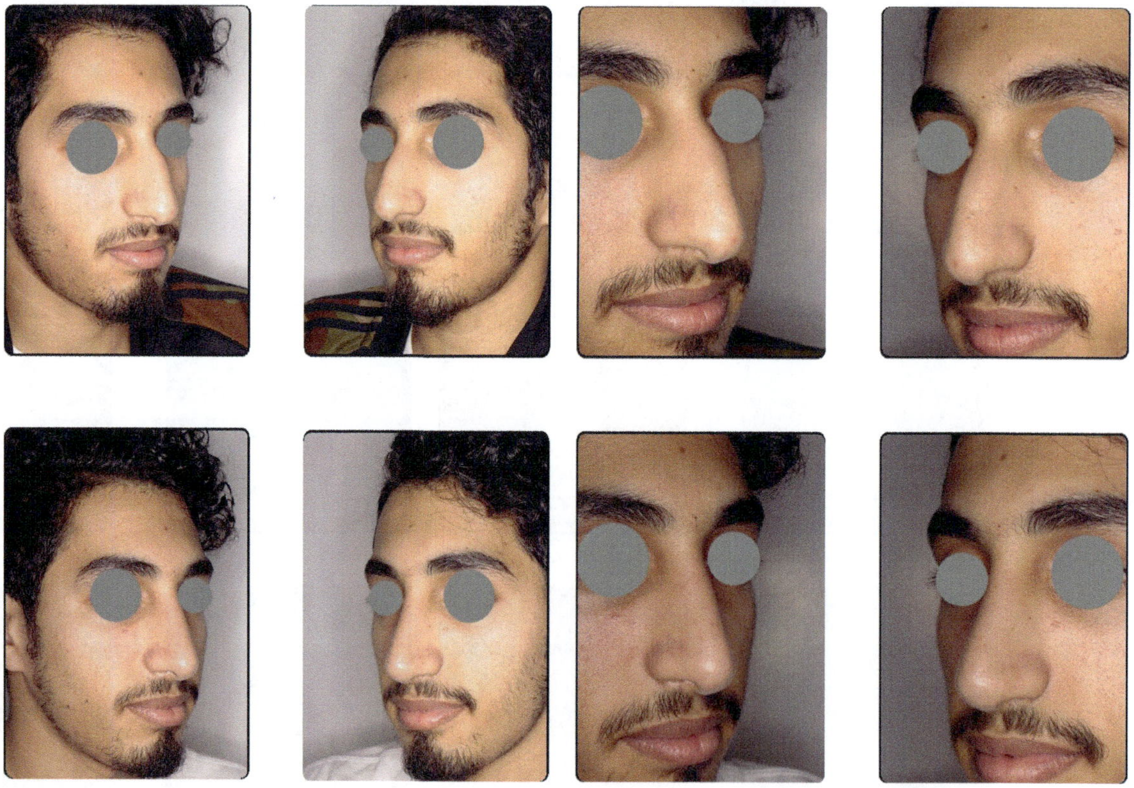

Right Oblique Cheek Margin Full Face	Left Oblique Cheek Margin Full Face	Right Oblique Cheek Margin Middle Third	Left Oblique Cheek Margin Middle Third

Preoperative

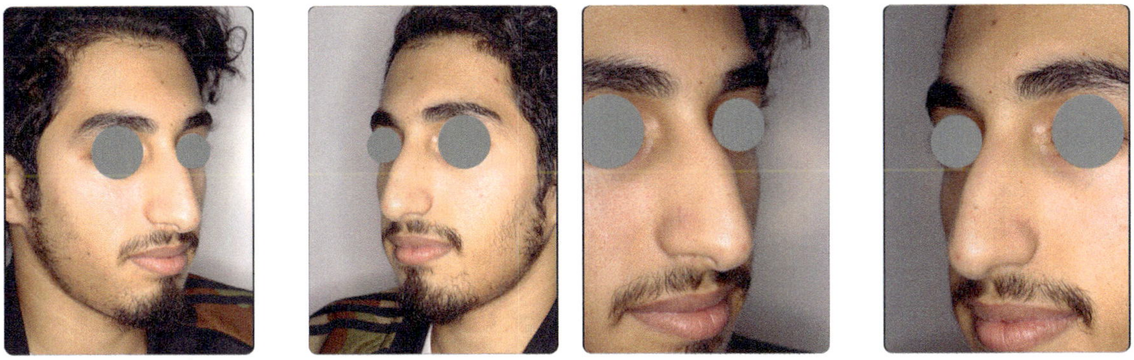

Postoperative

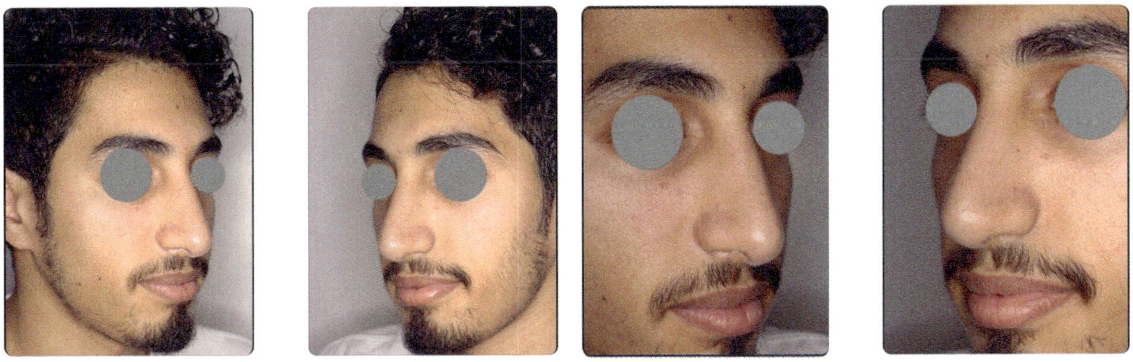

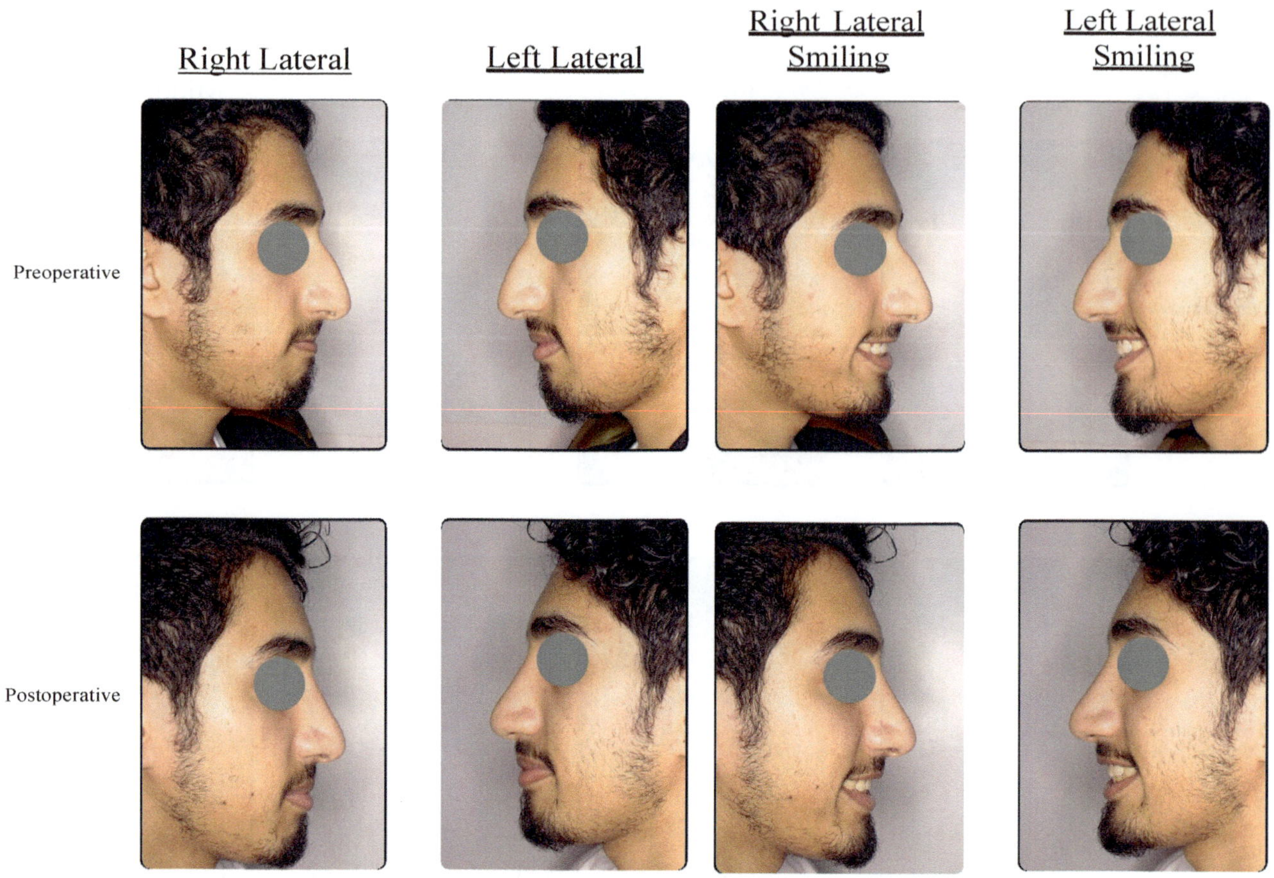
Right Lateral
Left Lateral
Right Lateral Smiling
Left Lateral Smiling
Preoperative
Postoperative

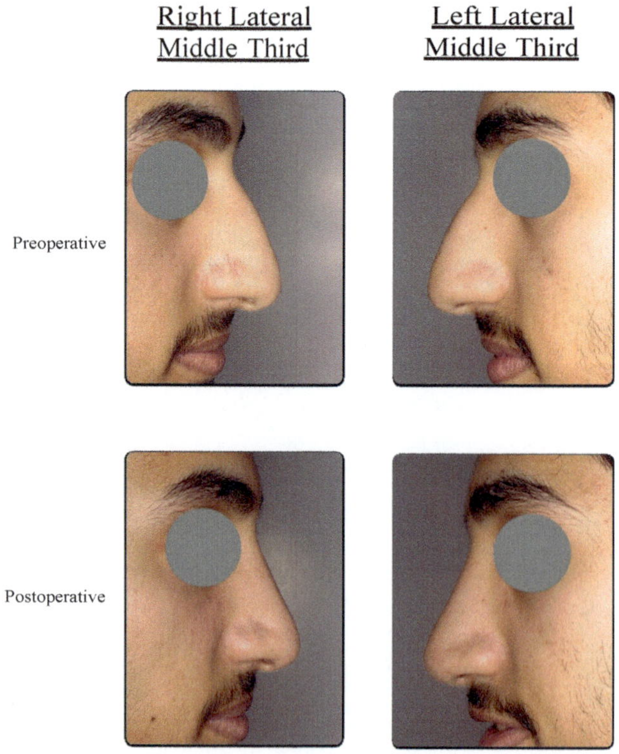
Right Lateral Middle Third
Left Lateral Middle Third
Preoperative
Postoperative

Part VI
Pediatric Rhinoplasty

Part VI: Clinical Case 1

46

Preoperative Assessment

1. **Frontolateral walls**
   Relatively bulky flat ill defined nasal tip (Frontal, Direct Dorsal, Backward Tilting, Basal and Nasal Aperture Views).
2. **Nasal septum**
   Nil of note.
3. **Bony pyramid**
   Wide base of boney pyramid (Frontal, Direct Dorsal and Backward Tilting Views).
4. **Alar base**
   Wide and bulky alar base, due to long inferior and thick posterior segments of the rim sill folds successively. The nasal openings are wide with transverse long axes, as commonly seen in African noses. (Basal and Nasal Aperture Views).

Aims of Surgery

1. To improve definition of the nasal tip.
2. To improve definition of nasal dorsum by narrowing and elevating the bony pyramid.
3. Reduction of the bulk and width of the alar base transforming the horizontal axes of the nasal openings into more vertical openings.

Surgical Plan

1. **Frontolateral walls**
   DDD excluding the weak triangle to reduce the size and bulk of the nasal tip and supratip area.
2. **Nasal septum**
   Nil of note.
3. **Bony pyramid**
   Osteotomies and medialization of the lateral bony walls to reduce the width and increase the height of the bony pyramid.
4. **Alar base**
   Bilateral resection of the posterior and inferior segments of the rim-sill folds.

Surgical Procedure

As per Surgical Plan.

Post-Operative Analysis

1. **Frontolateral wall**
   a. Tip definition: the nasal tip is smaller with thinner and smoother overlying skin. It is more prominent and well identified from the alae nasi on both sides. The alae nasi come into view to become clearly visible and share in nasal aesthetics (Frontal, Direct Dorsal, Overhead, Backward Tilting and Basal Views).
   b. Tip projection: The nasal tip at the same level of the nasal dorsum with good aesthetic angle. This is coupled with good aesthetic nasolabial angle (lateral and oblique views).
   c. Tip light reflex is seen as one spot off the nasal tip. (Frontal and Backward Tilting Views).
2. **Medial Wall**
   Nil of Note.
3. **Bony Pyramid**
   a. Bony pyramid aesthetics improved: the nasal dorsum is straight and the sidewalls are smooth and narrow (all views except the Basal Views).
   b. Dorsal light reflex is seen as an uninterrupted line off the nasal dorsum (Direct Dorsal View).
4. **Alar Base**
   a. Superior alar groove aesthetics improved by defatting. The grooves become longer and deeper (Nasal Aperture, Lateral and Direct Dorsal grooves).
   b. Posterior alar groove aesthetics improved by defatting and excision of rim-sill folds. The posterior groove

M. H. A. Shafy, *Atlas of Clinical Cases in Rhinoplasty*,
https://doi.org/10.1007/978-3-031-07504-9_46

angles with the upper lip are wider. (Basal, Nasal Aperture and Lateral Views).

c. Alae nasi aesthetics improved after defatting. They are pulled medially, became better seen and are smaller in size. (Backward Tilting, Basal and Nasal Aperture Views).
d. Nasal aperture aesthetics improved by defatting and excision of the rim-sill folds:
   i. The size of nasal apertures became smaller.
   ii. The shapes of nasal apertures are more elegantly oval.
e. Marginal light reflex: seen at the inferior alar margins. (Nasal Aperture Views).

Commentary

a. Only three of the four areas of Rhinoplasty were addressed in this child i.e. the nasal tip, bony pyramid and alar base.
b. This is a growing nose. Surgical procedures were pursued in areas away from the growing parts of the nose. It did not affect the normal growth of the nose.
c. There are better definitions of the nasal tip and dorsum. Both became narrower, higher and well recognized. The nose is no longer bulky or flat on the face.

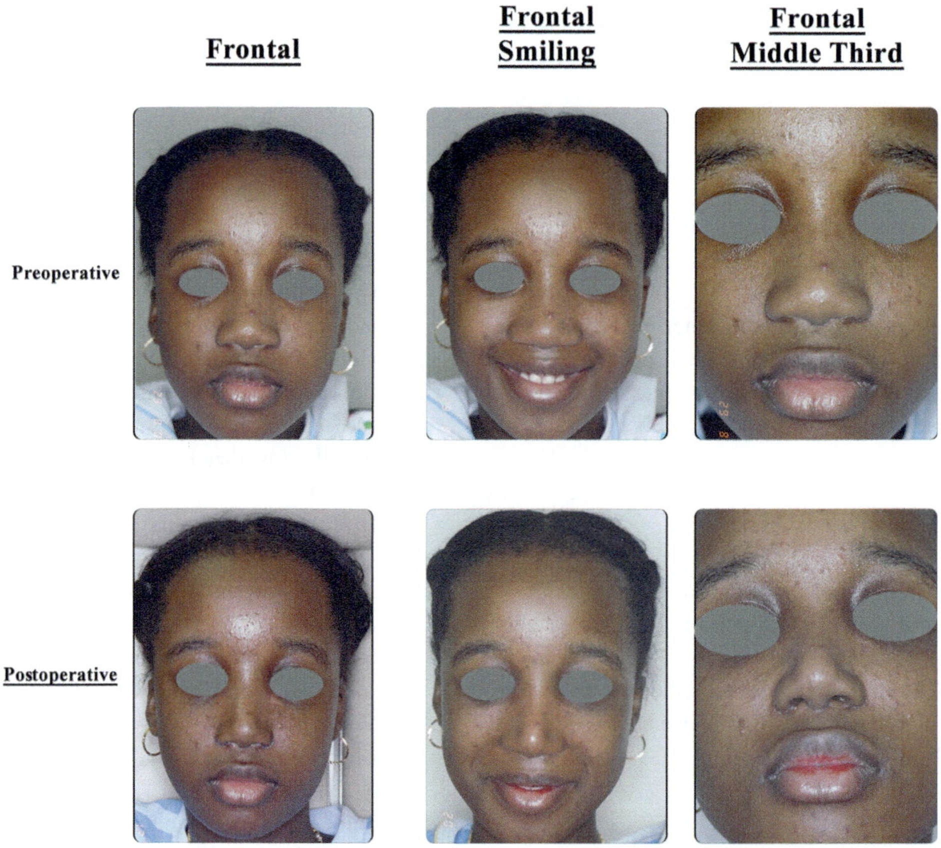

Direct Dorsal

Preoperative

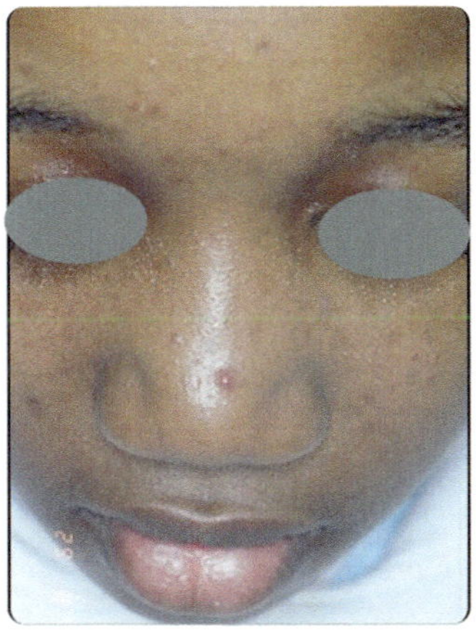

Postoperative

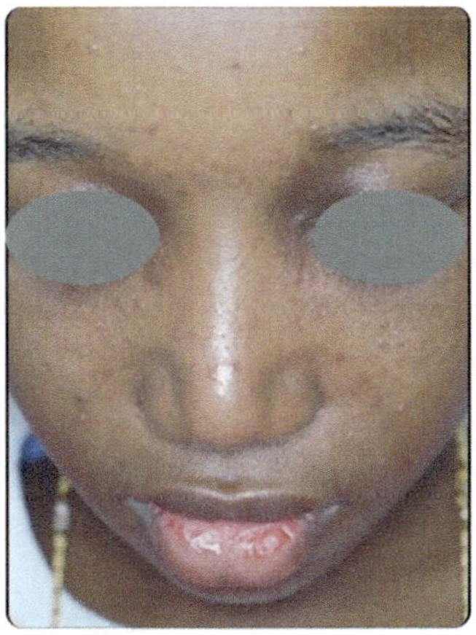

Backward Tilting

Preoperative

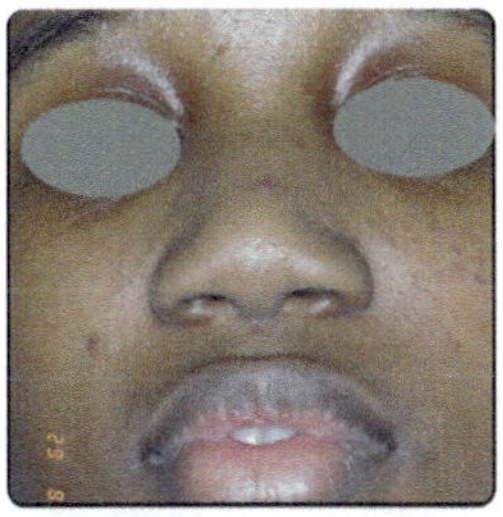

Postoperative

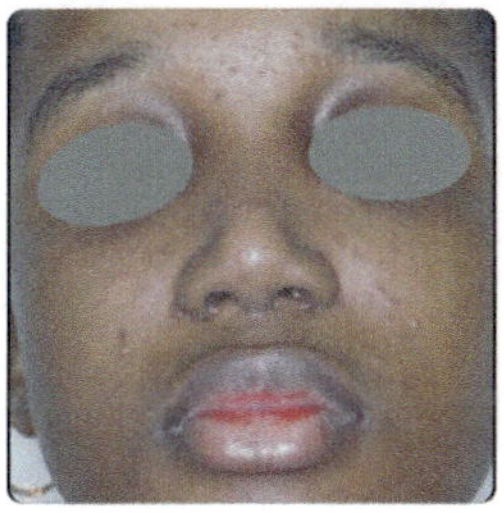

Basal

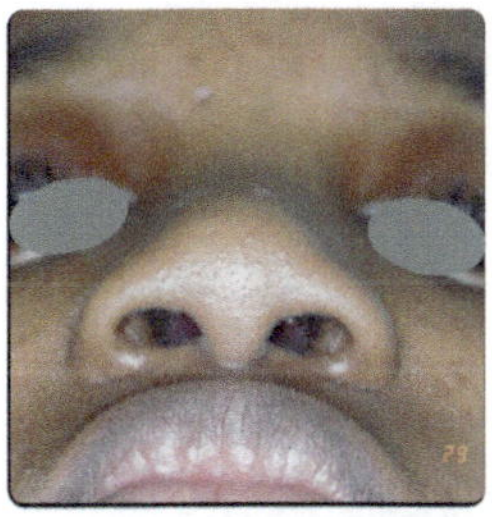

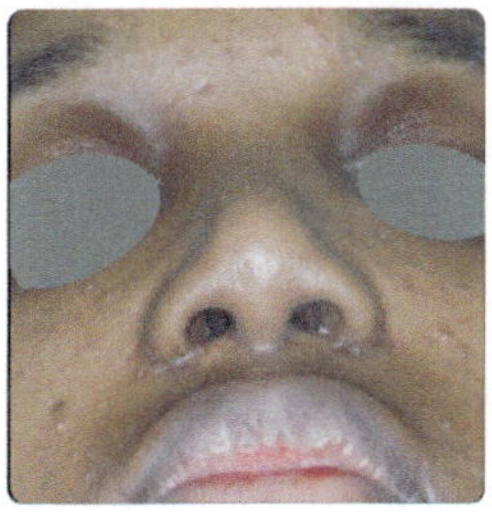

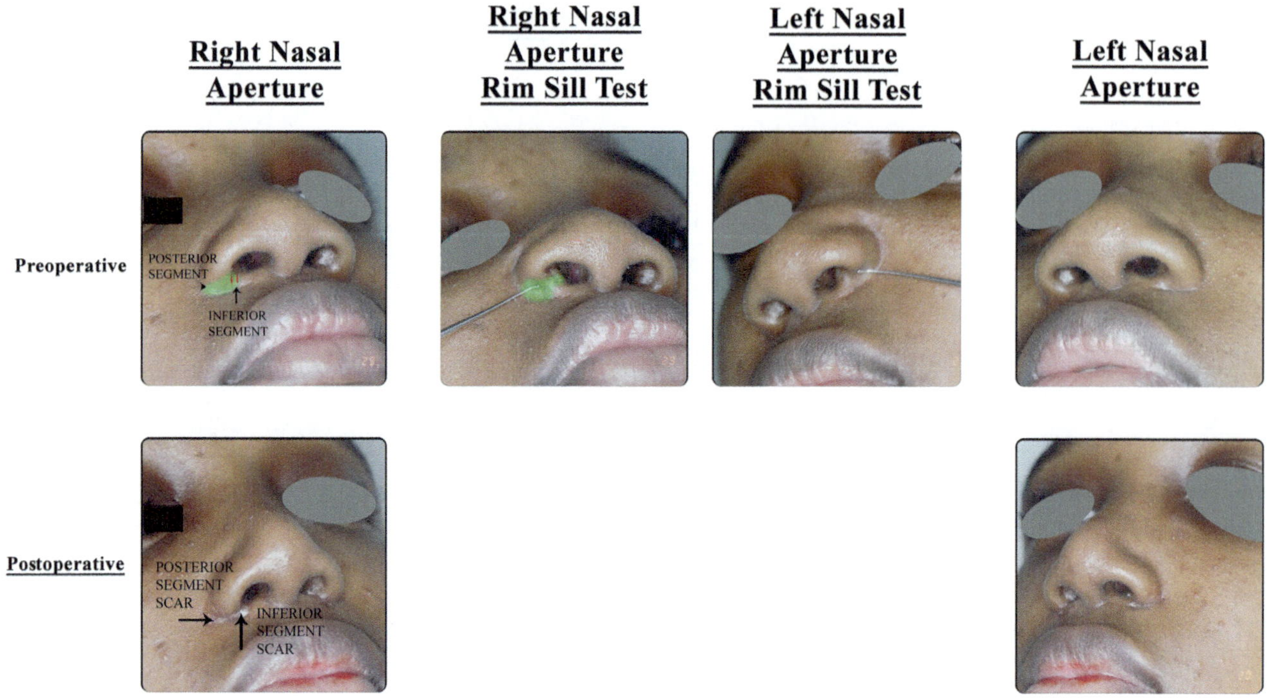

Note: These views, more than any other views demonistrates, postoperative narrower alar base, nasal tip and base of bony pyramids. Shape of the nasal apreture is oval, nasal tip is projected and the dorsum is higher.

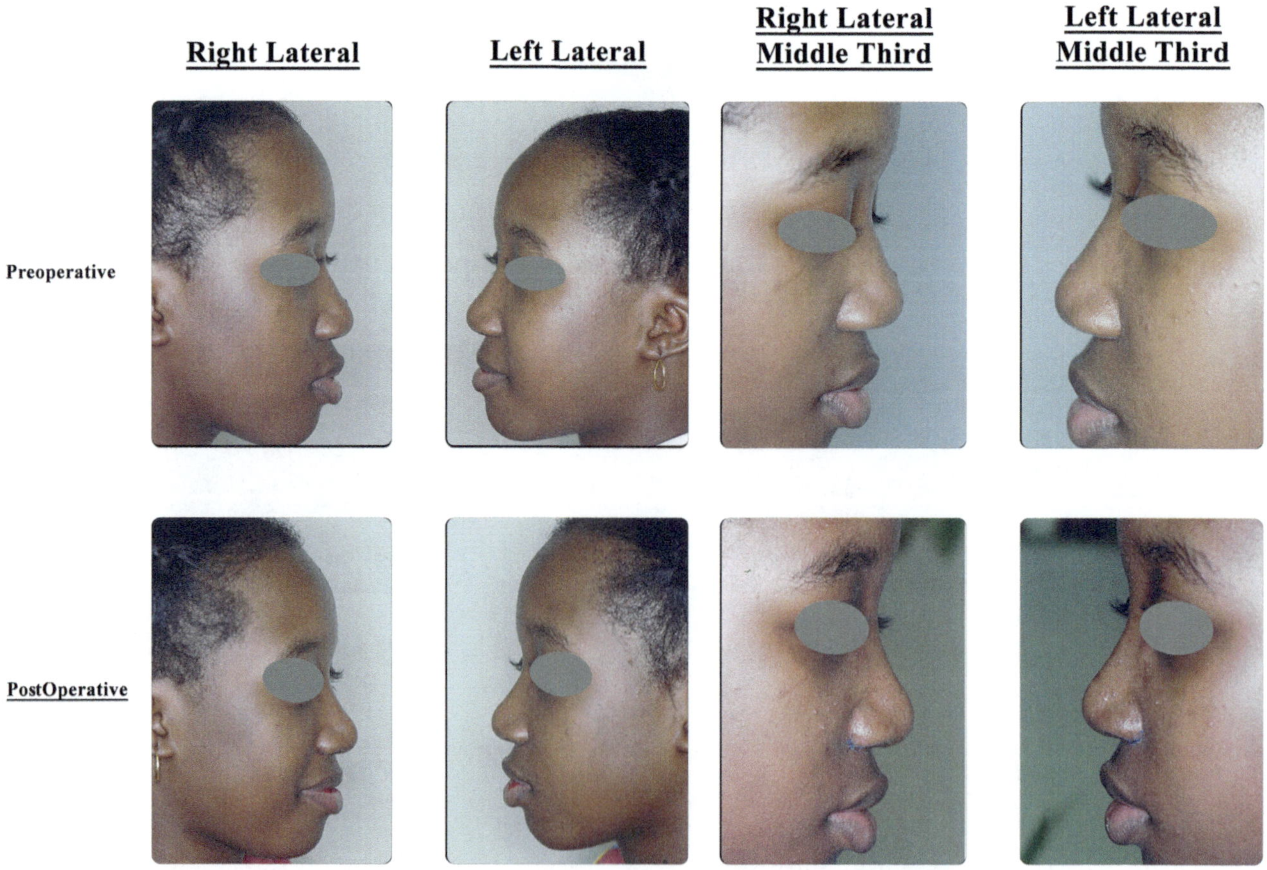

Part VI: Clinical Case 2

47

Preoperative Assessment

1. **Frontolateral walls**
   Relatively bulky nasal tip for a child. The nasal tip is small, flat and ill defined. (Frontal, Direct Dorsal, Backward Tilting and Nasal Aperture Views).
2. **Nasal septum**
   Nil of note.
3. **Bony pyramid**
   Wide base of bony pyramid (Frontal, Direct Dorsal and Backward Tilting Views).
4. **Alar base**
   The nasal openings look thick and wide with transverse long axes. The wide alar base is due to the long inferior segments while the bulky alae nasi is due to the thick posterior segments of rim-sill folds.

Aims of Surgery

1. Improve definition of the nasal tip.
2. Improve definition of nasal dorsum.
3. Reduction of the width and bulk of the alar base including the alae nasi. This will transform the horizontal axes of the nasal openings into more aesthetically pleasing vertical ones.

Surgical Plan

1. **Frontolateral walls**
   DDD excluding the weak triangle to reduce the bulk of the nasal tip and supratip area.
2. **Nasal septum**
   Nil of note.
3. **Bony pyramid**
   Osteotomies and medialization of the lateral bony walls to reduce the width and increase the height of the bony pyramid.
4. **Alar base**
   Bilateral resection of the posterior and inferior segments of the rim sill folds. The African alar base has a narrow inferior segments, that contribute to the aperture size, and thick posterior segments, that contributes to the nasal bulk (Basal, Nasal Aperature Views and illustrative artwork of the rim sill tests).

Surgical Procedure

As per Surgical Plan.

Post-Operative Analysis Note that the post operative photographs were taken nine years later, when the child became an adult of 21 years (she was 12 years old at the time of surgery).

1. **Frontolateral Walls**
   a. Tip definition improved i.e. the tip is slimmer and prominently well identified from the surrounding smaller alae nasi. (Frontal, Direct Dorsal, Overhead, Backward Tilting and Basal Views).
   b. Tip projection: the nasal tip is at the same level of the nasal dorsum with good aesthetic angle. This is coupled with good aesthetic nasolabial angle (lateral and oblique views).
   c. Tip light reflex is seen as one spot off the nasal tip. (Frontal and Backward Tilting Views).
2. **Medial Walls**
   Nil of Note.
3. **Bony Pyramid**
   a. Bony pyramid aesthetics improved: the nasal dorsum is high and the sidewalls are smooth strait and narrow (all views except the Basal Views).
   b. Dorsal light reflex is seen as a regular one line off the nasal dorsum (Direct Dorsal Views).

M. H. A. Shafy, *Atlas of Clinical Cases in Rhinoplasty*,
https://doi.org/10.1007/978-3-031-07504-9_47

4. **Alar Base**
   a. Posterior alar groove aesthetics improved by defatting and excision of the rim-sill folds (Backward Tilting, Basal and Nasal Aperture Views).
   b. Alae nasi aesthetics improved by defatting and excision of the posterior and inferior segments of the rim-sill folds. The alae nasi are pulled medially and remain of reasonable size after nine years. They are not as winging as they appeared before. They become more visible and smaller in size. (Backward Tilting, Basal and Nasal Aperture Views).
   c. Nasal aperture aesthetics improved after defatting and resection of the rim-sill folds:
      i. The size of nasal opening continuing to be small after nine years.
      ii. The shape transformed from thick walled rounded with transverse axes to thin walled ova with vertical axes of nasal openings.
   d. Marginal light reflex are clearly seen at:
      i. Inferior alar margins (Nasal Aperture Views).
      ii. Nasal sill bands (Oblique Views).
      iii. Lateral crural prominences (Lateral Views).

Commentary

a. Only three of the four Rhinoplasty areas were addressed in the following manners:
   i. The frontolateral walls: defatting of the two hypodermal layers. The lower lateral cartilages were not touched i.e. no direct surgery to the cartilaginous walls was necessary.
   ii. The bony pyramid: medial, lateral and superior osteotomies i.e. at the midline between the two nasal bones, at the roots of the frontal processes of maxillae and at the superior end of nasal bones successively.
   iii. Alar base: only the rim-sill folds were strictly excised.

b. This is a growing nose. The operation was performed when the child was 12 years old. The surgical procedure were pursued in areas away from the growing parts of the nose. The post-operative photos were taken nine years later when she was 21 years old. The child enjoyed a nose that she dreamed of having in her sensitive growing teenage. The nasal dorsum and the lower lateral cartilages continued growing to their normal adult sizes. In the meantime, the nasal tip and dorsum maintained their remarkable definitions. The nose did not revert to its original common African shape after growing. Furthermore the nose maintained its own original shape and image i.e. the same nasal print.
c. In all three areas the location of surgery avoided the growing cartilages and the germinal centers of the bones. This is a limited surgery which had an impressively favorable short and long term results. The surgery deals with the transitional tissues between the basic skeletal structures of the nose i.e. the rim-sill folds and the two subdermal fatty layers. The bony pyramidal work was clean cut osteotomies in safe locations.
d. Excising the rim-sill folds reduced the extent of alar flare on smiling. Widening of nasal apertures on smiling is very much smaller post-operatively, even with a larger, grown-up nose nine years after surgery (Frontal smiling views).
e. The child's family live in a remote area, they never came back for immediate post operative follow-up. It was only nine years later that she came for a consultation of another medical condition.

Frontal | **Frontal Smiling**

Preoperative Age 12

Postoperative Age 21

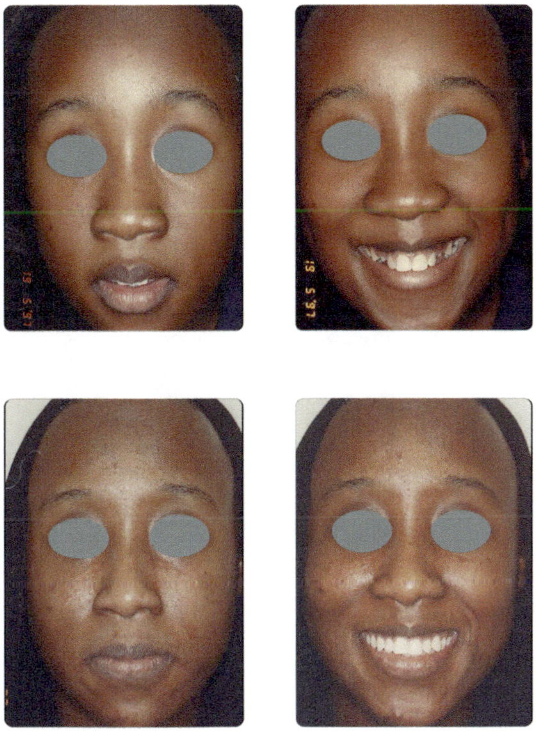

Direct Dorsal | **Direct Dorsal Smiling**

Preoperative Age 12

Postoperative Age 21

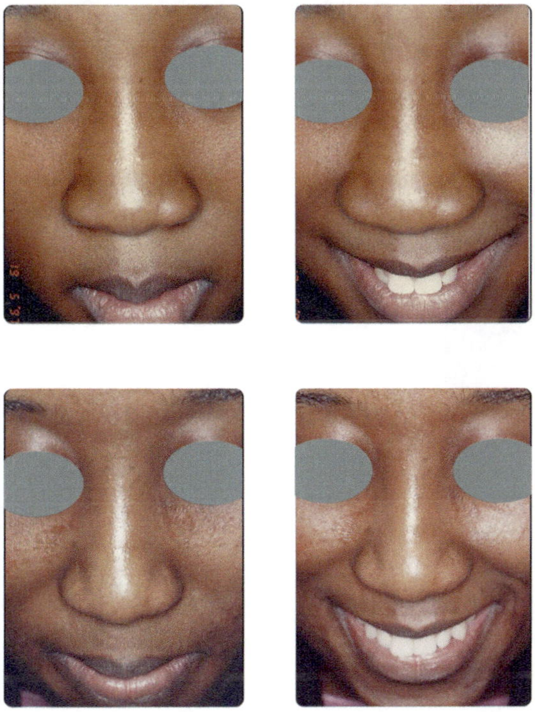

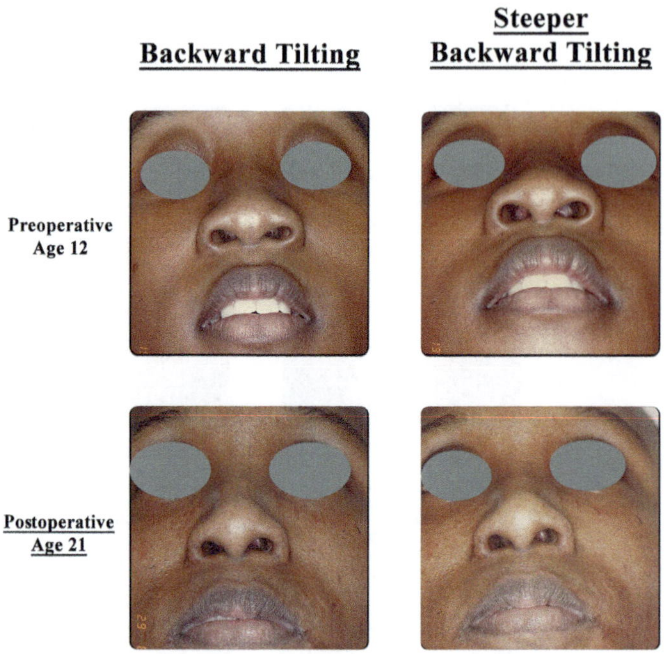
Backward Tilting
Steeper Backward Tilting
Preoperative Age 12
Postoperative Age 21

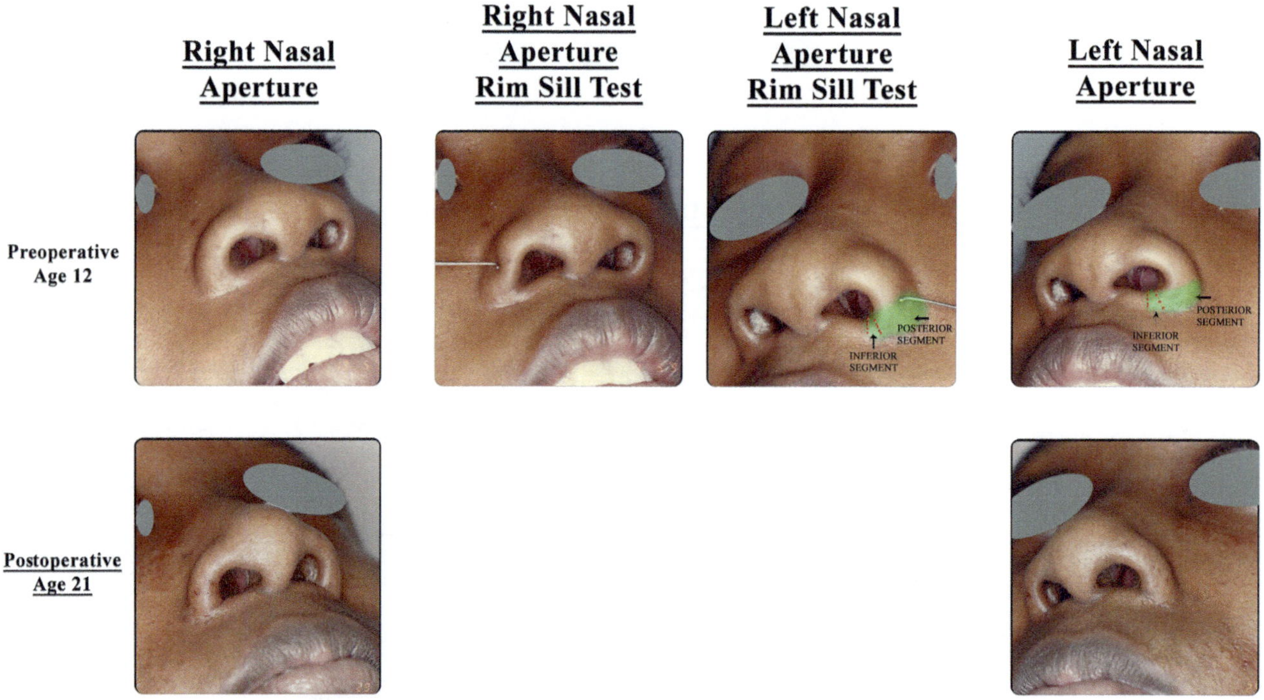
Right Nasal Aperture
Right Nasal Aperture Rim Sill Test
Left Nasal Aperture Rim Sill Test
Left Nasal Aperture
Preoperative Age 12
Postoperative Age 21
POSTERIOR SEGMENT
INFERIOR SEGMENT
POSTERIOR SEGMENT
INFERIOR SEGMENT

Right Oblique Mid Cheek Full Face | **Left Oblique Mid Cheek Full Face** | **Right Oblique Mid Cheek Middle Third** | **Left Oblique Mid Cheek Middle Third**

Preoperative Age 12

Postoperative Age 21

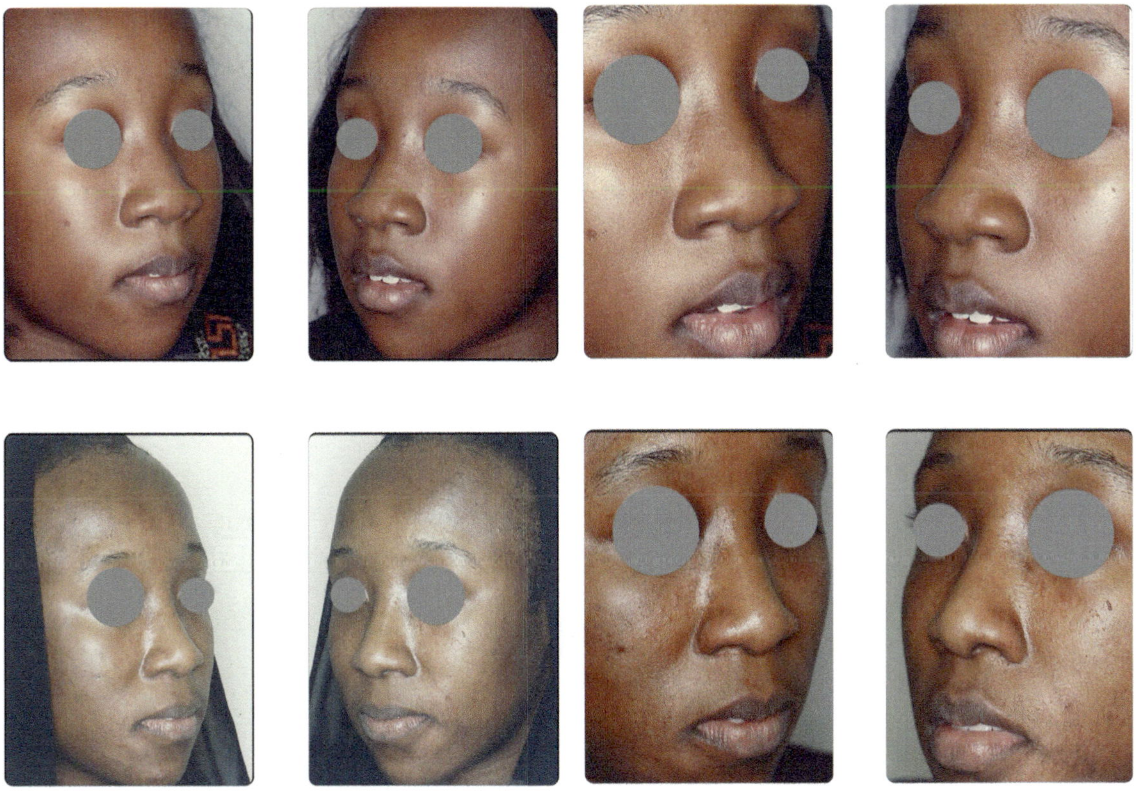

Right Oblique Cheek Margin Full Face | **Left Oblique Cheek Margin Full Face**

Preoperative Age 12

Postoperative Age 21

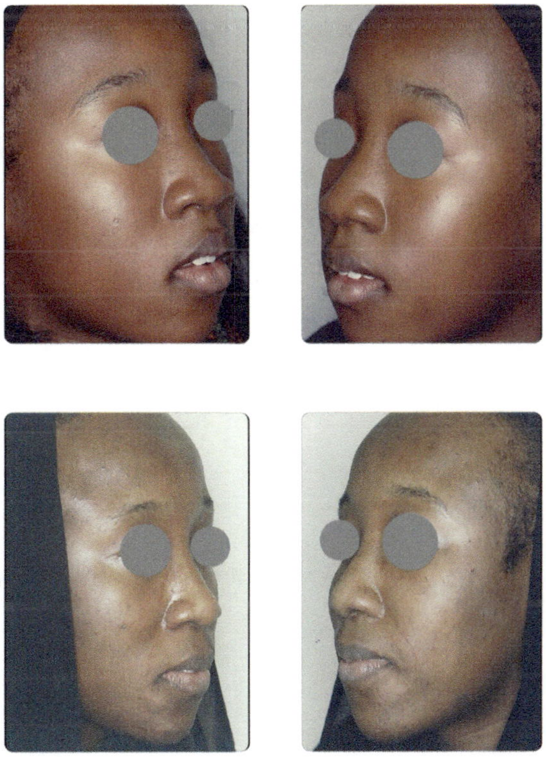

Right Lateral | **Left Lateral** | **Right Lateral Smiling** | **Left Lateral Smiling**

Postoperative Age 21

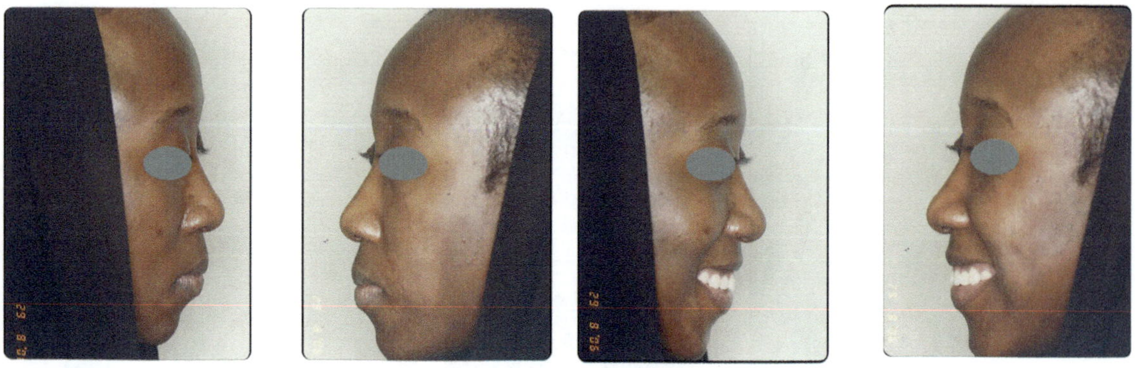

Right Lateral Middle Third | **Left Lateral Middle Third**

Preoperative Age 12

Postoperative 21

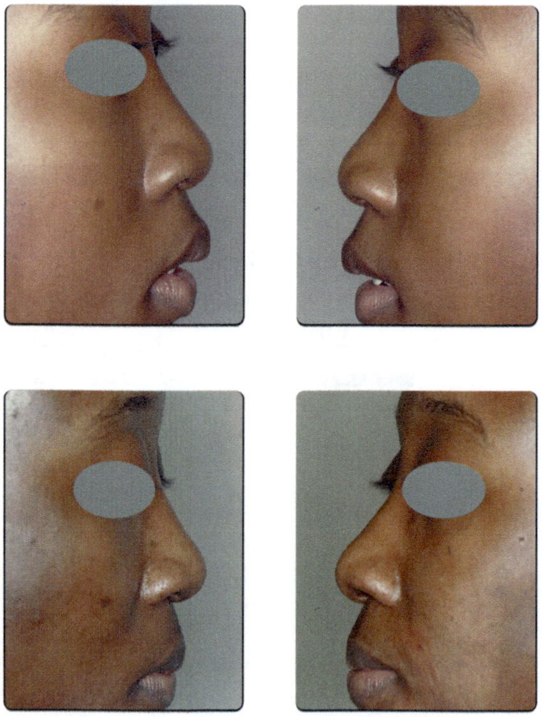

48 Part VI: Clinical Case 3

Preoperative Assessment

1. **Frontolateral walls**
   The child had a strikingly long nasal tip. The tip felt cystic on gentle palpation. The diagnosis of the presence of a subdermal cyst was verified by CT scan and ultrasound studies (Frontal, Oblique and Lateral Views).
2. **Medial Wall**
   Nil of note.
3. **Bony pyramid**
   Nil of note.
4. **Alar base**
   Nil of note.

Aims of Surgery

Removal of the cystic swelling without interfering with the normal anatomical structures of the nose.

Surgical Plan

1. **Frontolateral walls**
   a. An attempt of internal removal of the cyst.
   b. External approach was considered should the internal approach fail.
2. **Media Wall**
   Nil of note.
3. **Bony pyramid**
   Nil of note.
4. **Alar base**
   Nil of note.

Surgical Procedure

a. Bilateral inter-cartilaginous incisions were made as close as possible to the lower margin of the upper lateral cartilage. This avoided cutting through the overlapping scroll area of the lower lateral cartilages. This is an important clinical point in the growing nose of a child.
b. Bilateral delivery of the lower lateral cartilages. The lateral crurae were intact and healthy. The fibrous bands between the dermis and the crural fatty capsules were severed. The two subdermal fatty layers were left intact i.e. no defatting process was necessary.
c. Meticulous dissection of the cyst using a round ended, strongly curved scissor. A strait sharp tip scissors is avoided. The cyst had a very thick wall and the skin was thinner than normal.
d. After removal of the cyst, the skeletal structure of the nasal tip was satisfactory but there was an excess of redundant skin over the tip.
e. Wide undermining of the skin all over the dorsum of the nose extending laterally for about 1 cm over the frontal processes of the maxillary bones.

Post-Operative Analysis and Commentary

The excess skin was not excised. The wide undermining of the skin allowed the redundant skin to be distributed laterally, leaving sufficient amount over the tip with no excess.

M. H. A. Shafy, *Atlas of Clinical Cases in Rhinoplasty*,
https://doi.org/10.1007/978-3-031-07504-9_48

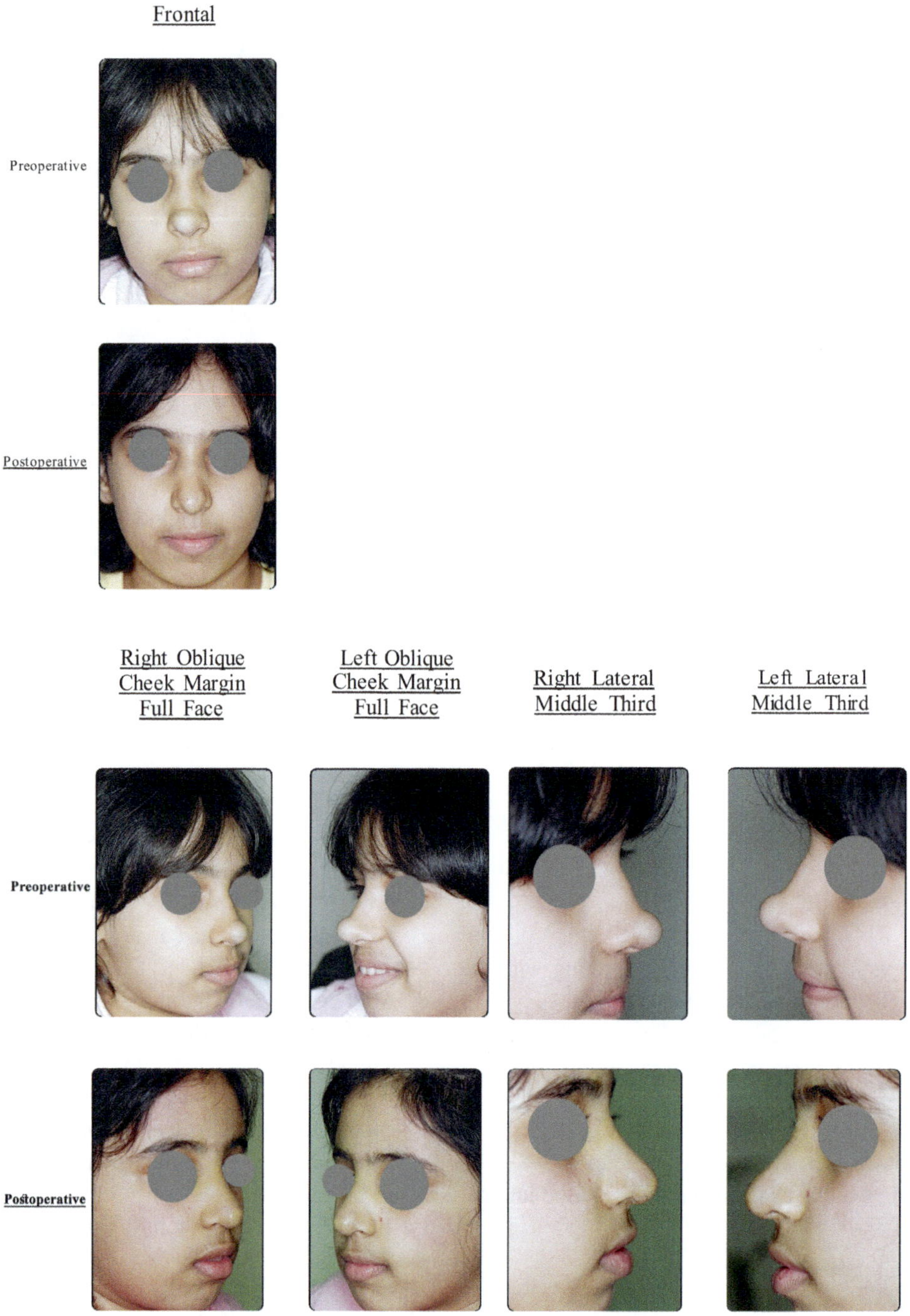
Frontal
Preoperative
Postoperative
Right Oblique
Cheek Margin
Full Face
Left Oblique
Cheek Margin
Full Face
Right Lateral
Middle Third
Left Lateral
Middle Third
Preoperative
Postoperative

Atlas Glossary

The concept of an Atlas is ideal for the surgery of Rhinoplasty. In this Atlas more than 4600 photographs of a wide range of clinical conditions that present for Rhinoplasty are displayed. These varieties of noses include; the large, bulky, crooked, deviated, oblique, fractured, finesse, secondary, ethnic, paediatric and special clinical conditions. In each case the nose and face are looked at from multiple different angles through the standard and the newly introduced specialized photographic views.

In the specialized views, each of the four anatomical subdivisions of the nose is clearly illustrated i.e. The frontolateral walls, the medial wall, the bony pyramid, including the mid-vault, and the alar base. Twenty-nine (29) photographs are taken to the nose and face pre-operatively and the same post-operatively.

A guide is written for assessment of the pre-operative photographs followed by the analysis of the post-operative photographs.

Successes, difficulties as well as pitfalls are discussed and illustrated photographically.

The art of displaying the pre-operative and post-operative **photographs** is quiet simple and easy for the eyes in order to clearly and immediately see the results. The aim that all photographs can be **seen at a glance**. **The texts** are well organized, simple, scientific and stereotyped so that they are **read at a glance.** The principle theme of this Atlas is:

SAG—Seen at A Glance
RAG—Read at A Glance

M. H. A. Shafy, *Atlas of Clinical Cases in Rhinoplasty*,
https://doi.org/10.1007/978-3-031-07504-9

GPSR Compliance

The European Union's (EU) General Product Safety Regulation (GPSR) is a set of rules that requires consumer products to be safe and our obligations to ensure this.

If you have any concerns about our products, you can contact us on ProductSafety@springernature.com

In case Publisher is established outside the EU, the EU authorized representative is:

Springer Nature Customer Service Center GmbH
Europaplatz 3
69115 Heidelberg, Germany

Batch number: 10793418

Printed by Printforce, the Netherlands